STENTS – STATE OF THE ART
AND FUTURE DEVELOPMENTS

Editor:
Dieter D. Liermann, M.D.
J.W. Goethe University Hospital
Frankfurt am Main, Germany

Stents – State of the Art and Future Developments

ISBN 0-921317-52-2

Polyscience Publications, Inc.
Morin Heights, Canada
in Conjunction with
Boston Scientific Corporation
Watertown, MA USA

Printed in Canada

Second Printing, June 1995

Dedicated to my teacher
in Interventional Radiology
Professor Jürgen Kollath

PREFACE

In 1969, Charles Dotter was the first to describe a new technique to preserve a patent lumen by the percutaneous implantation of a spiral stent. Several authors have reported experimental use with several stent devices and since 1983 have published clinical results using different stent types. Many indications remain for stent implantation in different organ systems as an alternative to surgical and non-surgical methods. The rapid development and research on stents has broadened the indications for stent implantation to the aorta, supraaortic, renal, and abdominal arteries, anastomosed arteries of different transplant organs, transjugular intrahepatic portacaval shunts (TIPS), pancreatic or bile ducts, and the respiratory and genitourinary tracts. In this book, basic research on stents, stent materials, stent extraction, and myointimal hyperplasia are discussed. Long-term results with stent implantation and comparative studies between stenting and other interventions, such as percutaneous transluminal angioplasty or surgery, are also presented. The future of stents represented by alternatives such as temporary, bioresorable, and covered or coated stents; the combination of stents with grafts, chemical, or pharmaceutical agents; and various methods to prevent or reduce myointimal proliferation including endovascular irradiation and radioactive stents are summarized in the almost 60 articles presented in this book.

I would like to thank all of the authors who have reported on their experiences and research with stent implantation for the treatment of occlusions and stenoses. Collectively, these contributions provide both a helpful and a comprehensive overview that will allow their colleagues to compare the different stent types, the advantages and disadvantages of stent implantation, indications for stenting, and the results following stent implantation.

Dieter Liermann, M.D.

STENTS – STATE OF THE ART AND FUTURE DEVELOPMENTS

TABLE OF CONTENTS

PART I. VASCULAR STENTS

PART II: NONVASCULAR STENTS

Pancreatic Duct and Bile Duct

Gastrointestinal Tract

PART I

VASCULAR STENTS

Endoluminal Stent-Grafts for Intrathoracic and Abdominal Aortic Aneurysms

James May, Geoffrey White, Richard Waugh, Weiyun Yu, John Harris

Department of Surgery, University of Sydney and
Department of Vascular Surgery, Royal Prince Alfred Hospital, Sydney, Australia

Endoluminal repair of abdominal aortic aneurysms was undertaken in 14 patients. Six were considered able to undergo standard open repair, but the remaining eight had co-morbidities which caused them to be rejected for operation at other centers. Complications resulted in endoluminal repair being converted to an open repair in six patients; the remaining eight patients had endoluminal repairs. No deaths occurred in the hospital following the operation. During follow-up, however, two patients in the endoluminal repair group died due to cardiac causes, while one patient in the endoluminal converted to open group died from liver failure. In addition, one patient with a large false aneurysm in the right proximal subclavian artery had this successfully repaired with an endoluminal stent-graft.

INTRODUCTION

Great interest in endoluminal repair of aortic aneurysms has been generated by the first reported use of this technique in humans by Parodi et al in 1991 (1). There have, however, been few clinical reports in the surgical literature following this seminal contribution. We present our early experience with this technique and document some of the problems which we have encountered.

MATERIALS AND METHODS

Endoluminal repair was attempted in 14 patients with abdominal aortic aneurysms. All patients were male and had an average age of 72 years. Six were considered physically fit for standard open repair of their aneurysm, while the remaining eight had been rejected for open repair at another medical center. Table 1 lists the co-morbidities of these eight patients.

The morphology of the aneurysms allowed the patients to be divided into two groups. In one group of six patients, the aneurysms were confined to the aorta and had

Table 1. Co-Morbidities in Eight Patients Who Had Been Rejected for Open Repair

Poor left ventricular function and renal impairment	2
Renal failure requiring dialysis	1
Advanced coronary artery disease	1
Viral myocarditis	1
Chronic obstructive airways disease requiring oxygen for 16 hours/day	1
Chronic liver disease (Hepatitis C) with thrombocytopenia	1
Hostile abdomen	1

proximal and distal necks which made them suitable for repair with an endoluminal tube graft. In the other group of eight patients, there were no distal necks to the aneurysms and the common iliac arteries were either ectatic or frankly aneurysmal. These patients were suitable for an endoluminal aortofemoral graft combined with a femorofemoral crossover graft. An additional patient, aged 79 years, presented with a large expanding false aneurysm in the proximal right subclavian artery.

Endovascular repair of aneurysms with materials currently used in vascular surgery was approved by the Institutional Review Board and informed consent was obtained from each patient. Laboratory and clinical experience with the use of intraluminal grafts for subclavian and aortic aneurysms has previously been reported by the authors (2-5).

Endoluminal Repair Technique

A balloon-expandable stainless steel stent was used in combination with a PTFE or Dacron graft in 12 patients. The grafts were delivered into the aorta through a sheath introduced through the femoral or iliac arteries and anchored proximally with a stainless steel stent under radiographic control in the manner described by Parodi et al (1). In four patients the graft was tubular and confined to the aorta. In the remaining eight patients, a tapered aorto-iliac or aortofemoral graft was used in combination with a femorofemoral cross-over graft and contralateral iliac artery interruption as described by May et al (5) (Figure 1). Two of the 14 patients who did not have balloon-expandable stent grafts were treated with the Endovascular Grafting System (Endovascular Technologies, Menlo Park CA). This is a catheter-based system in which the graft is delivered into the aorta via a sheath in the femoral artery and anchored by two self-expanding Z-stents which are attached to the ends of the graft. The patient with the aneurysm of the subclavian artery was treated with a balloon-expandable stent and PTFE graft delivered through a sheath in the brachial artery (2) (Figure 2).

RESULTS

Successful endoluminal repair was achieved in 8 of the 14 patients with abdominal aortic aneurysms. The remaining six patients required conversion to the standard open aneurysm repair. All but one of these open repairs were carried out at the time of the failed endoluminal repair. Regardless of which type of operation was used, no patients died or lost a limb during hospitalization. There have been two deaths related to cardiac causes and one death due to liver failure/bleeding peptic ulcer during follow-up. The patient with an endoluminal repair of his subclavian aneurysm is still alive and well with normal circulation in the right arm 15 months after the operation.

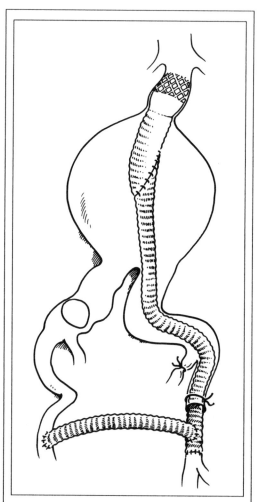

Figure 1. Tapered endoluminal aortofemoral graft combined with femorofemoral cross-over graft. Note the detachable balloon placed in the right common iliac artery to exclude the aneurysm from the general circulation.

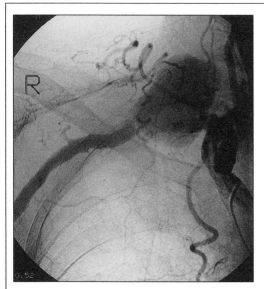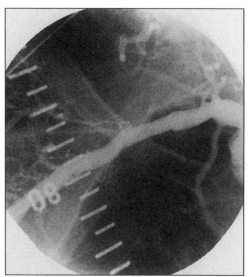

Figure 2. Pre-operative angiogram *(left)* demonstrating a large false aneurysm in the proximal right subclavian artery. Post-procedure angiogram *(right)* demonstrating normal flow through the subclavian artery and no leakage of contrast into the aneurysmal sac.

Complications

Complications which led to abandonment of the endoluminal repair in favor of an open repair were access problems (N=2), balloon malfunction (N=1), and stent migration (N=3).

Access Problems

A 29 Fr delivery sheath was introduced into the femoral artery. This sheath is almost 10 mm in diameter which was too large to be accepted by the 7-mm diameter external iliac artery in one patient. The disparity was known prior to operation but it was hoped that the artery could be dilated. We have subsequently avoided this problem by instituting a policy of not attempting sheath insertion into arteries less than 10 mm in diameter.

The second patient with an access problem readily accepted the introducing sheath into the aorta, but the bifurcated Dacron graft with balloon and stent could not be packaged in a sufficiently low profile to allow its insertion into the introducing sheath. This problem should have been identified in the laboratory prior to surgery. This problem has been eliminated in all subsequent cases by trial package of the stent-graft device in advance of the operation.

Balloon Malfunction

In one patient the stent-graft device was delivered without difficulty into the appropriate position below the renal arteries. The stent was also centered correctly between the radiopaque markers of the 30-mm diameter balloon. Upon inflation, however, the balloon expanded preferentially at the upper end. Attempts to make the lower end of the balloon inflate were unsuccessful and thus the stent, with its attached graft, was pushed distally into the aneurysm. Attempts to rectify the situation were unsuccessful and the endoluminal repair was abandoned in favor of an open repair.

Stent Migration

Stent migration is a serious problem and was observed on three occasions. Early in our experience, a stent-graft device was delivered into the appropriate position within the neck of the aneurysm. When the balloon was inflated, however, insufficient upward pressure was maintained on the shaft of the balloon and successive ventricular contractions pushed the balloon with its trapped stent distally into the aneurysm. This stent migration resulted in a leak at the upper end of the graft which did not seal off over a 3-week period and subsequently required conversion to an open repair. This problem has been minimized but not entirely eliminated by reducing the systolic arterial pressure to 80 mm Hg prior to inflation of the balloon and the application of firm upward pressure on the shaft of the balloon at the time of inflation.

Two additional patients had successful placement of stent-graft devices in the correct position in the neck of the aneurysm. Problems were experienced, however, in removing the deflated balloon through the distal 10-mm diameter portion of the tapered graft in each case. Although the balloons have a low profile of 4.5 mm in diameter before inflation, the diameter of the balloon following deflation on these two occasions was in excess of 10 mm. Unsuccessful attempts were made to reduce the diameter of the balloons by applying negative pressure. Unsuccessful attempts were also made to recover the balloons by withdrawing them into 21 Fr Teflon sheaths passed into the aorta through the dacron grafts. The amount of force required to free the balloons in these two patients produced excessive traction on the grafts and dislodged the stents from the neck into the body of the aneurysm. Both required conversion to an open repair.

CONCLUSIONS

We conclude from this study that endoluminal repair of aortic aneurysms is feasible. It is clear, however, that there is a long learning curve in acquiring the skills required with this technique. Although complications have reduced the overall success rate and have required conversion of endoluminal repair to an open repair in 6 of the 14 patients, none appear to have suffered any ill effects from the abandoned attempt. For those poor-risk patients with large aneurysms who have been previously rejected for operation, this approach would appear to be their only hope and thus, justified under the circumstances.

REFERENCES

1. Parodi JC, Palmaz JC, Barone HD. Transfemoral intraluminal graft implantation in abdominal aortic aneurysms. Ann Vasc Surg 1991;5:491-499.
2. May J, White GH, Waugh R, Yu W, Harris JP. Transluminal placement of a prosthetic graft-stent device for treatment of subclavian aneurysm. J Vasc Surg (accepted for publication).
3. May J, White GH, Yu W, Harris JP. Advantages and limitations of intraluminal grafts for thoracic and abdominal aortic aneurysm. Angiology 1993;Suppl 4:21.
4. White GH, Yu W, May J. Experimental endoluminal grafts and coated stents. Angiology 1993;Suppl 4:26.
5. May J, White GH, Yu W, Waugh R, Harris JP. Treatment of complex abdominal aortic aneurysms by a combination of endoluminal and extraluminal aorto-femoral grafts. J Vasc Surg (accepted for publication).

Endovascular Stent-Grafting for Treatment of Thoracic Aortic Aneurysms

Michael D. Dake and Charles P. Semba

Department of Radiology, Stanford University Medical Center, Stanford, CA USA

INTRODUCTION

Standard treatment for thoracic aortic aneurysms is a surgical graft replacement. Endovascular stent-grafts offer an alternative treatment approach that may be less invasive and less expensive, with a lower risk and a shorter hospital recuperation period than traditional operative therapy. The idea of transluminally-placed endovascular stent-grafts was initially conceived by Dotter (1). A number of investigators followed his proposal with feasibility research using experimental animal models of abdominal aortic aneurysms (2-7). Recently, the clinical use of endovascular stent-grafts was described for the treatment of abdominal aortic aneurysms, subclavian artery aneurysms, arteriovenous fistulas, and femoral occlusive disease (8-11).

This chapter describes our initial clinical experience with a transluminally-placed, self-expanding stent-graft for the treatment of descending thoracic aortic aneurysms. This preliminary experience suggests that endovascular stent-grafts may provide a safe and effective therapy to manage highly selected patients with aneurysms of the descending thoracic aorta.

MATERIALS AND METHODS

Our first patient in a current series of 18 was treated in July, 1992. All of the patients had aneurysms originating distal to the left subclavian artery and terminating above the celiac access. The aortic pathology was due to a variety of etiologies; however, atherosclerosis was responsible for most of the aneurysms. Almost all of the patients had previously undergone an operation for the treatment of cardiac or thoracic aortic pathology.

Table 1 details the imaging protocol prescribed for evaluation of all patients pre- and post-procedure. In particular cases, magnetic resonance (MR) imaging and/or intravascular ultrasound were employed to supplement the protocol exams.

Table 1. Imaging Protocol			
	Chest Radiograph (PA/LAT)	Spiral CT	Arteriography
Pre-Procedure	X	X	X
Intraoperatively			X
Post-Procedure	X	X	X
2 Months Post-Procedure	X		
6 Months Post-Prodecure		X	X
1 Year Post-Procedure	X	X	X
2 Years Post-Procedure and Annually Thereafter	X	X	

The endovascular stent-graft used in all patients was composed of individual Z-shaped wire stent bodies (at least 2.5 cm in length) linked together to form a stainless steel endoskeleton of a suitable length to bridge the aneurysm. This cylindrical framework was covered with a skin of woven Dacron graft (Meadox Medicals Inc., Oakland NJ). The crimp to the graft was ironed out to reduce the overall diameter of the stent-graft prior to attaching the graft to the stent by a series of interrupted polypropylene sutures (Figure 1).

The stent-grafts were custom fabricated for each individual patient with the appropriate diameter, length, taper, and curvature based upon measurements derived from spiral computed tomography (CT) and arteriography.

The delivery system to accommodate these stent-grafts consisted of a 24 Fr O.D. Teflon sheath, a graduated dilator, and a valve closure apparatus attached to the proximal operator end of the sheath to provide hemostasis. The dilator and sheath combination were introduced over a heavy-duty 0.89 mm (0.035 inch) guidewire which was positioned across the aneurysm. A solid Teflon mandril was used as a pusher device to ad-

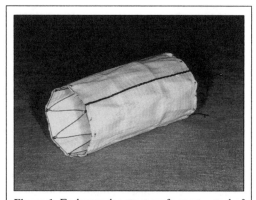

Figure 1. Endovascular stent-graft constructed of Z-shaped individual stainless steel stent bodies covered with a woven Dacron graft. The crimps in the graft have been ironed out to reduce the overall diameter of the device. The graft material is secured to the underlying stent framework by a series of interrupted polypropylene sutures.

vance the stent-graft within the sheath. All procedures were performed in the operating rooms of Stanford University Hospital with the patient supine or in a right lateral decubitus position, under general anaesthesia, on a radiolucent table. The operative field was prepared in anticipation of an eventual thoracotomy. A portable fluoroscopic image intensifier capable of video playback and hard copy image archiving was utilized in association with a mechanical contrast media injector to facilitate intraprocedural aortography. Image guidance for the stent-graft procedure was provided by fluoroscopy and supplemented in all cases by transesophageal ultrasound imaging to confirm optimal positioning of the stent-graft within the sheath prior to deployment and to assess the adequacy of the endovascular "repair" following device expansion.

In all cases, the initial technical step was placement of a pigtail angiographic catheter within the proximal aortic arch to permit preliminary aortography. If the aneurysm involved the transverse arch in close proximity to the left subclavian artery origin, the catheter was placed via the left brachial artery. In these cases, the catheter served as a conspicuous marker of the left subclavian artery and could be used for aortography to assess relationships between the device and aortic arch anatomy immediately antecedent to deployment. In patients with aneurysms involving the descending thoracic aorta exclusively, preliminary aortography was performed via a transfemorally-placed catheter, which was subsequently removed for insertion of the sheath/dilator system. After the initial arteriography of the thoracic aorta, intravenous administration of sodium heparin 300 IU/kg was given.

After the sheath was placed across the aneurysm and the dilator was removed, the stent-graft was introduced from its loading cartridge into the sheath by advancing the Teflon pusher. Once the device was appropriately located proximal to the aneurysm, a sodium nitroprusside solution was administered intravenously to decrease the mean arterial pressure to 50-60 mm Hg. Lowering the mean arterial pressure just prior to releasing the device reduced the risk of downstream migration during initial deployment due to arterial flow contacting the partially expanded stent-graft. After checking the fluoroscopic and transesophageal ultrasound images, the stent-graft was deployed by holding the pusher stationary and withdrawing the sheath. This allowed rapid deployment of the self-expanding prosthesis.

In 11 patients, a femoral artery was surgically isolated and a transverse arteriotomy was performed to allow insertion of the 24 Fr delivery system. In five patients with small and/or diseased iliac arteries which could not accommodate the delivery system, the 24 Fr sheath and dilator were inserted via direct puncture of the infrarenal abdominal aorta. In two other cases, the 24 Fr delivery system was introduced in conjunction with surgical resection of an abdominal aortic aneurysm. In both of these procedures, the delivery system was advanced via the abdominal aortic graft, using one limb of a bifurcated graft or via a 10-mm Dacron side-arm attached to the aortic segment of the graft.

After deployment, successful exclusion of the aneurysm was evaluated by aortography and transesophageal ultrasound imaging. In four cases, a second stent-graft prosthesis was deployed to completely exclude flow within the aneurysm. In two cases the second device was immediately deployed under the same anaesthetic; in two other cases, it was necessary to bring the patient back for a second procedure requiring a repeat endobronchial intubation and anaesthesia. Following the procedure, the patient was initially taken to the intensive care unit for post-operative monitoring.

RESULTS

The stent-graft was successfully deployed in all cases. Complete thrombosis of the aneurysm surrounding the stent-graft was achieved in 16 of the 18 patients (Figure 2). Three other patients initially had a small patent proximal tract communicating with the aneurysm. In all cases, these channels subsequently thrombosed within 2 months of the procedure. The mean maximum transverse diameter of the aneurysms was 6.0 cm (range, 5.0 to 8.0 cm). In these 18 cases, the mean diameter of the implanted stent-graft was 3.5 cm (range, 3.0 to 4.5 cm) and the average length of the device was 10.0 cm (range, 5.0 to 16.0 cm).

In the 18 patients treated thus far, there has been one death. This occurred in an 83-year-old man with an aneurysm of the aortic ductus diverticulum. The aneurysm off the transverse arch was successfully excluded during an uneventful procedure; however, the patient subsequently developed severe respiratory compromise in association with an episode of post-operative aspiration. This eventually resulted in bilateral pneumonia, respiratory failure, and death 23 days after the procedure.

There has been one episode of transient paraplegia. This occurred in a 67-year-old woman after stent-grafting of a 10-cm long descending thoracic aortic atherosclerotic aneurysm. The procedure was performed in conjunction with surgical resection of an abdominal aortic aneurysm and re-implantation of a renal artery and the inferior mesenteric artery. Immediately post-procedure, the patient was able to move all extremities, however, 36 hours post-operatively she became paraplegic. This was associated with cardiogenic shock and renal failure. The latter two resolved completely with supportive care, although marked distal lower extremity muscle weakness persisted 3 months after stent-grafting. There have been no instances of stroke, distal embolization, or infection. The only other significant early morbidity was pleuritic pain and left pleural effusion which were noted in four patients. These symptoms were self-limited and spontaneously regressed in all cases within 1 week after the procedure.

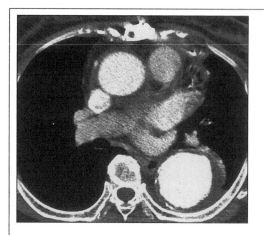
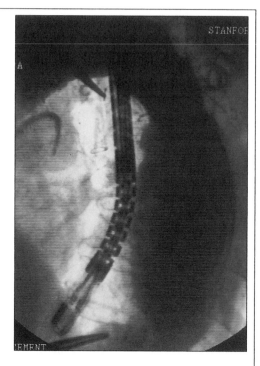
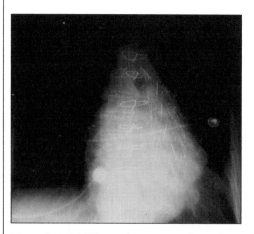
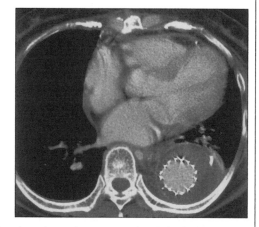

Figure 2. Axial CT scan demonstrates large descending thoracic aortic aneurysm (*top left*). Interoperative aortogram prior to stent-grafting shows a large fusiform degenerative aneurysm of the descending thoracic aorta (*top right*). Chest radiograph after stent-graft deployment demonstrates the position of the device within the thorax (*bottom left*). Note distorted contour of the cardio-mediastinal silhouette due to the large aneurysm. Axial CT scan after stent-graft procedure demonstrates patent prosthesis with surrounding thrombus within the aneurysm (*bottom right*). No evidence of contrast media leak into the aneurysm was noted.

One patient with a large aneurysm of the aortic ductus diverticulum required surgery following the stent-graft procedure to restore flow to the left subclavian artery. The aneurysm originated from the inferior aspect of the transverse arch with only a short segment neck of about 1 cm between the left subclavian artery origin and the aneurysm. Re-implantation of the subclavian artery into the left carotid artery or bypass from the left carotid artery to the subclavian artery prior to stent-grafting was contemplated; however, the added complexity of an additional procedure was less than attractive in this elderly woman with multiple co-existing medical problems. Following deployment of the stent-graft, completion aortography showed good flow in the left subclavian artery, and pressures performed through a catheter placed via the left brachial artery failed to document a pressure gradient across the left subclavian artery origin. Three days after the procedure, the patient experienced numbness and tingling in her left hand. Repeat arteriography demonstrated a clot within the proximal left subclavian artery. A trial of transcatheter-directed thrombolysis with urokinase did not completely dissolve the clot, and re-implantation of the left subclavian artery into the left carotid artery was required. The patient recovered uneventfully and is currently asymptomatic without any untoward effects related to the stent-graft procedure or subsequent surgery.

The mean current follow-up is 10 months with a range of 2 to 22 months. Follow-up using the imaging protocol described earlier has been performed in all patients. All stent-grafts are widely patent without evidence of aneurysm recurrence, stent-graft migration, false aneurysms, or significant change in the dimensions of the aneurysm sac in the 17 patients treated electively. In one patient with a complex extensive chronic type A dissection acutely complicated by a large descending false aneurysm, operative intervention was required 4 months after stent-grafting to treat continued expansion of the ascending aorta, arch, and the entire descending thoracic aorta. In addition, it was necessary to replace the aortic valve. This case illustrates the perplexing challenge posed by patients with thoracic aortic aneurysms due to aortic dissection. It is well-recognized from experience with standard resectional surgery that thoracic aneurysms secondary to aortic dissection are more lethal than atherosclerotic aneurysms, with a higher incidence of early rupture and a greater operative mortality (12-13). These complex cases provide a stiff challenge with a unique set of technical concerns. Presently, it is unclear if endovascular stent-grafting will be able to effectively manage this difficult group of patients, especially those with dissection and thoracic aneurysms.

DISCUSSION

Irrespective of the exact etiology, there are a number of general technical issues to consider when designing an endovascular stent-graft for treatment of thoracic aortic aneurysms. These considerations include:

- **Basic Stent Design**
  - Flexible or rigid stent
  - Deployment: balloon-expandable, self-expandable, or a combination
  - Stent location: proximal, proximal and distal, or throughout
  - Attachments: hooks or friction seal
  - Graft material: woven Dacron, knitted Dacron, or PTFE
  - Delivery system: Balloon catheter, sheath/pusher, capsule

- **Graft Material**
  I. *Characteristics*
  - Porosity
  - Capacity for radial expansion
  - Profile/thickness
  - Pliability
  - Dilation with time

  II. *Other Considerations*
  - Crimping

- Velour coating
- Collagen impregnation/pre-clotting

- **Technical Problems**
  - Device delivery to target
  - Misplacement of prosthesis
  - Reliable deployment
  - Migration

- **Anatomical Factors**
  - I. *Route of Delivery - Iliac Arteries*
  - Tortuosity
  - Significant atherosclerosis
  - Small caliber vessels

  - II. *Target Vessel Morphology*
  - Aortic arch curvature
  - Proximity to great vessels
  - Adequacy of focal necks
  - Correlation of proximal and distal neck sizes
  - Luminal contour

It is beyond the scope of this paper to individually discuss each of these factors. Indeed, the field of endovascular stent-grafting is rapidly developing. As technical and design advances progress the spectrum of applications and the relative indications and contraindications for stent-graft repair of thoracic aortic aneurysms will evolve.

Table 2 summarizes the clinical and anatomical conditions we currently consider in the selection of patients with thoracic aortic aneurysms for stent-graft procedures. Further investigation is clearly required before consequences of various prosthetic structural designs can be understood to determine the relative desirability of various stent-graft features. Similarly, the advisability of endovascular stent-grafting as a treatment option for all types of aortic pathologies has not yet been established. Indeed, the most challenging investigative hurdle for this new technology awaits additional follow-up. Establishing the ultimate safety, durability, and efficacy of transluminally placed endovascular stent-grafts for the treatment of thoracic aortic aneurysms and other pathological lesions will require dedicated investigation of the long-term effects of this procedure in larger numbers of patients.

Table 2. Selection Criteria for Stent-Graft Procedures in Patients with Thoracic Aortic Aneurysms

---

Characteristics of Aortic Aneurysms Precluding Stent-Graft Procedures

- Ascending Thoracic Aorta
- Significant Branch Vessel Involvement
- No Focal Neck(s)
- Markedly Tortuous
- Adjacent Organ Compression
- Inadequate Access
- ? – Mycotic
- ? – Marfan Syndrome

Characteristics of Aortic Aneurysms Amenable to Stent-Graft Procedures

- Transverse Aortic Arch
- Descending Thoracic Aorta
- Abdominal Aorta
- Atherosclerotic/Degenerative
- Traumatic
- Post-Operative
- Dissection-Related
- Giant Penetrating Ulcer

REFERENCES

1. Dotter CT. Transluminally placed coil spring endarterial tube grafts: long-term patency in canine popliteal artery. Invest Radiol 1969;4:329-332.
2. Laborde JC, Parodi JC, Clem MF, et al. Intraluminal bypass of abdominal aortic aneurysm: feasibility study. Radiology 1992;184:185-190.
3. Chuter TAM, Green RM, Ouriel K, Fiore W, DeWeese JA. Transfemoral graft placement. J Vasc Surg 1993;18:185-197.
4. Mirich D, Wright KC, Wallace S, et al. Percutaneously placed endovascular grafts for aortic aneurysms: feasibility study. Radiology 1989;170:1033-1037.
5. Lawrence DD, Charnsangavej C, Wright KC, Gianturco C, Wallace S. Percutaneous endovascular graft: experimental evaluation. Radiology 1987;163:357-360.

6. Balko A, Piansecki CJ, Shah DM, Carney WI, Hopkins RW, Jackson BT. Transfemoral placement of intraluminal polyurethane prosthesis for abdominal aortic aneurysms. J Surg Res 1986;40:305-309.

7. Yoshioka T, Wright KC, Wallace S, Lawrence DD, Gianturco C. Self-expanding endovascular graft: an experimental study in dogs. AJR 1988;151:673-676.

8. Parodi JC, Barone HD. Transfemoral intraluminal graft implantation for the abdominal aortic aneurysms. Ann Vasc Surg 1991;5:491-499.

9. May J, White G, Waugh R, Yu W, Harris J. Transluminal placement of a prosthetic graft/stent device for treatment of subclavian artery aneurysm. J Vasc Surg 1993;18:1056-1059.

10. Marin ML, Veith FJ, Panetta TF, et al. Percutaneous transfemoral stented graft repair of a traumatic femoral arteriovenous fistula. J Vasc Surg 1993;18:298-301.

11. Cragg AH, Dake MD. Percutaneous femoropopliteal graft placement. Radiology 1993;187:643-648.

12. Moreno-Cabral CE, Miller DC, Mitchell RS, et al. Degenerative and atherosclerotic aneurysms of the thoracic aorta. J Thorac Cardiovasc Surg 1984;88:1020-1032.

13. Pressler V, McNamara JJ. Thoracic aortic aneurysm. Natural history and treatment. J Thorac Cardiovasc Surg 1978;79:489-498.

Tantalum-Dacron Coknit Stent for Endovascular Treatment of Aortic Aneurysms: A Preliminary Experimental Study[1]

Philippe Piquet[1], Pierre-Henri Rolland[2], Jean-Michel Bartoli[1],
Pierre Tranier[1], Guy Moulin[1], Claude Mercier[1]

[1]*Services de Chirurgie Vasculaire et de Radiologie, Hôpital de la Timone and the INSERM –
Laboratoire de Chimie Biologique, Université d'Aix-Marseille II, France*
[2]*Faculté de Pharmacie, Université d'Aix-Marseille II, France*

Purpose: *The purpose of this study was to evaluate the efficiency of intraluminal tantalum-Dacron coknit stents for the treatment of artificial aortic aneurysms in minipigs.*
Methods: *Replacement of the infrarenal abdominal aorta with Dacron artificial aneurysm graft was performed in eight minipigs. After 2 weeks, balloon-expandable coknit stents were inserted through the femoral artery to the site of the artificial aneurysm in seven minipigs. One animal was kept as a control. Coknit stent/artificial aneurysm complexes were explanted at various intervals from 24 hours to 12 weeks and underwent gross examination, followed by scanning electron and light microscopy studies.*
Results: *Aortography performed at the time of stent placement displayed immediate exclusion of the aneurysm in every case. In follow-up studies, all coknit stents remained patent until the time of explant. Scanning electron microscopy studies revealed apparent endothelialization of the entire coknit stent lumen at and after 6 weeks.*
Conclusion: *Tantalum-Dacron coknit stents are efficient in the treatment of artificially created aneurysms in minipigs and facilitate the creation of an endothelialized new vascular wall. Clinical application of this coknit stent can be considered but necessitates retaining the same stent structure in diameters greater than 20 mm and the development of a suitable delivery system.*

Graft-replacement therapy for abdominal aortic aneurysm was introduced by Dubost et al (1) in 1951. Since then, the results of abdominal aortic aneurysmectomy have steadily improved, and early mortality rates of less than 5% have been reported after elective treatment (2-6). It is therefore generally accepted that elective aortic replacement aneurysmectomy must be performed for an aneurysm larger than 5 cm in diameter (7,8). There is, however, a group of patients at high risk for surgery because of associated heart, lung, and kidney diseases, or because of advanced age (9). For these patients, an alternative to direct aortic reconstruction is suitable. Acute induced thrombosis of the aneurysm with simultaneous axillobifemoral bypass has been proposed (10), but it has such poor short- and long-term results that the method is considered inefficient and unusable (11,12). Technologic progress in recent years has made it possible to consider transfemoral placement of aortic prostheses (13). The clinical application of this technique has been reported with a Dacron graft attached to both necks of the aneurysm by two Palmaz™ stents (Johnson & Johnson Interventional Systems, Warren NJ) (14). We have tested in minipigs a new kind of endovascular prosthesis that is a balloon-

[1] Reproduced from Piquet P, Rolland PH, Bartoli JM, *et al.* Tantalum-Dacron coknit stent for endovascular treatment of aortic aneurysms: a preliminary experimental study. J Vasc Surg 1994;19:698-706, with permission from Mosby-Year Book Inc.

expandable stent that serves as a framework for the development of a new aortic wall. The following is the report of our findings.

MATERIAL AND METHODS

Experimental Aortic Aneurysm Model

Eight Pitman-Moore minipigs of both sexes weighing 40 to 69 kg were used in this study. A segment of the infrarenal aorta was replaced with a fusiform-shaped conduit made of crimped, woven Dacron (Bard Vascular Systems Division, Billerica, MA). Measurements of this artificial aortic aneurysm were 3 cm in maximum transverse diameter and 4 cm in length. The diameter at both ends was 1 cm, and the overall length of the graft was 10 cm, to be adjusted before placement. After initial sedation with 15 mg/kg ketamine, minipigs were anesthetized with urethane-chloralose mixture (25% to 5% 1.5 ml/kg) and then intubated and ventilated with nitrous oxide and oxygen. Minipigs were placed in the supine position. A midline incision provided a transperitoneal approach to the infrarenal abdominal aorta. After administration of heparin (100 IU/kg), the infrarenal aorta was cross-clamped and then resected, sparing 1 cm below the renal arteries and 1 cm above the aortic trifurcation. The corresponding lumbar arteries were ligated and divided. The aneurysmal Dacron graft was cut at the right length and then was inserted and anastomosed end-to-end to the aorta with continuous 5.0 polypropylene sutures (Prolene; Ethicon, Somerville, NJ). The abdomen was closed in standard fashion. Ampicillin 20 mg/kg was given daily for 3 days. Two weeks healing time was allowed before transfemoral placement of the intraluminal prosthesis.

Endovascular Prosthesis Placement and Follow-up

The endovascular prosthesis (Boston Scientific A/S, Jyllinge, Denmark) is a modification of the balloon-expandable stent first designed by Strecker et al (15) (Figure 1). It is made of 0.10 mm outer diameter tantalum wire coknitted with four strands of texturized Dacron fiber. The tantalum is left exposed at both ends to facilitate fixation of the coknit stent on the carrying balloon catheter. The stent is fixed onto the balloon by two silicone sleeves that overlap the stent at each end. As the balloon is inflated, the sleeves roll back to release the stent. The coknit stents were 6 or 8 cm in length and 10 mm in expanded diameter. Each stent was mounted on a 10 mm diameter PENTA II high-pressure (10 ATM) polyethylene balloon catheter (Boston Scientific A/S). For placement of the coknit stent, each animal was anesthetized as previously described. After administration of heparin (100 IU/kg), the right femoral artery was surgically approached, and a 12 Fr introducer sheath with a hemostatic valve (Medicorp, Nancy - Brabois, France) was inserted through the femoral artery. Aortography was performed to visualize the aneurysm graft status. Radiopaque forceps were placed on surgical drapes to mark the proximal and distal ends of the aneurysm for fluoroscopic control. The coknit stent was inserted though the introducer sheath over a 0.035-inch guidewire (Terumo Corporation, Tokyo, Japan) and advanced through the arterial lumen under fluoroscopic guidance to the site of the aneurysm. Once the stent was properly positioned, the balloon was inflated, releasing the coknit stent. Angiography was then performed to assess the immediate post-placement results.

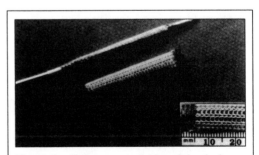

Figure 1. Balloon-expandable endoluminal prosthesis mounted on balloon catheter, than expanded. (*Insert*: close-up of expanded stent with scale).

After introducer sheath removal, the puncture site in the femoral artery was sutured with 6.0 polypropylene. The groin incision was closed in a standard manner. Calcium heparin (300 IU/kg daily) was given subcutaneously for 2 days.

Treatment of the aneurysm by means of a coknit stent was undertaken in seven animals. The artificial aneurysm was not treated in one minipig that was kept as a control to evaluate the fate of the Dacron artificial aneurysm. Abdominal CT scanning was performed in two minipigs 2 weeks after stent-graft implantation. The animals were killed by intravenous injection of potassium chloride with the pigs receiving anesthetic at 24 hours (one minipig), 1 week (one minipig), 3 weeks (one minipig), 6 weeks (two minipigs), 9 weeks (one minipig), and 12 weeks (one minipig). The control animal was killed after 9 weeks. Before death, aortography was performed in all minipigs by means of a left femoral artery catheterization. The intraluminal diameters of the coknit stents were measured and compared with immediate post-placement angiographic results. An iterative laparotomy was performed, and the segment of aorta with the aneurysmal graft containing the coknit stent was removed. The samples were sectioned longitudinally into two halves and photographed. Both halves were then fixed with ice-cold 2.5% buffered glutaraldehyde for 1 hour. One half of each specimen then was transversely sectioned into six portions that were identified according to their position from proximal to distal, dehydrated in progressive acetone and dried by the critical point method with acetone and liquid carbon dioxide. After sputter coating with 30 nm gold coating layer (ion sputter JEOL JFC-110; JEOL Ltd., Akishima, Japan), scanning electron microscopy of these fragments was performed with the use of a JEOL JSM 35 CF microscope (JEOL Ltd.).

Histologic examination was performed on the remaining half of each stent-graft complex after being divided into three parts, thereby defining proximal, central, and distal portions. Because tantalum is too resistant to provide adequate histologic slides, even when cut with a diamond knife, the histologic analysis was carried out after removing the coknit stent strands under microscopic guidance. After identification, the specimens were further fixed in Bouin's fluid for 24 hours, dehydrated in progressive alcohol, and embedded in paraffin. Four-micrometer transverse sections were obtained and stained alternatively with hematoxylin, eosin, and Safranin (Sigma Chemical Co., St. Louis MO) for general observation, Masson-green-trichrome for collagen and connective tissue and Darrow orcein for specific staining of elastic tissue. For the control animal, the aortic segment with the Dacron artificial aneurysm was explanted and similarly treated for macroscopic and histologic observation. Throughout the course of these experiments, animal care was in compliance with regulations in the "Guide for the Care and Use of Laboratory Animals" (The National Institutes of Health publication No. 80-23, revised 1985) and "Principles of Laboratory Animal Care", formulated by the National Society for Medical Research.

RESULTS

Recovery after placement of the artificial aneurysm graft was uneventful for all of the animals. Aortography performed before the coknit stent implant confirmed patency of the Dacron aneurysm graft in every case. Similarly, aortography demonstrated the patency of the aneurysmal graft in the control animal before explantation. The maximum transverse diameter of the aneurysms measured on angiography ranged from 28 to 30 mm (mean, 29 mm). One stent was placed in five animals. Two stents were placed overlapping in the additional two minipigs, as a result of low placement of the initial stent. All femoral arteries used as access routes for stent-graft placement were patent at the conclusion of the procedure. There were no technical problems associated with stent deployment. In all cases, coknit stent placement resulted in immediate exclusion of the aneurysm from the aortic blood flowpath. No extravasation of contrast media outside of the stent lumen was observed. We used an 80 mm long coknit stent in one animal; the distal portion of the stent extended into the right common iliac artery, immediately excluding the left common iliac artery. The animal recovered without any functional impairment of the left hind limb. Computed tomography (CT) scanning on two minipigs at 2 weeks confirmed total exclusion of the aneurysms by the coknit stents (Figure 2). The artifact created by the highly radiopaque tantalum prevented examination of the stent. However, the transverse sections clearly revealed that the artificial aneurysm surrounding the stent was full of thrombotic material. The maximum transverse diameter of the Dacron aneurysm measured on CT scanning was reduced with respect to the original 30 mm (2.7 cm in one case, 2.6 cm in the other). *In vivo* three-dimensional CT scanning reconstructions showed the flexible coknit stent to be fully expanded to 10 mm along the length of the artificial aneurysm itself. The stent ends

were slightly constricted by the Dacron aneurysm graft necks (Figure 2).

Angiographic follow-up on all seven stented animals documented coknit stent patency at the time of explant. No change in stent lumen diameter was noted for six of the minipigs (Figure 3). Angiography on the seventh minipig at 9 weeks displayed an apparent moderate narrowing of the stent lumen along the length of the artificial aneurysm.

Gross examination at 24 hours of the explanted stent and artificial aneurysm graft revealed a homogeneous layer of fresh red thrombus filling the space between the coknit stent network exterior and the internal wall of the artificial aneurysm graft. The flow surface consisted of a thin and transparent lining embedding the texturized Dacron stent fibers. A fibrin-like material filled the gaps between the meshes of the stent. On the 1- and 3-week explants, the coknit stent inner surface was increasingly covered by a fine layer of a translucent and shiny material. In the 6-, 9-, and 12-week explants, the coknit stent inner surface was covered with what appeared to be a continuation of the bright and opaque intimal

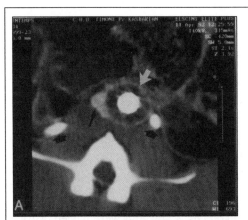 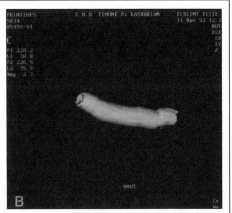

Figure 2. *In vivo* computed tomography scan with intravenous contrast injection 15 days after stent implantation. **A,** Transverse section through middle third of stent-graft complex. Artificial aneurysm graft is visible in form of linear opacity *(white arrow)*. Thrombosis of aneurysm sac is clearly hypodense, without enhancement after intravenous contrast injection. Coknit stent is well centered; hyperdensity of tantalum prevents any visualization of aortic lumen and causes small artifacts radiating outward from stent. Ureters are shown by *arrows.* Inferior vena cava is shown by *long arrow.* **B,** Three-dimensional reconstruction of aortic coknit stent obtained from 5 mm adjacent slices with correct computed tomography range slice-by-slice application. Note that both proximal and distal ends of stent were slightly narrowed by Dacron aneurysm graft necks.

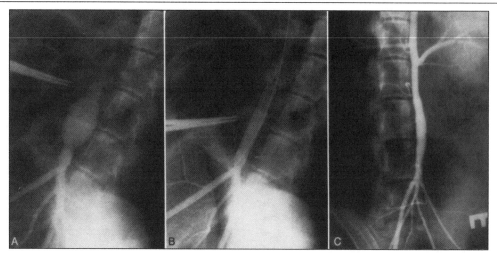

Figure 3. **A,** Arteriogram of aortic artificial aneurysm before implantation of coknit stent. **B,** Angiography after stent placement shows complete exclusion of artificial aneurysm from aortic blood flow. **C,** Arteriogram at 3 weeks after stent placement.

layer of the native aorta. Originating from the stent ends, this layer at 12 weeks occupied more than 75% of the total length of the explanted stent-grafts, whereas the luminal central portion still consisted of the opalescent layer through which the stent meshes were discernible (Figure 4). Concomitantly the thrombus filling the artificial aneurysmal space began to undergo resorption with, at 12 weeks, a dark-brown compacted appearance including off-white fibrotic cores. No significant intimal thickening was found obstructing blood flow through the stents.

Twenty-four hours after stent placement, scanning electron microscopy (SEM) analysis revealed that the flow surface consisted of a thin film of fibrinous material anchored onto the texturized Dacron strands of the stent, thereby forming a continuous alveolar-like network along the entire length of the stent (Figure 5). In the 1- and 3-week explants, this film thickened, further embedding the intraluminal stent strands, forming an acellular

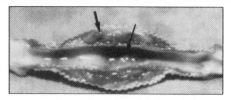

Figure 4. Macroscopic view of stent-graft complex explanted at 12 weeks. Note continuation of bright and opaque intimal layer of native aorta from both ends of coknit stent. Central portion of inner surface remained pale and opalescent *(long arrow)*, as it had been throughout entire length of stent at 3 weeks. Stent meshes were still discernible in this segment. Also note advanced staging of thrombus and off-white fibrosclerotic cores filling up aneurysmal space *(arrow)*.

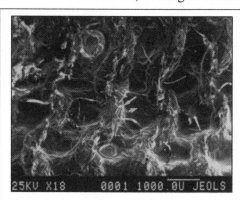

Figure 5. Photomicrograph of acellular fibrin lining making up flow surface of stent-graft complex explanted at 24 hours. Note alveolar-like network appearance of thin film of fibrin *(arrow)* anchored to bulging texturized Dacron strands of stent *(long arrow)* (SEM, original magnification x18; *white bar*: 1 mm).

luminal surface. High-magnification SEM study demonstrated that the lining was a microporous, mesh-like structure of fibrin strands. From 1 to 3 weeks, the intimal structure of the inner wall of the stent progressively consisted of more organized, compacted and flattened fibrin fibers layering, thereby smoothening, the flow surface. This fibrin layering paved the way for apparent endothelialization of the entire stent-graft lumen observed at 6 weeks after implantation (Figure 6). From SEM observations, the thickness of the proximal and distal portions of the neointima increased uniformly, measuring 115 ± 45, 220 ± 38, 230 ± 50, 280 ± 82, 320 ± 65, and 350 ± 70 μm at 24 hours, 1, 3, 6, 9, and 12 weeks, respectively. In the central part of the stent, the thickness of the wall remained less than 250 μm. At higher magnification, on and after 6 weeks, SEM showed that the stent lumen was covered with cells

with the morphologic appearance of endothelial cells (Figure 7).

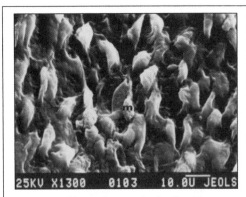

Figure 7. Photomicrograph of cells with appearance of endothelial cells covering flow surface of stent-graft proximal portion, explanted at 6 weeks (SEM, original magnification x1300; *white bar:* 10 μm; *m:* monocyte-macrophage).

Histologic examination of the stent-graft explants revealed that the aneurysmal space was filled with blood that from 24 hours up to 12 weeks after stent implantation had the usual appearance of an arterial thrombus. The histologic analysis at and after 6 weeks showed the existence of a neowall on the internal side of the coknit stent (Figure 8). At 12 weeks this neowall in the central portion of the explant consisted of a fibrinoid neointima whose cellular lining had the histologic appearance of an endothelium. In the

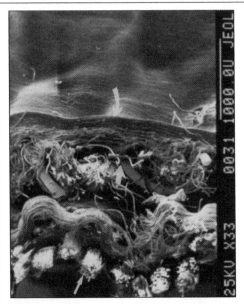

Figure 6. Photomicrograph of longitudinal section of stent-graft complex (proximal portion), explanted at 6 weeks (lumen on top). Edge of stent-graft complex simultaneously shows presence of Dacron artificial aneurysm fibers *(arrow)*, coknit Dacron-tantalum stent *(large arrow)* with endothelialized fibrin layers *(curved arrow)* (SEM: original magnification x33; *white bar:* 1 mm).

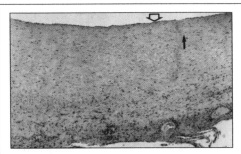

Figure 8. Histologic appearance of neointima at 6 weeks (lumen on top, thrombus at the bottom). Note parallel fibrin laminae infiltrated by myofibroblasts *(thin arrow)* and covered by apparent endothelium lining *(arrow head)*. (Masson-trichrome; original magnification x50).

proximal and distal parts of the explant the neowall consisted of a fibroproliferative intima coated with cells with the histologic appearance of endothelial cells, lined on the outside with a fibrocellular layer evoking a medial structure (Figure 9). In the control animal the analysis of the Dacron artificial aneurysm did not show significant thrombus formation. The inner wall of the Dacron graft was covered with a thin film of fibrin deposit.

DISCUSSION

Although experimental models of elastase-induced aortic aneurysms have been described in rats (16), satisfactory models do not exist for larger animals such as dogs or pigs. As previously described (17), we used surgical interposition of an artificial aneu-

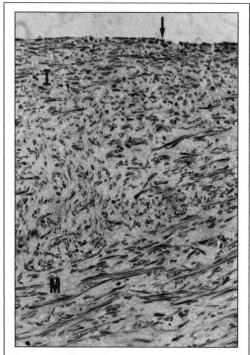

Figure 9. Histologic appearance of neovessel wall at 12 weeks (lumen on top). Neointima *(I)* is formed by cicatricial cell proliferation with luminal surface that is covered by clearly defined endothelium *(arrow)*. Note presence of elastic fibrils and of myofibroblasts in neomedia *(M)*. (Masson-trichrome; original magnification x125).

rysm conduit that has a configuration similar to the one found in human infrarenal aortic aneurysms that was not the case in other models described in the literature (13,18). The endoprosthesis we used was made of 0.1 mm tantalum wire coknited with Dacron fibers. The coknit stent was inserted through the femoral artery up to the infrarenal aorta, and then successfully deployed. This was the case in all the animals. Stent implantation was monitored in all cases by immediate exclusion of the artificial aneurysm from the aortic blood flow. Coknit stents remained patent in all animals, with a maximum follow-up of 12 weeks. Texturized Dacron fibers provided a suitable media to promote controlled fibrin deposition that excluded the aneurysmal space while avoiding luminal thrombosis. The fibrin fibers and trapped blood plasma proteins served as a natural substrate for a rapid (6 weeks or less) and complete apparent endothelialization of the lumen of the graft. Therefore this study established the feasibility of placing the present endoprosthesis in an artificially created aneurysm in the minipig, allowing the exclusion of the aneurysmal space from the aortic flow by formation of a new aortic wall from the tissues of the host.

Other types of endoprostheses have been proposed for treating aortic aneurysms. The endoprosthesis proposed by Balko et al (13) is made of polyurethane on a frame of nitinol and has been used in sheep but has not been further developed. Laborde et al (17) have studied in dogs an endoprosthesis made of a knitted Dacron tube attached at both ends to balloon-expandable Palmaz stents. As in our study, endoprostheses were implanted in artificially created Dacron aortic aneurysms. Early occlusion caused by a twisted intraluminal graft was observed in two dogs. The remaining six dogs had a patent bypass at 6 months with a kinking of the graft in four of them. SEM studies showed apparent endothelialization of only the stent portion of the bypass luminal surface. Lawrence et al (19) have developed an endoprosthesis made of a Dacron tube covering two self-expanding metal stents, connected at each end to two other stents that were not covered. Because of the non-expandable character of the Dacron, these authors noted a tendency to wrinkle, promote thrombosis or fibrogenesis, and eventually narrow the lumen. Dacron was then replaced by expandable nylon, and the graft was supported by self-expanding Gianturco stents and was tested in the normal and aneurysmal dog aorta (18,20). Of six animals whose aorta had been made aneurysmal, the endoluminal treatment was only successful in four cases. In the other cases, the endoprosthesis was placed too proximal, leading in one case to occlusion of both renal arteries and death of the animal.

The tantalum-Dacron coknit stent we tested in our study, measuring 10 mm in expanded diameter, was effective in treating artificial aneurysms in animals. In human abdominal aortic aneurysms, the diameter of the proximal aorta near the renal arteries, measured by ultrasonography, is a mean of 2.14 cm (7). Clinical application of the coknit stent for treatment of abdominal aortic aneurysm will necessitate having the properly sized endoprosthesis. However, before clinical observation, it is of course impossible to predict whether the histologic changes that occurred in the minipig will also occur in man. To favorize the same evolution, the human stent will have the same structure as the one used in this animal study. Surgical femoral access could be considered, allowing placement of large transfemoral introducer sheaths. Furthermore, transposition of the coknit stent to human application requires certain characteristics in patient selection to be successful. The anchoring of the device is the same as used in the vascular Strecker stent (15). The balloon inflates to permanently deform the tantalum wire of the stent into intimate contact with the necks of the aneurysm. Clotting within the aneurysm will add additional support to the body but the primary anchoring occurs at the necks. Consequently, ideal candidates will present infrarenal aortic aneu-

rysms with sufficient top and bottom necks to ensure stent anchorage. Relatively straight iliac arteries are suitable to facilitate stent advancement to the aorta. The presence of accessory renal arteries or a patent inferior mesenteric artery contraindicates stent placement. Finally the fate of patent lumbar arteries and the outcome of the thrombosed aneurysmal sac will not be known until clinical application is performed.

REFERENCES

1. Dubost C, Allary M, Oeconomos N. Resection of aneurysm of the abdominal aorta: reestablishment of the continuity by a preserved human arterial graft, with result after five months. Arch Surg 1952;64:405-408.

2. Crawford ES, Saleh SA, Babb JW, et al. Infrarenal abdominal aortic aneurysm: factors influencing survival after operation performed over a 25-year period. Ann Surg 1981;193:699-709.

3. Reigel MM, Hollier LH, Kazmier FJ, et al. Late survival in abdominal aortic aneurysm patients: the role of selective myocardial revascularization on the basis of clinical symptoms. J Vasc Surg 1987;5:222-227.

4. Bernstein EF, Dilley RB, Randolph HF. The improving longterm outlook for patients over 70 years of age with abdominal aortic aneurysms. Ann Surg 1988;207:318-322.

5. Johnston KW. Multicenter prospective study of nonruptured abdominal aortic aneurysm, part II: variables predicting morbidity and mortality. J Vasc Surg 1989;9:437-447.

6. AbuRahma AF, Robinson PA, Boland JP, et al. Elective resection of 332 abdominal aortic aneurysms in a southern West Virginia community during a recent five-year period. Surgery 1991;109:244-251.

7. Cronenwett JL, Murphy TF, Zelenock GB, et al. Actuarial analysis of variables associated with rupture of abdominal aortic aneurysms. Surgery 1985;98:472-483.

8. Nevitt MP, Ballard DJ, Hallett JW. Prognosis of abdominal aortic aneurysms: a population-based study. N Engl J Med 1989;321:1009-1114.

9. Johnston KW, Scobie TK. Multicenter prospective study of nonruptured abdominal

aortic aneurysms, I: population and operative management. J Vasc Surg 1988;7:69-81.

10. Leather RP, Shah D, Goldman M, Rosenberg M, Karmody AM. Nonresective treatment of abdominal aortic aneurysms. Use of acute thrombosis and axillo-femoral bypass. Arch Surg 1979;114:1402-1408.

11. Inahara T, Geary GL, Mukherjee D, Egan JM. The contrary position to the nonresective treatment for abdominal aortic aneurysm. J Vasc Surg 1985;2:42-48.

12. Schwartz RA, Nichols WK, Silver D. Is thrombosis of the infrarenal abdominal aortic aneurysm an acceptable alternative. J Vasc Surg 1986;3:448-455.

13. Balko A, Piasecki GJ, Shah DM, et al. Transfemoral placement of intraluminal polyurethane prosthesis for abdominal aortic aneurysm. J Surg Res 1986;40:305-309.

14. Parodi JC, Palmaz JC, Barone HD. Transfemoral intraluminal graft implantation for abdominal aortic aneurysms. Ann Vasc Surg 1991;5:491-499.

15. Strecker EP, Berg G, Schneider B, et al. A new vascular balloon-expandable prosthe-

sis: experimental studies and first clinical results. J Intervent Radiol 1988;3:59-62.

16. Anidjar S, Salzamann JL, Gentric D, Lagneau P, Camilleri JP, Michel JB. Elastase-induced experimental aneurysms in rats. Circulation 1990;82:973-981.

17. Laborde JC, Parodi JC, Clem MF, et al. Intraluminal bypass of abdominal aortic aneurysm: feasibility study. Radiology 1992;184:185-190.

18. Mirich D, Wright KC, Wallace S, et al. Percutaneously placed endovascular grafts for aortic aneurysms: feasibility study. Radiology 1989;170:1033-1037.

19. Lawrence Jr DD. Charnsangavej C, Wright KC, Gianturco C, Wallace S. Percutaneous endovascular graft: experimental evaluation. Radiology 1987;163:357-360.

20. Yoshioka T, Wright KC, Wallace S, Lawrence Jr DD, Gianturco C. Self-expanding endovascular graft: an experimental study in dogs. Am J Roentgenol 1988;151:673-676.

Long-Term Results Following Treatment of Iliac Artery Stenoses and Occlusions with Flexible Tantalum Stents

E.P. Strecker[1], B. Hagen[2], D. Liermann[3], I. Boos[1]

[1]Department of Radiology, Diakonissen Hospital Rüppurr, Karlsruhe, Germany
[2]Department of Radiology, Martin Luther Hospital, Berlin, Germany
[3]Department of Radiology, J.W. Goethe University Hospital, Frankfurt am Main, Germany

INTRODUCTION

Stent therapy of stenoses and occlusions of the iliac arteries has proven to be a valuable adjunct to percutaneous transluminal angioplasty (PTA), presenting long-term patency rates between 64 and 95% for balloon- or self-expandable stents (1-4). Although long-term patency rates are favorable, the success of stent therapy is diminished by acute thrombotic stent occlusions and late restenoses.

A long-term clinical study will provide more information about the success of stent therapy; the knowledge of risk factors will enable the interventional radiologist to prevent complications. This prospective multicenter study discloses new information about the benefits of iliac artery stenting with special regard to complications and risk factors, especially for long iliac artery occlusions.

PATIENTS AND METHODS

The technical properties of the balloon-expandable tantalum stent (Strecker™, Boston Scientific Corp., Denmark) and the insertion technique have previously been described in detail (5,6). Briefly, the stent, balloon-expandable and implantable through an introducer sheath, consists of a cylindrical, electropolished tantalum filament knit with a wire diameter of 0.1 mm. This prosthesis is flexible and elastic within certain limits in both the expanded and non-expanded states. The loosely connected wire loops give the stent an inherent flexibility, allowing the introduction of the catheter stent assembly through curved arteries, and the implantation into arteries leading over the hip or knee joint (Figure 1).

Correct positioning of the stent in the area to be treated is facilitated by the fact that shortening of the stent during dilatation will be compensated by the design, with longitudinal compression of the overlapping loops in the non-expanded state. In addition, the stent is visible under fluoroscopy due to the radiodensity of tantalum, which in this regard is superior to the stainless steel prostheses.

Recently improved catheter-stent assemblies with a 5 Fr-PTA-catheter and a balloon width up to 7 mm can be introduced through a 6.5 Fr-introducer sheath (Peter von Berg, Kirchseeon, Germany), whereas wider stents (9 mm) will need an 8 Fr-sheath and stents with a diameter of 11 mm will need a 10 Fr-introducer sheath. Available stents have a length of 4 or 8 cm.

Two hundred thirty-nine patients with atherosclerotic disease treated with iliac artery stents were included in this study. In 150 patients lesions of the common iliac artery were stented, including 25 patients who received kissing stents to treat atherosclerotic disease of the aortoiliac bifurcation (Figure 2). Lesions of the external iliac artery were treated in 89 patients. There were 56 occlusions (maximum length, 20.0 cm; mean, 6.8 cm), and 183 stenoses (maximum length, 16.0 cm; mean, 2.7 cm). In 33 patients, two or more stents (maximum of four) were implanted consecutively, from proximally to distally, with their ends overlapping by a few millimeters.

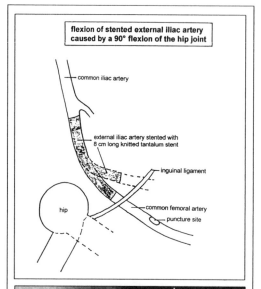

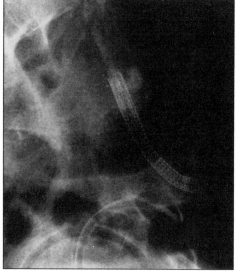

Figure 1. Iliac arteries appear to have a straight course in the anteroposterior view. However, in the lateral view, the external iliac artery curves increasingly with hip flexion. Therefore, in the case of a long (8 cm) stent requirement, only flexible stents can be implanted into this anatomical site.

Indications for iliac artery stenting were insufficient PTA results due to dissection (39%), elastic recoil (37%), and acute occlusion post-PTA (2%). Long artery occlusions were regarded as primary indications (25%).

During the preceding PTA procedure, herapin 5000 IU was administered intra-arterially as a bolus, and in the case of stent implantation, an additional 2000-5000 IU were given depending on the patient's weight, the duration of the procedure, and the length of the treated arterial site. Immediately post-implantation, heparin was given intravenously by a perfusor to increase the partial thromboplastin time to two or three times normal. Heparin treatment lasted up to 3 days; aspirin 100 mg was given daily ad infinitum to prevent thrombus formation by innibiting platelet aggregation.

Clinical symptoms before and after treatment were determined on the basis of Fontaine's classification. The Doppler sonographic ankle-arm indices (AAI) were evaluated immediately prior to treatment, 2 days after, 6 months later and, finally, at yearly intervals. Digital subtraction angiography controls were performed when clinical symptoms of the AAI deteriorated during the follow-up period.

RESULTS

Primary Results

Stents were successfully implanted in all cases. The Doppler AAI increased significantly immediately after stenting by more than 0.15 mm Hg in all patients. Eighty-three percent of the patients showed an improvement of their clinical symptoms, 16% remained clinically unchanged, and one patient showed a deterioration of clinical symptoms within the first weeks after stenting. Patients showing no improvement of their clinical symptoms required therapy for additional lesions located more distally.

Complications

Thrombotic stent occlusion occurred within the first 10 days after stenting in 11 patients. Such occlusion was treated with local fibrinolysis in eight patients. Distal embolization of thrombus material to distal arteries was seen in seven patients, which was also treated with local fibrinolysis or aspiration thrombectomy in six. The incidence of early thrombotic stent occlusion and peripheral thromboembolism was especially high in patients with long arterial occlusions. When there was an immediate partial stent compression because the arterial wall recoil effect was too strong, balloon dilation was eventually repeated with a shorter and wider balloon over a longer time period of 1 to 5 minutes. In one case, two stents were implanted in an overlapping fashion to obtain a higher stent stability.

Surgical intervention was required in three patients with acute thrombotic occlusion and in one of the patients with distal embolization. Nine patients developed a sizeable hematoma at the puncture site and required prolonged bed rest. Three patients developed a false aneurysm, which was treated by compression with the head of a color Doppler in two cases. The remaining patient required surgical intervention. One patient in whom arterial rupture occurred during balloon inflation underwent immediate bypass surgery after bleeding was stopped by dilation of a PTA balloon at the ruptured site.

A comparison between patients with iliac stenosis and those with iliac occlusion showed that the incidence of acute thrombotic stent occlusion and distal embolization was especially high in patients in whom iliac artery occlusion indicated stenting. Moreover, acute thrombotic stent reocclusion occurred significantly more often in patients with poor runoff vessels (more than 50% stenosis of the common or superficial femoral artery).

Follow-Up and Long-Term Results

The longest post-implantation observation time was 72 months (mean, 20 months). In 41 patients, deterioration of the Doppler AAI was observed during the follow-up period. In 28 cases this was due to stent restenosis (more than 50% of the diameter)

angiographically proven between 2 and 18 months after stent implantation. Seven patients underwent bypass procedures, 19 patients were successfully treated with a repeat PTA, and 2 patients with only mild symptoms did not receive any therapy. In the remaining 13 patients, angiography revealed patent iliac stents, but also hemodynamically-relevant atherosclerotic disease located more distally. Life table analysis showed a 54-month cumulative patency rate of 81.5% for iliac artery stents when acute complications such as thrombotic stent occlusion within the first 10 days after stent placement were included. The separation of stented stenoses and stented occlusions reveals a 4-year primary patency rate of 82.9 and 76.3% for iliac stenoses and iliac occlusions, respectively; the difference between both patency rates was statistically significant ($p < 0.01$) (Figure 3).

DISCUSSION

In recent years stent therapy has proven to be a valuable support for the interventional radiologist performing PTA of the aortic bifurcation and iliac arteries (1-4). Long occlusions of the iliac arteries or the aortic bifurcation have been added as new stent indications (5-9). As an endoluminal mechanical support, the stent counteracts the mechanical recoil of the elastic components still remaining after PTA. Furthermore, wall dissection or intimal flaps are able to reduce the lumen of the arteries or even to occlude them. Vascular stenting provides successful treatment of such complications followed by good long-term success rates. Our stent study included 239 patients and revealed a 54-month primary patency rate of 81.5% (Figure 4), which is superior to the success rate published by Johnston (10) of 667 patients treated solely with PTA (Figure 5). It must be emphasized that our cohort includes only patients suffering from very severe arterial lesions not responding to PTA treatment, thus representing a group even less favorable than the PTA group. Richter also confirmed our results and

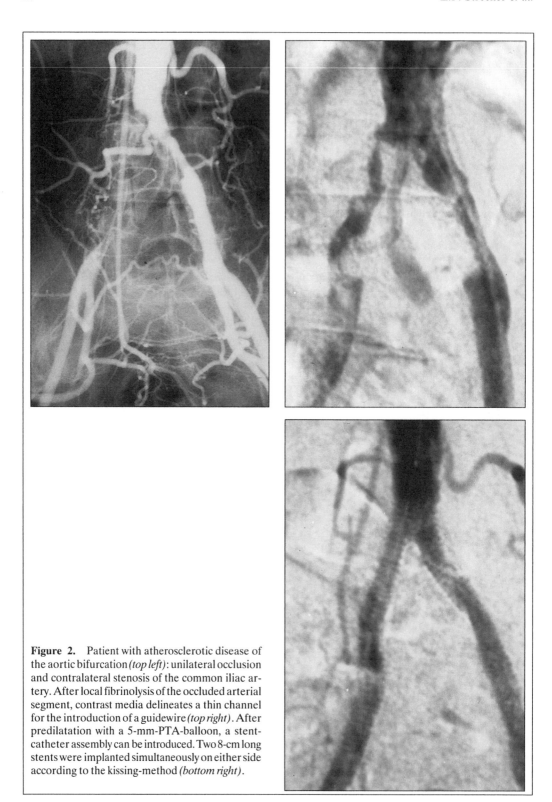

Figure 2. Patient with atherosclerotic disease of the aortic bifurcation *(top left)*: unilateral occlusion and contralateral stenosis of the common iliac artery. After local fibrinolysis of the occluded arterial segment, contrast media delineates a thin channel for the introduction of a guidewire *(top right)*. After predilatation with a 5-mm-PTA-balloon, a stent-catheter assembly can be introduced. Two 8-cm long stents were implanted simultaneously on either side according to the kissing-method *(bottom right)*.

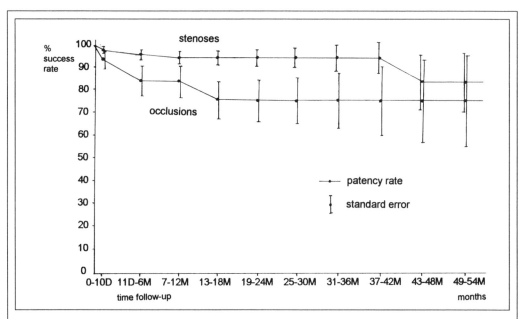

Figure 3. Cumulative patency rates over a follow-up period of 54 months: stented stenoses (183 patients) versus stented occlusions (56 patients).

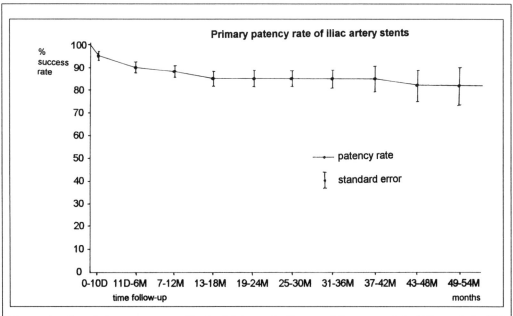

Figure 4. Cumulative patency rate (Kaplan-Meier method) over a follow-up period of 54 months for 239 stented iliac arteries, including stenoses and occlusions.

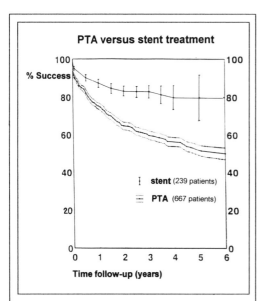

Figure 5. Iliac artery occlusions and stenoses: Patency rate of iliac arteries having been stented primarily in artery occlusions or secondarily after failed PTA versus patency rate of iliac arteries solely treated with PTA (data of Johnston [10]) over an observation time of 6 years. There is a significantly higher success rate for stented lesions.

described a superior patency rate for stented iliac arteries versus arteries solely treated with PTA (11).

PTA has revealed insufficient results when used as the sole treatment of long occlusions of the iliac arteries and the aortic bifurcation. This is due to the high incidence of acute collapse of the thrombotic material into the previously opened arterial segment, accompanied by acute thrombosis. Therefore, because of early recurrence, iliac artery occlusions were not felt to be suited for PTA therapy. Stent therapy, however, offers a new treatment modality of long iliac artery occlusions (7-9), providing a long-term success rate of 76.3% in our study. This patency rate is not as favorable as in stenotic lesions (Figure 4),

which is mainly explained by the higher incidence of acute thrombotic occlusions within the first 10 days after stent implantation. Occlusions are usually longer than stenoses and result in more extensive wall injury. More metallic stent material is introduced and the surface of thrombotic material fragmented beyond the stent meshes additionally increases thrombogenicity. Furthermore, thrombotic material might protrude backwards into the lumen, causing thrombosis. Therefore, a thoroughly performed anticoagulation becomes necessary after stenting of iliac artery occlusions.

Local fibrinolysis represents another modality used to reopen long iliac artery occlusions and has been advocated for the sole treatment of these arteries. Generally performed using the cross-over technique, the fibrinolytic agent is injected from the contralateral side through a catheter into the thrombus. For a complete dissolution of the thrombus, however, 3 to 24 hours are necessary and control angiographies must be performed repeatedly. Since there is a risk of systemic side effects causing severe hemorrhaging, patients must be thoroughly monitored. Local fibrinolysis is a stressing and time-consuming method and often, PTA or stent treatment also has to be performed in order to achieve success (12).

When combined with vascular stenting, however, local fibrinolysis might prove helpful. As performed initially, it can provide a thin channel, enabling the radiologist to pass a guidewire through the obstructed segment (Figure 2). After underdilatation with a 5 Fr-PTA-balloon, a stent can then be introduced and dilated. A complete predilatation with a PTA balloon would increase the risk of peripheral thromboembolism. Peripheral thromboembolism and acute stent thromboses, representing the main complications occurring after stent implantation into long arterial occlusions, can be treated successfully with local fibrinolysis or aspiration thrombectomy.

CONCLUSIONS

In conclusion, stent therapy offers new areas for vascular interventions like the re-opening of long arterial occlusions in the area of the aortic bifurcation and the iliac arteries.

REFERENCES

1. Strunk HM, Schild HH, Dueber C, et al. Reobstruction after iliac artery stent placement: frequency and methods of treatment (abst. 1088). Radiology 1993;189(Suppl P):293.
2. Strecker EP, Hagen B, Liermann D, Schneider B, Wolf HR, Wambsganss J. Iliac and femoropopliteal vascular occlusive disease treated with flexible tantalum stents. Cardiovasc Intervent Radiol 1993;16:158-164.
3. Palmaz JC, Richter GM, Nöldge G, et al. Intraluminal stents in atherosclerotic iliac artery stenosis: preliminary report of a multicenter study. Radiology 1988;168:727-731.
4. Zollikofer CL, Antonucci F, Pfyffer M, et al. Arterial stent placement with use of the Wallstent: midterm results of clinical experience. Radiology 1991;179:449-456.
5. Strecker EP, Kuhn FP, Liermann D, et al. Strecker flexible tantalum stent. In: Kim D and Orron DE, eds. *Peripheral Vascular Imaging and Intervention*. First Edition. St. Louis: Mosby Year Book, Inc.; 1992;541-552.
6. Strecker EP, Hagen B, Liermann D, et al. Treatment of atherosclerotic occlusive disease of the aortic bifurcation with balloon expandable tantalum stents. Eur Radiol 1993;3:536.
7. Palmaz JC, Encarnacion CE, Garcia OJ, et al. Aortic bifurcation stenosis: treatment with intravascular stents. JVIR 1991;2:319.
8. Vorwerk D, Günther RW. Mechanical revascularization of occluded iliac arteries with use of self-expandable endoprostheses. Radiology 1990;175:411-415.
9. Rees CR, Palmaz JC, Garcia O, et al. Angioplasty and stenting of completely occluded iliac arteries. Radiology 1989;172:953-959.
10. Johnston KW. Iliac arteries: reanalysis of results of balloon angioplasty. Radiology 1993;186:207-212.
11. Richter GM. Erste langzeitergebnisse der randomisierten 5-Jahres-Studie: iliacale stentimplantation versus PTA. Vasa Suppl 1992;35:192.
12. Hausegger KA, Lammer J, Klein GE, et al. Percutaneous recanalization of pelvic artery occlusions — fibrinolysis, PTA, stents. Roefo Fortschr Geb Röntgenstr Neuen Bildgeb Verfahr 1991;155:550.

Further Analysis of a Randomized Trial Comparing Primary Iliac Stenting and PTA

Goetz M. Richter[1], Gerd Nöldge[1], Thomas Roeren[1], Matthias Brado[1],
J. R. Allenberg[2], Guenter W. Kauffmann[1]

[1]Department of Diagnostic Radiology, University Hospital Heidelberg, Germany
[2]Department of Vascular Surgery, University Hospital Heidelberg, Germany

INTRODUCTION

Several different stent designs are commercially available for various vascular regions to treat vessel wall collapse (elastic recoil), occlusive intimal flaps, and dissecting membranes secondary to previous angioplasty. These have also been used to treat both late morphologic and clinical failures resulting from restenosis after angioplasty.

There is no proof, however, regarding whether primary vascular stenting is associated with better morphologic and clinical results compared to traditional balloon angioplasty in iliac arteries. Our early experience with the Palmaz balloon-expandable stent was accumulated under a multi-institutional pilot study protocol accepted by the Federal Drug Administration (FDA) (1,2). We soon realized that demonstration of better morphologic and clinical efficacy of stents compared to angioplasty could not be achieved by comparing results of iliac artery stenting with historic results of balloon angioplasty (3). Therefore, a randomized trial of primary balloon-expandable stenting versus traditional balloon angioplasty in atherosclerotic iliac artery disease was begun in July 1987. Herein, we provide a further update on the early and long-term results of this study.

MATERIAL AND METHODS

Stent Characteristics

The Palmaz™ iliac stent (Johnson & Johnson Interventional Systems Co., Warren NJ) used in this study consists of a single segment, tubular stainless steel mesh, surgical grade 316L, with a wall thickness of 120 μm. The circumference of this stent type consists of four slots that are 4.5-mm long. The number of slots in the longitudinal extension depends on the length of the stent. Its diameter in the non-expanded state measures 3.1 mm. Radial compression of the stent over a balloon catheter decreases its diameter and the stent attaches onto a 7 Fr balloon catheter. A vascular stent should oppose circumferential compression forces, and both elastic and plastic force may function in this regard. The Palmaz stent is a non-flexible, rigid stent type that employs plastic forces to the vessel wall after expansion. The diameter of the stent is dependent on the balloon size used for delivery. The stent type used in this study had an optimal diameter within the range of 7 to 16 mm. Hence, the expansion ratio ranged between 1:3 and 1:6. Vascular stents should have a maximum of biocompatibility without corrosion problems. The design of the Palmaz stent avoids any crossing points with metal riding over metal which might otherwise be a source of fretting corrosion. In addition, the Palmaz stent is the only commercially available device for which fatigue studies simulating a foreseeable lifelong workload have been positively carried out.

Study Enrollment

With few exceptions (acute and subacute occlusions) the inclusion criteria of this randomized trial were virtually identical to those of the previously mentioned multi-institutional trial (1). Briefly, the inclusion criteria were as follows:

- Clinically symptomatic occlusive iliac artery disease in stages IIa, IIb, III, or IV according to Fontaine's classification.
- Focally stenotic common or external iliac artery disease involving less than 50% of the total vessel length.
- Unilateral or bilateral stenotic lesions of the aortoiliac junction.
- Acute or subacute iliac artery occlusion of less than 6 months.
- Transstenotic gradient of > 10 mm Hg measured as mean arterial pressure.

Exclusion criteria included:

- Long segment disease involving more than 50% of the total length of the iliac arteries.
- Multifocally or totally diseased iliac artery involving more than four isolated treatment sites.
- Untreated and hemodynamically-significant isolated aortic lesion.
- Chronic iliac artery occlusion (longer than 6 months duration).
- Lesion within the area of the arterial puncture site.
- Lesion below the inguinal ligament or extending up to 1 cm higher than the inguinal ligament.
- Contraindication to anticoagulation treatment or contrast media application.
- Women of childbearing potential.
- Severe mental disorientation or drug addiction preventing proper follow-up studies.
- Septic status.

Pre- and Post-Interventional Examinations

Before intervention, the following non-invasive tests were performed: bilateral segmental ABI-index measurement (ankle/brachial Doppler peak systolic pressure index) including the distal forearm, proximal thigh, distal thigh, proximal calf, and ankle; segmental pulse quality measurement (0 = none, + = diminished, + + = normal); tread-mill walking test (3.5 km/h, 10° angulation); evaluation of skin changes; clinical examination of the venous system of the extremities; and an electrocardiogram. Laboratory tests included red and white blood cell counts, evaluation of blood sedimentation time, anticoagulation status, renal function, and screening for risk profile (cholesterol level, diabetes, etc.).

Similar non-invasive and laboratory tests were performed 1, 3, 6, and 12 months after the intervention and at 12-month intervals thereafter. Invasive angiographic studies, including measurement of the mean arterial transstenotic pressure gradient, were performed 6 and 12 months after the intervention and at 12-month intervals thereafter.

Patients with Additional Peripheral Artery Disease

Prior to study enrollment, the relevance of the iliac artery lesion was specifically evaluated during the decision making process. When additional peripheral lesions appeared to require treatment, it was determined which lesion to treat first and by which method. For the final evaluation of success, the entire treatment concept had to be completed to avoid creating inappropriate failure rates from failure of the additional intervention alone. A patient was not considered a failure if an additional bypass was performed after successful iliac intervention and the bypass occluded. In this case, the patient was withdrawn from the study and censored as a success for the given interval period.

Interventional Technique

The principles of stenting with the Palmaz stent have been published in great depth (e.g., 1,2). Angioplasty and local arterial lysis were performed according to standard technical protocols using routine catheter technology. When elastic recoil or inappropriate initial results were found after angioplasty, prolonged balloon inflation and larger balloons were applied to improve success rates.

Antiplatelet medication (aspirin 100 mg) was begun 1 day before the intervention and continued for 3 months. Anticoagulation therapy was only given during the intervention by intraarterially injecting heparin 5000 IU immediately prior to angioplasty or stent placement. In a few selected patients with a combination of iliac intervention and peripheral bypass surgery, oral anticoagulation therapy was established after successful completion of the surgical procedure.

RESULTS

Stenting

A total of 123 patients underwent stent placement. Their age, risk profile, and clinical stage distribution are summarized in Figure 1. The vast majority of patients had severe claudication, categorized as stage IIb according to Fontaine's classification. Seven percent of patients had less severe symptoms, qualifying them as stage IIa; these patients

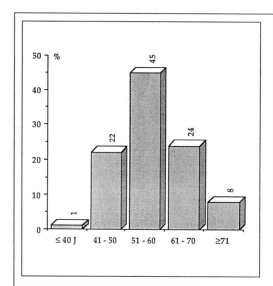

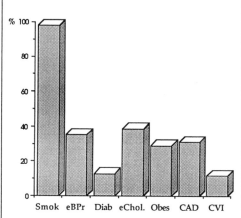

Smok = history of smoking (minimum 20 packs/year)
eBPr = hypertension according to WHO classification of elevated blood pressure
Diab = insulin dependent diabetes
eChol = elevated blood cholesterol levels (> 120 mg%)
Obes = obesity (weight exceeding: body length in cm −100 + 20% of body length in cm −100)
CAD = coronary artery disease
CVI   = cerebrovascular insufficiency

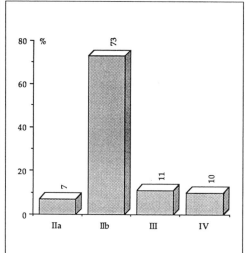

Figure 1. Characteristics of patients in stent group. Age distribution *(top left)*, risk profile *(top right)*, and clinical stage of atherosclerotic artery disease *(bottom left)*.

received treatment because they needed reasonably good walking ability for professional reasons. Severe leg ischemia of stage III or IV was apparent in 21% of the patients. The most frequent risk factor among all patients was smoking (98%), and approximately one-third of the patients had hypertension, hypercholesterolemia, symptomatic coronary artery disease, and were obese.

Tables 1 and 2 display early and long-term technical, hemodynamic, and clinical results for both stenting and PTA. In 121 of 123 patients the stent was correctly deployed (technical success, 98.4%). The mean transstenotic pressure gradient dropped below 5 mm Hg after intervention in 120 patients. In the total cohort it dropped from an average of 29.4 to 1.4 mm Hg. A large hematoma developed after stenting in four patients which necessitated surgical intervention. Early thrombosis was found in another patient and was successfully treated by lysis. Thus, the total complication rate was 4.1%. A life table analysis (Table 2) shows a 91.6% clinical success rate (persistence of clinical improvement by at least one clinical stage) in the latest interval of 4 to 5 years.

PTA

Percutaneous transluminal angioplasty was performed in 124 patients. Their age, risk profile, and clinical stage distribution are summarized in Figure 2. As observed in the stent group, the vast majority of patients had severe claudication (72%) categorized as stage IIb according to Fontaine's classification, while 10% had less severe, stage IIa symptoms. Fourteen percent of the patients in the PTA group had severe leg ischemia in stage

Table 1. Early Results With Both Interventions (<30 Days)

Procedure	Success			Major Complication[d]
	Technical[a]	Hemodynamic[b]	Clinical[c]	
Stent	98.4%	97.6%	97.6%	4.1%
PTA	91.9%	91.9%	89.5%	6.5%

[a] Technical success is defined as stent deployment precisely at target site without residual stenosis.
[b] Hemodynamic success is defined as a residual mean transstenotic pressure gradient < 5 mm Hg.
[c] Clinical success is defined as an improvement by ≥ 1 clinical stage.
[d] Major complication is defined as an event necessitating surgery or other vascular repair (e.g., lysis).

Table 2. Late Clinical Results With Both Interventions

Procedure	Cumulative Success Rate			
	1-year	2-year	3-year	4-year
Stent	95.2%	93.4%	92.1%	91.6%
PTA	88.1%	85.1%	79.5%	74.3%

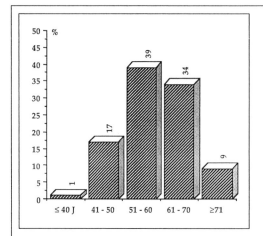

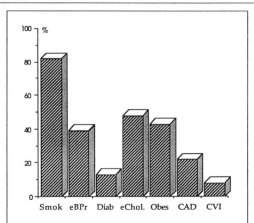

Smok = history of smoking (minimum 20 packs/
               year)
eBPr = hypertension according to WHO classi
               fication of elevated blood pressure
Diab = insulin dependent diabetes
eChol = elevated blood cholesterol levels
               (> 120 mg%)
Obes = obesity (weight exceeding: body length
               in cm −100 + 20% of body length in
               cm −100)
CAD = coronary artery disease
CVI   = cerebrovascular insufficiency

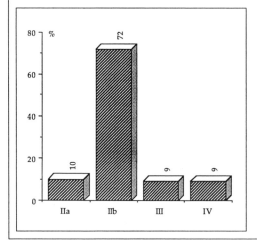

Figure 2. Characteristics of patients in PTA group. Age distribution *(top left)*, risk profile *(top right)*, and clinical stages of atherosclerotic artery disease *(bottom left)*.

III or IV. Smoking was the most common risk factor (84%), with approximately 40% of the patients having hypertension, hypercholesterolemia, and obesity. Approximately 25% of patients had symptomatic coronary artery disease.

Technical success was noted in 111 of the 124 patients (morphologic results corresponding to 70% of desired target diameter). The mean transstenotic pressure gradient dropped below 5 mm Hg after intervention in 111 patients while in the total cohort, it dropped from an average of 29.5 to 6.7 mm Hg. In three patients a large hematoma developed after PTA requiring surgical intervention. Severe lumen compromising dissection or early thrombosis was apparent in five pa-

tients, with four treated by reintervention (lysis plus stent placement) and three undergoing bypass surgery. Thus, the total complication rate is 6.5%. Life table analysis (Table 2) shows a 74.3% clinical success rate (persistence of clinical improvement by at least one clinical stage) in the interval from 4 to 5 years.

Statistic Evaluation

The hemodynamic success rate following stenting was superior to that following PTA (p < 0.0001). Technical success, early and long-term clinical success, and complication rates were significantly better after stenting compared to PTA with p-values of < 0.01 to 0.005.

DISCUSSION

The results of this comparison among comparable patient groups demonstrate that stenting is significantly superior to PTA in the immediate post-intervention interval in terms of technical, hemodynamic, and clinical effects. The better morphologic response noted with stenting was reflected both by a lower average residual transstenotic gradient (1.6 mm Hg versus 6.7 mm Hg after PTA) and less technical failures (2 versus 13 after PTA) following the intervention. This is due to increased elastic recoil, less pronounced plaque fracture, and a high incidence of lumen compromise from dissecting membranes and intimal flaps after angioplasty. Relevant dissections were not seen in any patient following stenting. This seems to justify the conclusion that the use of the balloon-expandable Palmaz stent with high resistance to hoop stress sufficiently opposes collapsing forces of the vessel wall while dissections from plaque fracture seem to be sealed in place. Therefore, the incidence of significant complications was also somewhat lower in the stent group. The early results in the PTA group compare well with historical observations and previously summarized results (3). Thus, the higher success level of stenting is not a reflection of bad PTA results but rather a feature of the intrinsic properties of this new device.

Similarly, long-term clinical results after stenting are characterized by statistically significantly less failure and better persistence of clinical success. Although there is a constant decline of cumulative success rates to a level of 91% at the interval from 4 to 5 years, this outcome compares favorably with historical groups. It might be speculated that more favorable long-term results after stenting are based on better morphologic repair such that after the period of biologic incorporation of the device, the resulting luminal restoration at the lesion site lowers the risk of restenosis as compared to balloon angioplasty.

REFERENCES

1. Palmaz JC, Richter GM, Nöldge G, Kauffmann GW, Wenz W. Die intraluminale Stent-Implantation nach Palmaz. Erster klinischer Fallbericht über eine ballon-expandierte Geläßprothese. Radiologe 1987;27:560-563.
2. Palmaz JC, Garcia OJ, Schatz RA, et al. Placement of balloon-expandable intraluminal stents in iliac arteries: first 171 procedures. Radiology 1990;174:969-975.
3. Becker GJ, Katzen BT, Dake MD. Noncoronary angioplasty. Radiology 1989;170:921-940.

Wallstents in Pelvic Arteries – Indications and Results

D.Vorwerk and R.W. Günther

Clinic of Radiological Diagnostics, RWTH Aachen, Germany

INTRODUCTION

Becker and colleagues have reported a mean technical success rate of 92% (range, 50 to 96%) for percutaneous transluminal angioplasty (PTA) of aortoiliac lesions. A 2-year patency rate of 81% and a 5-year patency rate of 72% were reported for iliac interventions in this trial (1). The complication rate following iliac PTA is reportedly low. Examination of the published results tends to create the impression that technical improvements in percutaneous procedures involving peripheral arteries are unnecessary. There is great demand for new techniques, however, since the success rate of the published series can, in some cases, be attributed to the selection of case material prior to percutaneous procedures, i.e., lesions which are easily accessible to percutaneous procedures or those in which unsatisfactory results would be expected. The proportion of the latter is surprisingly high amongst arteriosclerotic cases. Problematic lesions include chronic pelvic artery occlusions and lengthy, eccentric, and calcified lesions of the pelvic circulation.

Between November 1, 1987 and June 20, 1991, a total of 204 patients were treated by means of vascular endoprostheses at our clinic. Arterial lesions were noted in 177 patients, with the majority (152 patients) involving the aortoiliac arteries. The remaining 25 procedures involved femoropopliteal arteries.

MATERIALS AND METHODS

One hundred fifty-two lesions of the aortic and pelvic vessels were treated in 150 patients (28 women, 122 men). The mean age of all patients was 56.7 ± 8.3 years. In two patients the lesions were bilateral or in the aorta, while in 63 and 83 patients, the right or left pelvic circulation, respectively, was affected. The obstructions were located in the aorta (N=2), the common iliac artery (N=84), and the external iliac artery (N=38). Both the common iliac artery and the external iliac artery were affected in 28 patients.

The affected sections of the vessels were calcified in 74 patients; x-ray examinations showed the calcification to be severe in 48 patients and moderate in 26 patients. Nineteen lesions showed aortal plaques close to the outflow.

Additional hemodynamically-relevant stenoses were present in dependent flow areas in 105 lesions. The ipsilateral internal iliac artery was stenotic in 32 patients and was occluded in 29 patients such that it was no longer available for possible collateral circulation. Stenosis (N=19) or occlusion (N=35) of the ipsilateral femoropopliteal flow was also present in 54 patients. According to Fontaine's classification, 11 patients were in stage II, 129 in stage IIb, 5 in stage II, and 4 in stage IV. One patient was asymptomatic before treatment, but suffered an acute complication during diagnostic angiography and was immediately treated with stent implantation.

The mean lesion length was 4.3 ± 2.9 cm and the pre-treatment mean ankle-arm index of the extremity involved was 0.57 ± 0.15. Purely aortic lesions were stented in two patients; both patients had stage II bilateral claudication according to Fontaine after walking 180 or 50 m, respectively.

Iliac Stenoses

In 75 patients (63 men, 12 women) with a mean age of 57.2 ± 8.5 years, 77 iliac stenoses were treated with a self-expanding endoprosthesis (Wallstent™, Medinvent, Lausanne, Switzerland) after balloon dilatation. The mean length of the stenoses was 3.2 ± 2.1 cm.

Iliac Occlusions

Seventy-three patients with 73 pelvic artery occlusions were treated with stents after successful mechanical passage of the occluded segment. The aortic bifurcation was affected in 34 patients and the iliac bifurcation was affected in 19 patients. Lesions affected the entire length of the common iliac artery (N=16), the entire length of the external iliac artery (N=11), or the entire pelvic artery from the aortic bifurcation to the femoral artery (N=8). The mean lesion length was 5.4 ± 3.2 cm. The affected segments of the arteries were calcified in 23 patients; after x-ray examination, the calcification was classified as severe in 16 and moderate in 7. Ten lesions showed aortal plaques close to the outflow. According to the classifications used by the Standards of Practice Committee of the Society of Cardiovascular and Interventional Radiology (SCVIR), 28 patients (38%) had a morphological Class III lesion (occlusions under 5 cm). The mean occlusion length in these patients was 2.7 ± 1.1 cm (median, 2.65 cm; range, 1 to 4.9 cm). In 45 patients (62%), the occlusion was classified as Class IV (occlusion length > 5 cm), with a mean occlusion length of 7.1 ± 3 cm (median, 6.0 cm). Length varied from 5 to 22 cm in this latter group of patients.

RESULTS

Successful placement of the endoprostheses was accomplished in all patients and no procedures were prematurely discontinued. Placement of the endoprostheses involved overlapping of the aortic bifurcation in 47 patients and overlapping of the iliac bifurcation in 39 patients. Both bifurcations were crossed in 12 patients.

In total, 203 individual endovascular prostheses were implanted (1.3 prostheses per lesion). The mean length of the stented vessel segment was 5.6 ± 2.9 cm (range, 3 to 24 cm). A single stent was implanted in 107 lesions. In the case of 45 lesions, several overlapping endoprostheses with a mean length of 6.3 ± 4 cm were implanted. Two stents were required in 40 patients, three stents in 4 patients, and four stents in 1 patient.

Acute and Early Complications

In 15 cases (9 stenoses, 6 occlusions), the lesion was not completely bridged by the endoprosthesis despite appropriate stent length, making it necessary to implant a second stent. This second stent covered only a few millimeters and was always placed without complications. Acute complications occurred immediately after intervention in nine patients (5.9%) with the most frequent complication being embolization of thrombotic material (N=3). Within the first 3 months of stenting, an additional four patients (4%) showed early complications, with the most common also being rethrombosis in patients with occlusion (N=3). The proportion of occlusions treated in the group suffering acute and early complications was above average, i.e., 10 out of 14 patients. The complication rate for aortoiliac stenoses was 5%, while for iliac occlusions it was 13.7%. The percentage of complications requiring intervention was 8.2% for occlusions and 3.8% for stenoses.

Clinical Results

Following endoprosthesis implantation and discharge from hospital, the mean Doppler index was 0.91 ± 0.16 (range, 0.4 to 1.2).

According to Fontaine's classification, upon discharge 115 patients were stage I, 28 patients were stage IIa, and 5 patients were stage IIb. Discharge status was unknown for two patients. None of the patients suffered pain at rest following discharge. One hundred eleven patients improved by two stages and 36 patients improved by one stage. One patient was asymptomatic before and after treatment. Clinical findings after discharge remained stable in 117 patients up to the last available follow-up date.

Treatment of Reocclusions and Restenoses

Thirteen of the 16 patients with reobstructed stents were revised percutaneously. Two patients decided against any form of revascularization and one patient with predominantly contralateral complaints was first treated for a contralateral lesion.

Patency Rates

Using the Kaplan-Meier method, primary cumulative patency rates for iliac occlusions of 92 ± 9% after 6 months, 88 ±13.5% after 12 months, and 82 ± 16.6% after 24 months were noted. Calculation of the cumulative patency rate was based on angiographically-verified progressive findings as the decisive assessment factor. The cumulative patency rate in stenotic iliac arteries was 98 ± 5%, 96 ±8.5%, and 84 ± 21% after 6, 12, and 24 months, respectively. The secondary cumulative patency rate, i.e., after one reobstruction and percutaneous revision, in iliac occlusions was 97 ± 5% after 6 and 12 months and 95 ± 8% after 24 months. The angiographically-verified secondary patency rate for iliac stenoses after 6, 12 and 24 months was 100%. There was no significant difference between occlusions and stenoses (Log rank test) for either angiographically- or clinically-verified primary and secondary cumulative patency.

DISCUSSION

In the majority of cases, good technical success rates are achieved with metal endoprostheses in pelvic arteries. In our own series, technical success was achieved in all patients immediately after implantation of the endoprosthesis after successfully overcoming the lesion. Within the first 2 months, the technical success rate was 96%. Once the occlusion had been overcome with wire and catheterization, the sub-group of iliac artery occlusions also showed a success rate of 93.2%.

The complication rate in our patients was 9.2% (14/152), with only nine patients requiring further percutaneous or operative interventions. Stent thrombosis occurred in only one case (0.6%). Embolization of occlusive material occurred more frequently (N=3; 2%), but occurred only in the treatment of pelvic artery occlusions where it was the most common complication. Thanks to the small delivery apparatus for the Wallstent, i.e., 7 to 9 Fr, no inguinal hematoma or pseudoaneurysms occurred at the puncture site. These are reported as the most common complication following implantation of the Palmaz stent (2). Taking into account the relatively large proportion of pelvic artery occlusions in our own series with stent implantations and assuming a higher complication rate (3) for the treatment of such occlusions, stent implantation in the pelvic area does not appear to involve any particular risks to the patient.

The excellent PTA results recently reported appear to successfully compete with the results following iliac stent implantation and thus question the clinical necessity of the latter technique. A simple comparison of numbers, however, makes no allowance for the important factor of the type of lesion. Tegtmeyer and colleagues (4) reported on only 6 pelvic artery occlusions (3%) in their group of patients, while in the series of tests conducted by Johnston et al (5), occlusions accounted for 12%. In our own series of iliac stent implantations, the proportion of occlusions was 73 of 152 lesions (48%), and lesions of SCVIR classes III and IV — which are by definition barely accessible to simple balloon dilatation (6) — accounted for up to 63% of the stenoses and occlusions treated. Satisfactory long-term results were achieved even for severe lesions, despite the negative selection of case material. The problems associated with treatment of SCVIR III and IV lesions is underscored by the fact that in our series, all of the acute and early complications and 14 of the 16 cases of reobstruction involved lesions of those classes.

While the indication for percutaneous intervention must fundamentally be for clinical reasons, the use of metal endoprostheses depends upon technical aspects, usually bearing in mind the primary results after balloon dilatation. There is, therefore, no special clinical indication for stent application.

REFERENCES

1. Becker G, Katzen B, Dake M. Noncoronary angioplasty. Radiology 1989;170:921-940.
2. Palmaz J, Richter G, Nöldge G, et al. Intraluminal stents in atherosclerotic iliac artery stenosis: preliminary report of a multicenter study. Radiology 1988;168:727-731.
3. Ring E, Freiman D, McLean G, Schwarz W. Percutaneous recanalization of iliac artery occlusions: an unacceptable complication rate. Am J Roentgenol 1982;39:587-589.
4. Tegtmeyer C, Hardwell G, Selby B, Robertson R, Kron I, Tribble C. Results and complications of angioplasty in aortoiliac disease. Circulation 1991;83:I53-I60.
5. Johnston K, Rae M, Hogg-Johnston S, et al. 5-year results of a prospective study of percutaneous transluminal angioplasty. Ann Surg 1987;206:403-413.
6. Standards of Practice Committee of the Society of Cardiovascular and Interventional Radiology. Guidelines for percutaneous transluminal angioplasty. Radiology 1990;177:619-626.

The US FDA Trial of the Wallstent

E.C. Martin[1], B.T. Katzen[2], D.E. Schwarten[3]

[1]Miami Vascular Institute, Miami, FL USA
[2]Columbia Presbyterian, New York, NY USA
[3]St. Vincent's Hospital, Indianapolis, IN USA

INTRODUCTION

To gain approval to market a new stent in the United States, it is necessary to conduct a clinical trial with the device. Between August 1991 and January 1993, 226 patients were entered into a multicenter trial of an investigational stent. Indications for stent placement were restenosis within 90 days of an angioplasty procedure (17 patients), iliac occlusions (13 patients), and for the remainder of patients, angioplasty failure. This latter indication was defined as poor cosmetic results with a 30% or greater residual stenosis, a dissection longer than the dilated lesion, or a pressure gradient ≥ 5 mm Hg in the iliac artery. The exclusion criteria in this trial included single or multiple lesions longer than 10 cm, perforations or aneurysms caused by angioplasty, and patients unsuitable for anticoagulation.

PATIENTS

Iliac stents were placed in 130 patients while 91 patients had femoral stents placed. Five patients had placement of both femoral and iliac stents. The 91 patients with femoral stents form the basis of this report.

Ninety-one patients had femoral Wallstents placed in 118 lesions involving 96 limbs. All patients with femoral stents were heparinized with 5000 units during implantation and intravenous heparin was started 4 hours after the procedure. Concomitant treatment with coumadin was begun and heparin was continued until the prothrombin time was 1.5 times normal; this usually took 48 hours. Coumadin was continued for 6 months and aspirin was administered indefinitely.

In the femoral system, 77 stenoses and 41 occlusions were stented. The average length of the stenoses was 3.7 cm (range, 1 to 30 cm), while that of the occlusions was 9.1 cm (range, 1 to 30 cm). The stenoses were predominantly short, whereas the occlusions were approximately evenly distributed between 0 to 5 cm, 5 to 10 cm, and greater than 10 cm in length; the latter were considered protocol violations. The majority of patients had claudication. Seventy-five percent of patients were in the Society of Vascular Surgery grade I; at baseline, the mean ankle/brachial index (ABI) was 0.66 (SD $\pm$ 0.2).

RESULTS

As a result of stent placement, stenoses were increased in diameter from 1.5 to 5.4 mm and the occlusions were increased to 5.45 mm. The primary angiographic success rate was 96.4% and the mean ABI increased from 0.66 $\pm$ 0.2 to 0.96 $\pm$ 0.21. The primary clinical success rate was also analyzed using the Rutherford criteria. Using this criteria, +3 implies normalization with an ABI greater than 0.9 and no symptoms; +2 indicates an increase in ABI of 0.1 and an increase in category; and +1 represents either one of these criteria but not both. Using the Rutherford criteria of +2 and +3, the primary success rate was 88%. When the +1 criteria was included, the primary success rate was increased to 96%. There was no significant difference in the results between stenoses and occlusions.

The initial ABI increase to 0.96 fell to 0.92 after 6 months for both stenoses and occlusions. After a mean follow-up of 8 months, the ABI was 0.88 and 0.83 for stenoses and occlusions, respectively. Using the Rutherford criteria, no statistical difference was observed between stenoses and occlusions. Seventy-two percent of the occlusions were categorized as +2 or +3 while 79% were categorized as at least +1 after a mean of 8 months. This represents a deterioration in clinical status.

Angiographic follow-up has been achieved in 48 of the 91 patients and at 6 months, 11 patients had > 50% occlusion or stenoses; therefore, the 6-month angiographic patency rate was 77%. These results mirror those previously described by Sapoval (1) and Zollikofer (2).

The complication rate (16%) in our trial was typical of multicenter trials and only 2.7% of patients required surgery.

REFERENCES

1. Sapoval MR, Long AL, Raynaud AC, et al. Femoropopliteal stent placement: long-term results. Radiology 1992;184:833-839.
2. Zollikofer CL, Antonucci F, Markus P, et al. Arterial stent placement with use of the Wallstent: midterm results of clinical experience. Radiology 1991;179:449-456.

Have Stents Led to a Change in the Indication for Vasosurgical Reconstruction in Aortoiliac AOD?

H.-W. Menges and S. Rewerk

General Surgical and Vasosurgical Clinic
Diakonissenkrankenhaus GmbH, Mannheim, Germany

INTRODUCTION

Numerous established methods are available for vasosurgical reconstruction of aortoiliac flow. The methods with the best long-term results, however, also have the highest complication rates and involve considerable strain for the patient. Other interventional techniques have been developed which have a clearly defined place in the treatment of peripheral arterial occlusive disease (AOD). Those methods have met with rapid success because they have low complication rates and do not involve any great trauma or strain for the patient. Thus, they offer the patient a substantial increase in comfort compared with conventional vasosurgical reconstruction. This is particularly true for transluminal recanalization of the pelvic section. The excellent results with stent implantation can certainly be compared with those of vasosurgical reconstruction. As a logical further development of transluminal catheter dilatation, stent implantation has led to an indication for aortoiliac reconstruction.

FORMULATION OF THE PROBLEM

In contrast to practice in the United States, vasosurgery in Europe, and in Germany in particular, has taken a more restrictive attitude to endoluminal interventional techniques, at least with regard to their integration in operative therapy concepts. Although Charles Dotter stated in 1968 that "... the technique should be learned, used and improved by surgeons ..." (1) in his classic publication "Transluminal Dilatation of Atherosclerotic Stenosis", the new method was initially rejected by vascular surgeons on grounds of principle (2).

Although angioplasty has not led to a decrease in the total number of arterial reconstructions (3), the frequency of aortoiliac reconstructions — similar to renal artery stenoses — has nevertheless decreased since angioplasty and stent implantations offer lower risk and less stressful alternatives.

Patients with changes in the pelvic area often have a poor morbidity profile. According to ASA classification (American Society of Anesthesiologists), their allocation to a risk group which cannot be subjected to classic operative reconstruction of the pelvic section is above average owing to a number of concomitant cardiopulmonary diseases (4).

In the case of younger patients, the focus is on a different problem: the threat of impotency following orthotopic aortoiliac reconstruction. Although it is extremely difficult to assess the actual rate of impotence induced by the operation — the literature quotes rates of 20 to 80% (5,6) — this threatened complication increasingly causes younger patients to seek other therapeutic options. Understandably, the possibility of endoluminal reconstruction meets with substantially better acceptance (cf. Figure 1). This is all the more so considering that primary stent implantation can significantly improve the long-term results of catheter dilatation alone in the iliac area (7, 8).

MATERIALS AND METHODS

Our experience is based on 127 cases of angioplasty with stent implantation in the pelvic artery area. In 67 patients (Group I)

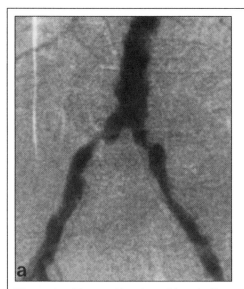 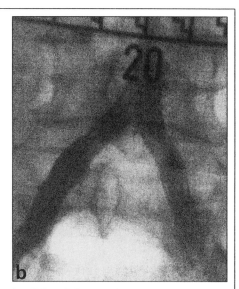

Figure 1. 54-year-old patient with typical buttock claudication *(left, a)*. DSA revealed severe aortic bifurcation/bilateral stenosis of the common iliac artery. The patient rejected direct aortic bifurcation reconstruction because of fears concerning impotence. Follow-up angiography after angioplasty using a "kissing balloon" technique with primary bilateral stent implantation *(right, b)*. The results showed optimal hemodynamic recanalization.

the stent was implanted percutaneously, while in 60 patients (Group II) it was implanted intraoperatively in connection with vasosurgical reconstruction. The two groups differed considerably in terms of age, sex, and risk factors. Group I contained 73.2% men with a mean age of 63 years. Group II was characterized by a substantially greater risk profile; all cases involved a multisectional disease and had an mean age of 70.9 years.

Both Strecker™ (Boston Scientific Corp., Denmark) and Palmaz-Schatz™ (Johnson & Johnson Interventional Systems Co., Warren NJ) stents were implanted. Patients were administered a minimum dose of a thrombocyte aggregation inhibitor after the procedure.

In 89.3% of the patients intraarterial pressure was measured before manipulation to verify the hemodynamic relevance of the stenosis and to document the recanalization result after angioplasty or stent implantation (Figure 2). This was especially important when it occurs as the relevance of a pelvic arterial

stenosis can be suppressed in combination with occlusion of the superficial femoral artery in particular. In such cases, stress should be simulated with drug-induced vasodilatation in order to verify the actual stenotic effect (Figure 2, right).

The method of intraoperative endovascular stent implantation was extremely simple. One prerequisite, however, was the availability of suitable x-ray equipment in the sense of a C-arm with integrated digital subtraction angiography (DSA) technology and the possibility of road mapping. The patient was given a regional anaesthetic and the anterior wall of the femoral bifurcation was exposed. The communal femoral artery was punctured using the Seldinger method before the arteriotomy. The guidewire was then passed through the affected segment of the vessel. Placement of the balloon catheter with the mounted stent was followed by pressure-controlled dilatation and expansion of the stent. After the catheter material had been extracted, the arteriotomy was ex-

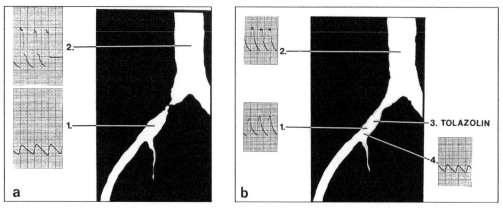

Figure 2. Technique of intraarterial pressure measurement in severe and angiographically less marked pelvic artery stenosis and/or ipsilateral occlusion of the superficial femoral artery (6). *(Left, a):* First measurement was taken post-stenotically (1) and the second in the aorta (2). In the event of significant difference in pressure (20 mm Hg), angioplasty was executed. *(Right, b):* No significant difference in pressure between the first measurement (1) and the second (2). Post-stenotic injection of a vasodilator (tolazolin) (3) and the measurement was repeated (4). Dilatation with stent implantation was executed only when the pressure differential was accented.

ecuted, including the puncture defect, and the remaining vasosurgical reconstruction completed.

RESULTS AND DISCUSSION

Arterial occlusive disease is characterized by its fateful course and virtually unalterable progression. Anyone who performs invasive therapy must realize that the vascular intervention methods available today may be clinically efficient but do not have any causal basis for their therapeutic effect. This consideration logically leads to the demand for a concept which can achieve a hemodynamic result appropriate to the patient's living circumstances, but without an excessive risk. By far the most frequent indication for endovascular stent implantation in aortoiliac AOD is isolated pelvic artery stenosis. We have excellent experience with stent implantation for this indication, as do other authors, and can record a primary success rate of 98%.

No long-term results are as yet available, however, in contrast to conventional vasosurgical reconstruction. However, vasosurgery has certainly lost ground with regard to the treatment of pelvic artery stenosis. In view of the minimally-invasive nature of the angioplastic method, a conventional operative approach can be justified in individual cases only, since the operation always involves a greater risk, a longer hospitalization stay, and higher morbidity.

In cases of solitary, unilateral pelvic artery occlusion, however, the indication is still a matter for discussion. If the occlusion is short, attempted recanalization with stent implantation may be justified. If the pelvic arterial occlusion is lengthy, we consider reconstruction by means of an extraanatomical cross-over bypass, since this involves less risk and is also probably less expensive. The morbidity and complication rates of this therapeutic approach are also just as low as those of stent implantation and the procedure guarantees a good hemodynamic result.

By far the most frequent indication for endovascular angioplasty in cases of aortoiliac AOD in our group was pelvic artery stenosis in combination with a contralateral pelvic artery occlusion, bring an unfavorable prognosis upon the patient. In such cases, an extraanatomical femorofemoral bypass is an excellent reconstructive instrument. Its hemodynamic results are satisfactory but depend to a great extent on an intact, nonstenotic donor vessel. If there is an impediment in the latter which affects the hemodynamic flow, the reduction in flow and pressure must be eliminated before bypass implantation. Retrograde, endovascular dilatation with stent implantation in the donor vessel has proved very successful in such cases (Figure 3). We prefer intraoperative stent implantation in these cases as we are able to operate in a virgin common femoral artery area and do not have to cope with the risk of prosthesis infection as a result of prior manipulation.

In emergency situations, too, we have found endovascular reconstruction very successful. In the case of an acute pelvic arterial occlusion, for example, emergency orthotopic bypass implantation has a high mortality and morbidity rate. If recanalization via a transfemoral Fogarty thrombectomy is unsatisfactory, and a bifurcation stenosis can be verified as the cause of the acute occlusion by means of intraoperative angiography, we now regard endoluminal bilateral angioplasty with stent implantation using the kissing balloon technique (Figure 4) as the gold standard. We know of cases in which only unilateral flow could be restored by means of the Fogarty catheter, but in which a hemodynamically-relevant residual stenosis remained and the contralateral flow could not be recanalized. Unilateral stent implantation in combination with the implantation of a cross-over bypass has proved successful (Figure 5) in these cases.

In principle, every situation in which a hemodynamically-active stenosis impedes inflow to a distal bypass reconstruction is suitable for endoluminal angioplastic treatment with stent implantation. This is particularly true for patients in whom a distal femoropopliteal reconstruction is combined with ipsilateral pelvic artery stenosis. Such stenoses are probably one of the main causes of unexplained femoropopliteal bypass occlusions (9). Elimination of these stenoses is imperative and an essential hemodynamic prerequisite for peripheral bypass implantation.

The combined use of an operative procedure with endovascular and transluminal angioplasty and stent implantation in the pelvic area has proved a sensible therapeutic approach, as has the percutaneous modification in the hands of the vascular surgeon. It gives polymorbid patients a therapeutic chance with minimal invasiveness and a satisfactory hemodynamic effect.

CONCLUSION

Endovascular angioplastic procedures have proved successful worldwide in the treatment of aortoiliac arterial occlusive disease. They have not only led to a fundamental change in indication for vasosurgical reconstruction in the pelvic region, but have provided new therapeutic opportunities for certain groups of patient. Experience gained on 127 patients has shown that in cases of circumscribed stenoses and short occlusions of the pelvic arteries, angioplastic treatment with primary stent implantation should be the preferred therapy. This is particularly true in the case of younger men with stenosis of the aortic bifurcation. In high risk patients with multisectional complaints, interventional techniques have considerably extended the range of therapies available if combined with conventional vasosurgical reconstructive methods. From a vasosurgical point of view, the following indications have emerged for such cases: intraoperative stent implantation of an iliac stenosis in planned ipsilateral femoropopliteal bypass; angioplastic treatment and stent implantation in stenosis of the inflow in cases of femoral bifurcation reconstruction; stent implantation in cases of a stenotic donor artery in femorofemoral bypass implantation; and incomplete recanalization in cases of acute Lériche syndrome. Since the results of aortoiliac stenting are comparable with the results of conventional vasosurgical reconstruction methods, the

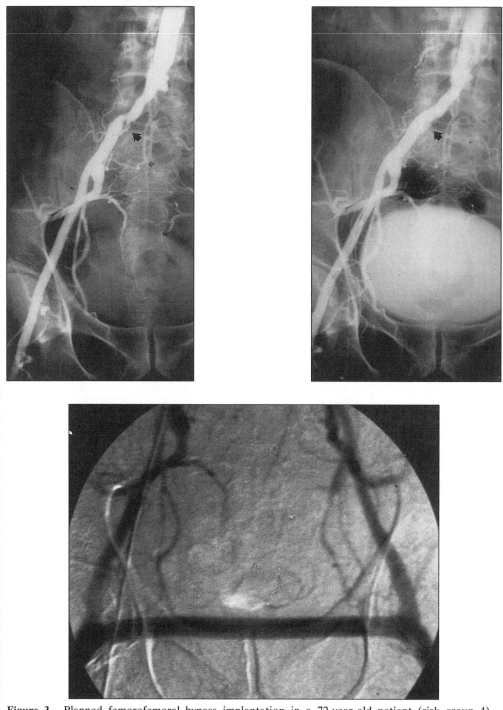

Figure 3. Planned femorofemoral bypass implantation in a 72-year-old patient (risk group 4). Hemodynamically-significant stenosis of the right common iliac artery with contralateral occlusion of the iliac artery *(top left)*. Follow-up angiogram *(top right)* after intraoperative transluminal angioplasty with stent implantation in preparation for femorofemoral bypass implantation *(bottom)*.

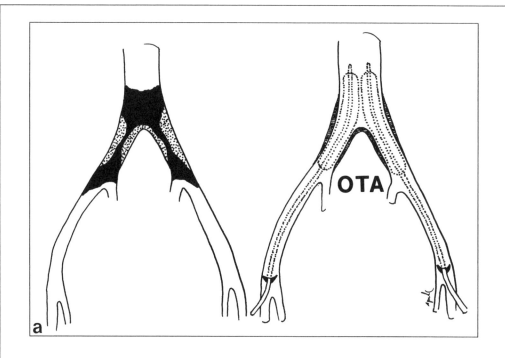

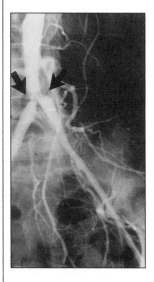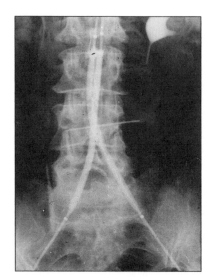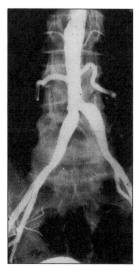

Figure 4. Therapeutic approach for acute bifurcation occlusion on the bottom of a bifurcation stenosis *(top, a)*. After thrombectomy, intraoperative transluminal angioplasty with stent implantation (OTA) in the bifurcation using the "kissing balloon" technique. Intraoperative angiography after pelvic artery thrombectomy revealed significant bifurcation stenosis *(bottom left)*. OTA with the dilatation catheters in "kissing balloon" position *(bottom middle)*. Angiographic control after OTA indicated complete elimination of the stenosis *(bottom right)*.

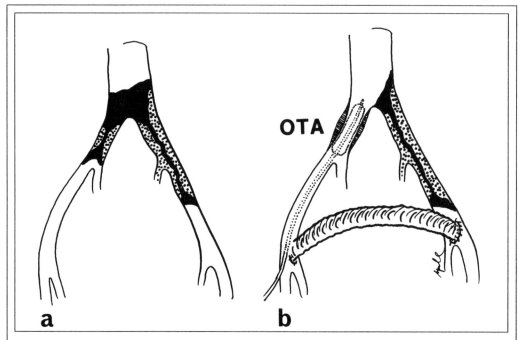

Figure 5. Therapeutic approach in a case of acute pelvic arterial occlusion on the bottom of a bilateral pelvic artery stenosis where only unilateral reconstruction succeeded by means of thrombectomy. The initial situation consisted of distal aortic and/or pelvic artery occlusion with existing stenoses *(left, a)*. Residual stenosis remains after Fogarty thrombectomy on the right. Angioplasty and stent implantation (OTA) of the residual stenosis of the right iliac artery (donor vessel) guarantees the required hemodynamic conditions for cross-over bypass implantation *(right, b)*.

decisive advantages of interventional procedures lie in the circumvention or minimization of the operative risk, in reducing operation duration in the case of combined treatment, and in shorter hospitalization stays.

REFERENCES

1. Dotter CT, Rösch J, Judkins MP. Transluminal dilatation of atherosclerotic stenosis. Surg Gynecol Obstet 1968;127: 794-804.
2. Vollmar J, Trede M, Laubach K, Forrest H. Principles of reconstructive procedures for chronic femoro-popliteal occlusions. Report on 546 operations. Ann Surg 1968;2:215-223
3. Menges H-W, Jaschke W, Trede M. Percutaneous transluminal angioplasty: the surgeons role. World J Surg 1988;12: 788-757.
4. Menges H-W, Schaupp W, Busch HP, Huck K, Trede M. Die Becken-arterienstenose: wann operieren — wann dilatieren? Indikationsstellung aus gefäßchirurgischer sicht. Angio 1986;8:237-244.
5. May A, Weese JA, Rob LG. Changes in sexual function following operation of abdominal aorta. Surgery 1969;65:41-47.
6. Sabri S, Cotton LT. Sexual function following aorta iliac reconstruction. Lancet 1971;2:1218-1220.
7. Richter GM, Roeren T, Brado M, Nöldge G, Landwehr P, Kaufmann GW. Prospektiv randomisierte Studie: Primäre Implantation von ballon-expandierten Palmaz-Stents versus traditioneller Ballonangioplastie bei AVK der Beckenarterien. In: Kollath J and Liermann D, eds. *Stents II.* Konstanz: Schnetztor Verlag; 1992; 31-38.
8. Gross-Fengels W, Friedmann G, Palmaz JC. Ballonexpandierbare Stents bei arteriellen

Veränderungen der Beckenstrombahn. Fortschr Röntgenstr 1991;155:349-356.

9. Flynn W, Harris JP, Rudo HD, Bergan JJ, Yao IST. Atheroembolism of cause of graft failure in femoral distal reconstruction. Surgery 1982;90:698-706.

Use of the Strecker Stent in Lower Extremity Arterial Vessels: A Long-Term Follow-Up

D. Liermann

Department of Radiology, J.W. Goethe University Hospital, Frankfurt am Main, Germany

INTRODUCTION

Surgery of iliac and peripheral vessel stenoses and occlusions shows acceptable results (1-4). However, the risk associated with anaesthesia remains and a significant rate of restenosis and occlusion is typical (5-13). New techniques (14) were developed for the interventional treatment of AOD (arterial occlusive disease) which made it possible to successfully recanalize even old and long occlusions without, however, being able to maintain vessel patency through percutaneous transluminal angioplasty (PTA) in all cases (15-22). This resulted in a significantly reduced success rate for PTA in our patient population which, in turn, caused us to search for a successful method of keeping the vessel lumen patent. After our own experimental studies, we decided to use a tantalum endoprosthesis initially in the iliac, femoral, and popliteal arteries. The objective of our study was to find out if, subsequent to an unsuccessful PTA, the tantalum stent (Strecker™; Boston Scientific Corp., Denmark) would improve flow in iliac, femoral, or popliteal vessels. In addition, it was necessary to compile indications for stents as an alternative for surgical or conservative procedures (23). Our material and methods correspond to those previously described for the use of tantalum endoprostheses.

INDICATIONS

This was the first study worldwide on the implantation of tantalum endoprostheses in peripheral human vessels. The study objective was to translate the results obtained from human cadavers and animals to the most problematic areas confronted clinically, e.g., adductor canal and distal superficial femoral arteries. The following indications were accepted for stent implantation: vessel reocclusion within a 6-month period after PTA, reocclusion during PTA, or occlusion due to iatrogenous vascular dissection during PTA. Unsatisfactory results after PTA were only accepted if recoiling of the stenosis was expected to produce significant flow obstruction and restenosis. Another prerequisite besides a sufficient circulation above the vascular region to be stented was a minimum of one patent tibial vessel.

STUDY POPULATION

The results obtained from a total of 101 patients with one or several tantalum endoprostheses are summarized. Twenty-four patients received stents in the proximal superficial femoral artery, 65 patients received stents in the adductor canal, 8 patients received stents in the popliteal artery, and four patients were implanted in the anastomosis between the popliteal artery and the distal end of an iliacopopliteal bypass. Four patients had stenoses and another 20 patients had occlusions of the proximal superficial femoral artery. Fifteen patients had stenoses and 62 had occlusions of the adductor canal or the popliteal artery. Using Fontaine's classification, 22 patients were in stage IIb, 67 patients were in stage III, and 12 patients were in stage IV prior to stent implantation.

Patients were between 38 and 92 years of age (mean, 69 years); 32 were female and 69 were male. Sixty-one patients were implanted with one stent, 26 patients were implanted with two stents, 10 patients received three stents, and 4 patients received four stents in the same vascular segment. The length of the occlusions ranged from 0.2 to 48 cm in the peripheral vessels (mean, 8.8 cm). The diameter of the implanted stents was between 4 and 8 mm.

Risk factors included diabetes (14.7%), high blood pressure (35.4%), and long-term nicotine abuse (89%). All patients were subjected to a strictly defined peri-interventional anticoagulation protocol (Table 1) as well as an accurate follow-up with periodical determination of ankle-arm indices (AAI) and walking range without pain before and after stent placement. AAI and walking range were determined 3, 6, 12, and 18 months post-stenting and at 6-month intervals thereafter. A routine intravenous digital subtraction angiography (DSA) was carried out after 6 and 12 months and then at yearly intervals after stent implantation or in the case of a significant AAI drop.

RESULTS

Follow-up examinations in patients with stented proximal femoral vascular arteries took place between 6 and 72 months (mean, 39 months) after implantation and between 6 and 62 months (mean, 36 months) in patients with stents in the adductor canal and popliteal vascular sections (Table 2). The group with proximal femoral vascular stents exhibited a patency rate of 82%, while the group of stent implantations in peripheral vascular sections showed a patency rate of only 46%. Stents in this latter group were mainly in the adductor canal or the popliteal artery.

Due to thromboses in the stented vascular regions in the first two cases of restenosis, a rigid peri-interventional anticoagulation therapy was set up. As expected, no histological thromboses were found during the remainder of the follow-up procedures in the case of restenosis or reocclusion but only intimal hyperproliferative wall reactions. The histological material was collected after preliminary examination via a Simpson atherectomy catheter which was applied for this purpose only. For different reasons, aspirin or Marcumar® therapy was interrupted in cases of thrombosis in a stented vascular section. Surprisingly, interruption of the Marcumar therapy for a duration of 3 weeks resulted in no side effects in a female patient 2 months after implantation of an endoprosthesis in the adductor canal. Histologic examination of the stenoses and occlusions that occurred mostly between 6 and 9 months post-stenting showed that all flow obstructions were caused by intimal

---

Table 1. Peri-Interventional Anticoagulation Protocol

I. Conservative therapy includes daily doses of aspirin 325 mg for most patients prior to intervention.

II. After sheath introduction, each patient is administered heparin 100 IU/kg body weight. Another heparin 5000 IU are applied after PTA and before stent placement. Complicated and long interventions require higher doses.

III. In the first 72 hours post-stenting, the patient is usually given heparin 1000 IU/hour through the perfusor. Depending upon laboratory parameters, higher doses can become necessary in order to prevent an early reocclusion.

IV. Long-term therapy with daily doses of aspirin and dipyridamole seems to be sufficient for iliac and proximal femoral vessels.

Table 2. Results After Arterial Stent Placement in 101 Patients

Femoral Arteries	89 patients	Mean Follow-Up	37.2 months (Range, 6 to 72 months)
Proximal	24 patients		Patency: 82%
Distal	65 patients		Patency: 46%
Popliteal Vessels	8 patients	Mean Follow-Up	38 months (Range, 6 to 72 months)
			Patency: 72%
Bypass Anastomosis	4 patients	Mean Follow-Up	26 months (Range, 6 to 53 months)
			Patency: 75%

hyperproliferative wall reactions. All cases of stenoses and occlusions were removed without any problems by PTA or laser treatment (Neodym Yag Laser). The re-PTA or laser application led to a relatively short recurrence-free interval compared to the time of the first recurrence and consequently to an earlier recurrence of restenosis (4 to 7 months). These restenoses were also treated by PTA or laser. In all patients a number of re-dilatations were necessary.

In 20 selected cases, a new therapy was applied subsequent to the re-PTA using endovascular afterloading with iridium 192. The first results were quite promising. All stented vascular sections in these patients were unobstructed 18 to 24 months after endovascular irradiation with single vascular wall doses of 12 Gy. Stents implanted across knee joints did not exhibit any signs of stent deformation or a higher restenosis rate.

Stent treatment of the peripheral vascular vessels resulted in an improvement of all patients' clinical condition. All cases having a clinical stage II (Fontaine) before stenting achieved stage I (Fontaine) after stent placement. In all cases with a clinical stage III or IV (Fontaine) before stenting, it was possible to attain stage II after stent implantation with one exception. The AAI follow-up for peripheral vessels before stent implantation (mean, 0.61) also showed a significant increase of the value to a mean of 0.90 after stent implantation. A different development was noted during further follow-up due to the numerous restenoses or reocclusions that developed by the mid-term examination at 35 months post-stenting. The group with restenoses showed an early AAI drop during the 6-month follow-up, whereas the group of patients without restenosis exhibited only an insignificant drop to a mean of 0.81. Each AAI drop required angiography to differentiate a restenosis in the stent from the formation of flow obstructions in the vessels above and below the stented region.

During the first clinical applications of the Strecker stents we had three problems concerning stent extraction because one of the fixing silicone rubber sleeves did not roll back after balloon inflation and thus did not release the stent despite proper expansion. We had another problem with the rupture of a balloon before the stent was completely expanded. Two of the stents were able to be extracted by carefully rotating and turning the balloon while withdrawing it. Two more had to be extracted using a procedure employing a long 10 Fr sheath (Cook, Europe). Following balloon deflation, the sheath was inserted with its tip just before the balloon-stent tandem and the tandem was then pulled into the sheath. In doing this we were able to apply our experiences gained in experimental stent extractions. After the necessary exchange of the sheath and catheter system via a guidewire, a new sheath was introduced and a new stent implanted without any problems. Due to a stent-vessel mismatch, one stent dislocation occurred in the iliac vascular system at 2 cm below the stenosis necessitating the placement of a larger diameter stent. A small hematoma occurred after stent implantation.

Recently, six stents had to be removed since the placement of a second stent caused dislocation due to an inadequately small diameter with a resulting deformation or due to hypercoagulation. This was done using the extraction set tested in experimental trials which consisted of a 5 Fr recovery forceps and a 9 Fr aspiration catheter. In one case, three stents with a length of 8 cm, 4 cm, and 4 cm, respectively, and a diameter of 6 mm had been placed in the popliteal segment. A second case had two stents of 8 cm each with a diameter of 6 mm in the adductor canal, while a third case had two stents of 8-cm and 4-cm lengths with diameters of 6 and 7 mm, respectively. In these and all other cases we were able to extract the stents using the set described above and no complications were noted at the follow-up examination after stent extraction. In the first case, the stents were successfully replaced by larger stents. In the other two cases where stents had been implanted to treat a long dissection which in turn caused hypercoagulation adverse to therapy, the stents were removed 24 hours later and the coagulation disorder was successfully terminated. A positive side effect subsequent to the extraction of the endoprostheses after 24 hours was the repositioning of a dissection under pressure from the stents and an unobstructed flow in these vascular sections. No surgery was required in any of these cases (Figures 1-3).

DISCUSSION

Experimental trials using Strecker stents with a diameter of 2 to 14 mm have already been successfully completed. Our own results obtained under clinical conditions substantiate these experimental results. The properties of these stents permit their placement in bent vessels and across joints. Very high patency rates (98%) have been documented for stent applications in larger diameter arteries such as the iliac artery or the superficial femoral artery at a mid-term follow-up after 20 months. The situation is more difficult for peripheral vessels. A lower flow and turbulence, especially near the adductor canal, can be considered as possible causes for the significantly worse long-term results of stent placement in peripheral vessels. Often, additional stenoses in the tibial region during generalized AOD further influence the distal flow. The follow-up shows a mean restenosis rate of 30% in the adductor canal. The group of patients with reocclusions treated by endoprostheses in the adductor canal even shows a mean restenosis rate of almost 40%. On the basis of these results, routine application of stents in distal vessels cannot be recommended.

The causes and pathogenesis of restenoses in atherosclerotic and non-atherosclerotic vessels after PTA have been extensively discussed (16,19,21,24-35). In canine studies, Barth et al (36) showed different diameters of the stented vascular regions at different time points after stent placement. The thickest intimal layer in the stent was 313 microns 8 weeks after implantation. Twenty-six weeks after implantation of the endoprosthesis, there was a significant decrease of the diameter of this layer to only 223 microns. However, these results from animal trials could not be translated to the situation of atherosclerotic vessels in humans. Possibly, after an intensive stage of hyperproliferation immediately after stent placement, transition to a less intense proliferation can be expected which still narrows the diameter of the stented vessel but does not lead to occlusion. This would explain why vessels with a relatively large diameter such as the iliac artery remain open, whereas smaller diameter vessels are occluded due to

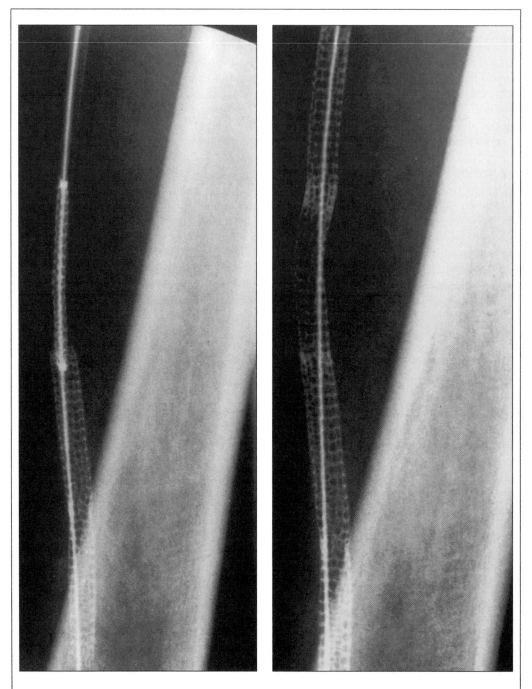

Figure 1. This figure indicates that there are now problems associated with implanting the Strecker stent in cases where it is necessary to implant several overlapping stents because the Strecker stent does not shorten upon expansion. *Left:* Two stents have already been implanted and a third is positioned. *Right:* Four stents have been successfully implanted using an overlapping technique.

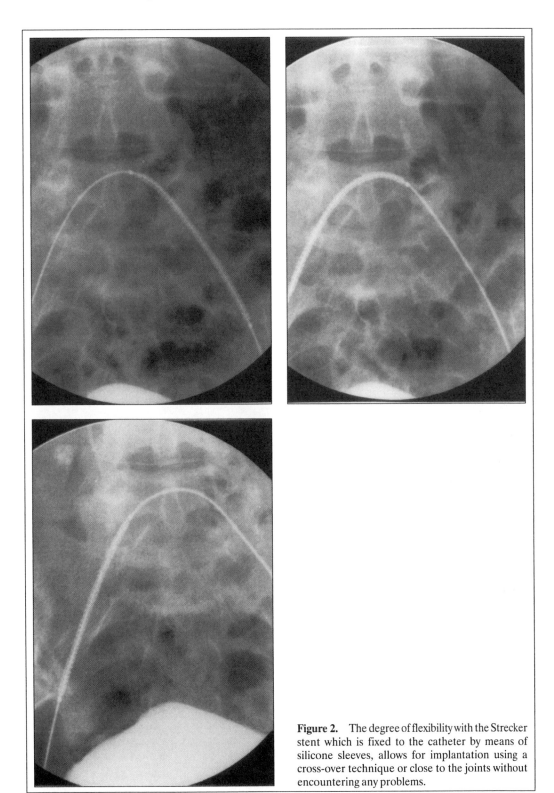

Figure 2. The degree of flexibility with the Strecker stent which is fixed to the catheter by means of silicone sleeves, allows for implantation using a cross-over technique or close to the joints without encountering any problems.

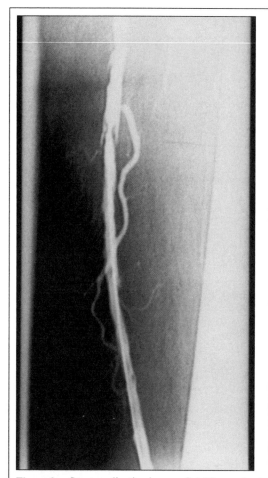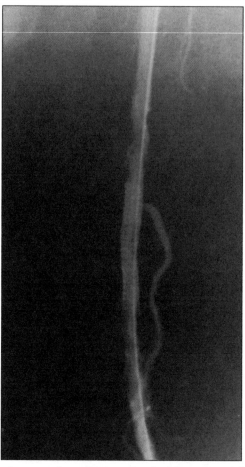

Figure 3. Stent application in superficial femoral artery in severe, short-distance stenosis with unsuccessful PTA, after recanalization of an occlusion leading to an extreme flow retardation with imminent reocclusion. The collateral artery overlapped by the stent remains open.

the very intense hyperproliferation in the beginning. A reduction of stent application in peripheral vessels seems to be necessary until this procedure can be safely applied in humans. It seems interesting that stent extraction in peripheral vessels in cases of dislocation or deformation does not pose a problem. What seems to be even more interesting, however, is that stents can be extracted in case of therapy-resistant hypercoagulation. Extraction led to the not insignificant side effect of repositioning two dissections caused by a recanalization of the occlusion. An only temporary placement of stents to treat dissections is highly interesting considering the

well-known problems caused by intimal hyperplasia after stent implantation.

Based on these results, the indications for stent implantation should follow the proposals given in Table 3. Further indications for stent implantation should be a Fontaine stage IIb to IV along with sufficient circulation in the proximal and distal vascular regions to be stented and at least one patent tibial vessel. Factors that will influence the further development of this procedure will be the thromboresistance and flexibility of the stent material as well as its long-term patency compared to PTA and surgical intervention. Also, the further development of methods to

Table 3.   Indication for Stent Implantation in Peripheral Vascular Systems

I. Acute dissection with subsequent vascular occlusion that cannot be sufficiently controlled by repeated, long-term use of PTA.

II. Reocclusion of a vascular segment that has been successfully opened by the same intervention through PTA, due to vascular wall deficiency.

III. As an <u>exception</u> in cases of persistent restenosis after PTA with an expected occlusion in the near future due to the considerable slowing down of blood flow.

reduce fibromuscular hyperproliferation after stent placement will be of utmost importance, as only the development and simultaneous application of these methods holds promise for a further extension of indications for stent placement in peripheral vessels.

REFERENCES

1. Denck H. Der akue Extremitätenverschluß. In: Heberer G and van Dongen RJAM, eds. *Gefäßchirurgie*. Berlin: Springer; 1987; 373-386.
2. van Dongen RJAM, Franke F. Chronische Verschlußprozesse der Unterschenkelarterien. In: Heberer G and van Dongen RJAM, eds. *Gefäßchirurgie*. Berlin: Springer; 1987;415-430.
3. Gall FP, Franke F. Chronische Verschlußprozesse der Arteria femoro-poplitea. In: Heberer G and van Dongen RJAM, eds. *Gefäßchirurgie*. Berlin: Springer; 1987; 404-414.
4. Trede M, Thiele HH. Aortoiliakale Verschlüsse; hohe Aortenverschlüsse. In: Heberer G, van Dongen RJAM, eds. *Gefäßchirurgie*. Berlin: Springer; 1987; 387-402.
5. Blaisdell FW, Hall AD. Axillary-femoral artery bypass for lower extremity ischemia. Surgery 1963;54:563.
6. Clowes AW, Gown AM, Hanson SR, Reidy MA. Mechanisms of arterial graft failure: 1. role of cellular proliferation in early healing of PTFE prostheses. Am J Pathol 1985;118:43-54.
7. Gresham GA. Atherosklerose: Ihre Ursachen und ihre potentielle Reversibilität. Triangel 1976;15:39-43.
8. Gruss JD. Der in-situ Bypass. In: Heberer G, van Dongen RJAM, eds. *Gefäßchirurgie*. Berlin: Springer; 1987;431-443.
9. Krüger BJ, Stockmann U, Witte C. Der axillo-femorale bypass: ein therapeutisches Verfahren bei Risikopatienten mit chronischer Verschlußkrankheit der Beckenarterien. Thoraxchirurgie 1971;19:493.
10. Pratschke E, Schäfer K, Becker HM. Der gekreuzte suprapubische femoro-femorale Bypass. Indikation, Operationsverfahren und Ergebnisse. Angio 1980;1,2:31-36.
11. Schlicht L. Zur Behandlung von Verschlüssen der Beinarterien mittels Kunststofftransplantaten. In: Hess V, ed. *Die obliterierenden Gefäßerkrankungen*. München: Urban & Schwarzenberg; 1959.
12. Upson JF. The comparative development of atherosclerosis in normal aorta, vascular grafts and endatherectomized aorta. J Surg Res 1963;3:384.
13. Vollmar, J. Rezidiveingriffe an der Aorta abdominalis und den Beckenarterien. Langenbecks Arch Chir Suppl, Kongressbericht 1991;514-518.
14. Vallbracht C, Kollath J, Roth FJ, et al. Grundlagen, Technik und Ergebnisse der Rotationsangioplastie. In: *Gefäßchirurgie im Fortschritt*. Stuttgart: Thieme Verlag; 1991;249-254.
15. Clowes AW, Reidy MA, Clowes MM. Kinetics of cellular proliferation after arterial injury. Lab Invest 1983;49:327-334.
16. Cox JL, Gottlieb AL. Restenosis following percutaneous transluminal angioplasty: clinical, physiological and pathological features. Can Med Assoc J 1986;134:1129-1132.
17. Faxon DP, Sanborn TA, Haudenschild CC. Mechanism of angioplasty and its relation to restenosis. Am J Cardiol 1987;60:5B-9B.

18. Ip JH, Fuster V, Badimon L, Badimon J, Taubman MB, Chesebro JH. Syndromes of accelerated atherosclerosis. Role of vascular injury and smooth muscle cell proliferation. J Am Coll Cardiol 1990;15:1667-1687.

19. Laerum BF, Vlodaver Z, Castaneda-Zuniga WR, Edwards E, Amplatz K. The mechanism of angioplasty. Fortschr Röntgenstr 1982;136:573-576.

20. Spaet TH, Stemermann MB, Veith FJ, Lejnieks I. Intimal injury and regrowth in the rabbit aorta. Medial smooth muscle cells as a source of neointima. Circ Res 1975;36: 58-70.

21. Wissler RW. Principles of the pathogenesis of atherosclerosis. In: Braunwald E, ed. *Heart Disease: A Textbook of Cardiovascular Medicine*. 2nd edition. Philadelphia: WB Saunders; 1984;1183-1204.

22. Zollikofer CL, Cragg AH, Hunter DW, Yedlicka JW, Castaneda-Zuniga WR, Amplatz K. Mechanism of transluminal angioplasty. In: Castaneda-Zuniga WR and Tadavarthy SM, eds. *Interventional Radiology*. Baltimore: Williams and Wilkins; 1992;249-298.

23. Blair JM, Gewertz BC, Moosa H. Percutaneous transluminal angioplasty versus surgery for limb-threatening ischemia. J Vasc Surg 1989;9:698-703.

24. Block, PC. Percutaneous transluminal coronary angioplasty. In: Connor WE and Bristow JD, eds. *Coronary Heart Disease: Prevention, Complications and Treatment*. Philadelphia: Lippincott; 1985;405-418.

25. Essed CE, Van den Brand M, Becker AE. Transluminal coronary angioplasty and early restenosis: fibrocellular occlusion after wall laceration. Br Heart J 1983;49:393-396.

26. Fallone BG, Wallace DS, Gianturco C. Elastic characteristics of the self-expanding metallic stents. Invest Radiol 1988;23:370-376.

27. Mabin TA, Holmes DR, Smith HC. Follow-up clinical results in patients undergoing percutaneous transluminal coronary angioplasty. Circulation 1985;71:754-760.

28. Palmaz JC, Garcia F, Sibbit SR, Chang P. Expandable intrahepatic portacaval shunt stent in dogs with chronic portal hypertension. AJR 1986;147:1251-1254.

29. Palmaz JC, Windeler SA, Garcia F. Atherosclerotic rabbit aortas: expandable intraluminal grafting. Radiology 1986; 160:723-726.

30. Rollins N, Wright KC, Charnsangavej C, Gianturco C. Self-expanding metallic stents: preliminary evaluation in an atherosclerotic model. Radiology 1987;163:739-742.

31. Rousseau H, Raillat C, Joffre F, Knight C, Ginestet MC. Treatment of femoropopliteal stenoses by "Wallstent" endoprosthesis. Radiology 1989;172:961-964.

32. Strecker EP, Berg G, Schneider B, Freudenberg N, Weber H, Wolf HRD. A new vascular balloon-expandable prosthesis: experimental studies and first clinical results. J Interv Radiol 1988;3:59-62.

33. Strecker, EP Liermann D, Barth KH, et al. Expandable tubular stents for treatment of arterial occlusive diseases: experimental and clinical results. Radiology 1990;175:97-102.

34. Triller J, Mahler F, Thalmann D. Die vaskuläre Endoprothese bei femoropoplitealer Verschlußkrankheit. Fortschr Röntgenstr 1989;150:328-334.

35. Wolf GL, Le Veen RF, Ring EJ. Potential mechanism of angioplasty. Intervent Radiol 1984;7:11-17.

36. Barth KH, Virmani R, Strecker EP, et al. Flexible tantalum stents implanted in aortas and iliac arteries: effects in normal canines. Radiology 1990;175:91-96.

First Clinical Experience with the Memotherm Vascular Stent

E. Starck

Department of Radiology, Red Cross Hospital, Frankfurt am Main, Germany

INTRODUCTION

The Memotherm® stent (Angiomed, Karlsruhe, Germany) is made of a shape-memory metal alloy (nitinol). Nitinol is a nickel-titanium-aluminum alloy in which the titanium's oxidation exudation is strongest. This is intended to seal off the alloying components by a coat of titanium oxide on the surface after mechanical processing for un-complicated use of the stents, even in persons allergic to nickel. The configuration is cut from sheet metal with a laser (wall thickness: 0.16 mm/femoral and 0.18 mm/iliac) so that no wire crossings result (Figure 1). Using the lowest possible amount of foreign material, this "low-profile, single-wall" construction facilitates placement into the intima without creating strong pressure, resulting in the best possible laminar flow without turbulences.

The equilibrium temperature of the shape-memory alloy was determined between the martensite point of 26°C and the austenite point of 35°C by means of production-engineering heat treatment. This means that at normal external temperatures, a compressed femoral stent has a diameter of 1.1 mm which spontaneously expands to 4 to 8 mm at body temperature (7 to 12 mm with an iliac stent, according to rhombus design). Current stent lengths range from 2 to 11 cm. During application, an outer sheath is removed which causes the stent to immediately expand in response to body warmth. Introducer sets up to 50 mm in length have a diameter of 6 Fr and can be placed via a 0.025-inch guidewire while sets from 50 to 120 mm (7 Fr) can be placed via a 0.035-inch guidewire. The single-hand operation introducer sets have distal and proximal platinum markers. Additional injection of contrast medium is possible at any time via a Y-shaped connector. The stents are sufficiently radiopaque and antimagnetic and there are no artifacts impairing resolution during CT and magnetic resonance imaging (MRI) examinations. Nitinol stents have a very low corrosion tendency (1-4). In order to keep thrombogenicity as low as possible, a special polishing process was developed which refines the surface to a rhombus depth of 0.18 μm and results in a mirror-like surface. This smooth surface finish and the negative electric charge are intended to reduce or prevent the formation of platelet-rich thrombi.

METHODS AND RESULTS

Stents were implanted during 14 (3%) of 482 angioplastic procedures performed between January and August 1993 prior to the introduction of Memotherm. Of these, 29% were iliac stents (femoral stents: > 60%; popliteal stents: only 7%).

Indications for stenting are rather strict, e.g., emergency procedures. Most are bail-

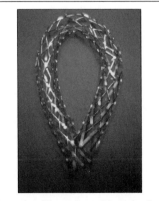

Figure 1. Memotherm Vascular Stent

out stent implantations, mainly in the case of residual stenoses with impaired perfusion following balloon dilatation in stages III and IV according to Fontaine's classification (i.e., a significantly decreased chance of limb salvage). Dissections or detached atherosclerotic plaque material with luminal obstruction following balloon dilatation may also be included. Coagulopathies of uncertain etiology (which cannot be specifically treated) are contraindicated, with hypercoagulation regarded as more serious than hypocoagulation, function-relevant obstructions of the inflow path, poor outflow, or missing intraluminal, distal connection of the lumen. Fresh, soft thrombotic or embolic material is primarily removed by aspiration and/or thrombolysis, even with iliac occlusions.

In my opinion, an infrainguinal aneurysm, whether partly or completely thrombosed, is an excellent indication for stent implantation since this will change perfusion to a degree where the aneurysm is completely thrombosed or, with a new lumen, thrombotic sections are cut off from the perfusion, thus avoiding embolization. The first such implantations were performed 3 years ago; short-term results proved the soundness of this concept. Changes in the stent material, however, made further stenting unfeasible. Kinking or disintegration occurred with the Strecker™ stent (Boston Scientific Corp., Denmark), i.e., numerous fatigue failures, especially in the popliteal region. In one case we bridged and secured the crumbled Strecker stent with two Wallstents™ (Medinvent, Lausanne, Switzerland). After 6 weeks the Wallstents were dislocated outside the aneurysm (due to their tendency to shorten), despite primarily correct, overlapping implantation.

The outstanding stability of the new stent material, its excellent flexibility and compressibility, self-expansion capability (which renders the stent undeformable by flexion), and extremely high elasticity (which makes fatigue failure improbable) prompted us to use it in three patients with popliteal aneurysms. While we achieved overall clinical success, reocclusion occurred in one patient 3 days after implantation due to outflow problems at the trifurcation below the stent. Recanalization of the occluded region by aspiration and lysis presented no problems. Recanalization of the stented vessel segment with the aspiration catheter alone (without dislocation or deformation) was easy, as opposed to our earlier experience with Strecker stents. After overdilation treatment of the trifurcation and subsequent anticoagulation with phenprocoumon (Marcumar®), the course corresponded to that in the other two patients who had a popliteal aneurysm stented but were not given Marcumar. No complications were noted.

DISCUSSION

Treatment of suprainguinal aneurysms by stenting alone (5) is not recommended. At present, it is not thought to be safe since the intravascular pressure wave is passively (measurably) directed toward the vessel wall and thus entails further growth and the risk of rupture despite ongoing thrombosis (6). This is highly improbable for the femoral and popliteal regions.

Further stent implantations were performed in two patients with iliac occlusions, one of which had an antegrade dissection caused by sounding of a severe stenosis. Pressure did not rise sufficiently following removal of the fresh thrombotic material by aspiration and subsequent balloon dilatation. The implantation of an 8 mm Memotherm stent (length: 8 cm) produced normal perfusion without an intravascular pressure gradient. Primary stent implantation in the case of iliac occlusion has been considered controversial (7,8). Iliac occlusions have the highest complication rate of all angioplasty procedures; on the other hand, primary stent implantations in case of stenoses give better long-term results (9). We treat fresh iliac occlusions primarily by thrombolysis, aspiration, and balloon dilatation. Only in case of insufficient rise in pressure or perfusion (as with the second patient) is stent implantation performed. Reocclusion also occurred 4 days after this procedure; however, it originated distally of the stent in the presence of poor outflow, which was demonstrated by a preceding angiogram. Furthermore, hypercoagulopathy with antithrombin III deficiency was diagnosed. As expected, the stented iliac region was included in a setting of complete occlusion and clinical deterioration. Following substitution of antithrombin III, the stented segment was easily recanalized by lysis and aspiration. Unlike earlier procedures, the outflow problems in the femoropopliteal region were treated not only by balloon dilatation but by placement of two additional Memotherm stents. After approximately 10 days, an infrapopliteal amputation had to be carried out due to progressive gangrene in the presence of existing muscular necroses, despite unchanged patency of the main flow path to the foot, including the stented regions.

In the long run we will give priority to the implantation of femoral stents, regardless of the restrictive indications due to unsatisfactory results mentioned above (10). In a special case, for instance, further heparin anticoagulation in order to ensure perfusion of the also dilated superficial artery was contraindicated because of an incomplete iliac rupture following transpopliteal puncture and balloon dilatation. Because of progressing thrombosis that also affected all tibial vessels, a transfemoral puncture had to be later performed. The freshly thrombosed vessels were recanalized by aspiration and a single dose of heparin. Two Memotherm stents (each 10-cm long) had to be implanted in order to definitively ensure perfusion of the superficial femoral artery. Rethrombosis did not occur despite the unavailability of further anticoagulation. In my opinion, this indicates a low thrombogenicity of the stent material. As of yet, there is no way to judge the extent to which the mirror-like surface and the negative charge will produce long-term reduction of intimal hyperplasia and better long-term results in comparison with conventional angioplastic therapy or surgical bypass operations. A marked increase in the relatively small share (presently 3%) of this rather simple angioplastic procedure will depend on it, as well as our decision to liberally treat restenoses and reocclusions by an expensive stent implantation rather than by repeated balloon dilatation.

CONCLUSION

Thanks to the excellent long-term results, stent placement in the iliac region is considered safe among the various procedures (7,9). I hope that the Memotherm stent, which has been substantially improved in many respects, will also bring about such improvements for therapy of the femoral region.

REFERENCES

1. Palmaz JC. Intravascular stents: tissue-stent interactions and design considerations. AJR 1993;160:613-618.
2. Cragg AH, De Jong S, Barnhart W, Landas S, Smith T. Nitinol intravascular stent: results of preclinical evaluation. Radiology 1993;189:775-778.
3. Baier RE, Meyer AE, Natiella JR, Natiella RR, Carter JM. Surface properties determine bioadhesive outcomes: methods and results. J Biomed Mater Res 1984;18:337-355.
4. Edie JW, Anderson GF, Zaytoun MP. Surface corrosion of nitinol and stainless steel under clinical conditions. Angle Orthod 1981;51:319-324.
5. Hagen B, Harnoss BM, Trabhard S, Ladeburg M, Fuhrmann H, Franck C. Self-expandable macroporous Nitinol stents for transfemoral exclusion of aortic aneurysms in dogs: preliminary results. J Cardiovasc Intervent Radiol 1993;16:339-342.
6. Reekers J. Persönliche Mitteilung 1993.
7. Vorwerk D, Günther RW, Keulers P, Wendt G. Complications and reobstruction after placement of an arterial stent: frequency and

methods of treatment. Radiology 1992; 185P:180.

8. Rominger M, Rauber K, Matthes B, Schulze A, Rau W. Interventionell-radiologisches Vorgehen bei längerstreckigen kompletten Beckenarterienverschlüssen. Fortschr Röntgenstr 1991;154:310-314.

9. Richter G, Nöldge G, Roeren T, et al. First long-term results of a randomized multicenter trial: iliac balloon-expandable stent placement vs. regular percutaneous angioplasty. Radiology 1990;177P:151.

10. Sapoval MR, Long AL, Raynaud AC, Beyssen BM, Fiessinger JN, Gaux JC. Femoropopliteal stent placement: long-term results. Radiology 1992;184:833-839.

Endoprostheses in the Treatment of Bypass Anastomoses

D. Liermann[1], J. Berkefeld[1], M. Zegelman[2], P. Satter[2]

Departments of [1]Radiology and [2]T.H.V. Surgery,
J.W. Goethe University Hospital, Frankfurt am Main, Germany

INTRODUCTION

Among the common vascular surgery procedures for the treatment of arterial occlusive disease, establishing a bypass or a graft to circumvent a vessel segment which can no longer be rehabilitated or reconstructed with other methods is the last resort (1). Other methods, such as the Forgaty balloon stripper procedure or a thromboendarterectomy using a ring stripper, have priority for many vessels. One reason is that a vascular replacement for a vessel segment can only be achieved if collateral vessels are sacrificed. The patient can do without these collaterals if the bypass remains open. Should, however, reocclusion of a bypass occur, the affected vessel area below it is in acute danger (2-8). Surgical revision of the bypass is necessary to save the dependent limb.

The causes of a bypass occlusion are extremely diverse. Bypass occlusion can occur because of a too-low dose of anticoagulation therapy. It can also be the result of congestion, with an increasingly slower flow in the bypass because of progressive atherosclerosis in the vessel segments below and the development of stenoses and occlusions. The kinking phenomenon during sitting, for example during long flights, leads to a slowing of blood flow and to thrombosis. Embolization from ulcerous vessel segments above the bypass or from the heart with known arrhythmias causes an occlusion (1,6,9-12). Formation of scar tissue with subsequent slow flowing, or hypertrophic growth of the vascular anastomosis can also contribute to occlusions between the bypass and the proximal or distal vessel segment (6,13-18).

If thrombosis has occurred, its elimination must be given top priority and the cause should also be eliminated to prevent further recurrences. A surgeon will be most willing to undertake a surgical intervention the first time a bypass occludes. This willingness will diminish as the amount of scar tissue resulting from several revisions becomes more and more insurmountable. Antegrade puncture for visualizing an occlusion, respectively for distending it towards the peripheral vascular region, has become established for such cases because it makes antegrade insertion of a 4 Fr lysis catheter into the fresh thrombosis through a wire possible as a second measure with only one puncture. An attempt is made to clear the bypass obstruction within the framework of the following local lysis therapy (2,19-21). If the clear cause of the thrombosis is found after elimination of the thrombus, it can often be removed by using percutaneous transluminal angioplasty (PTA) (19,22). In some cases, especially those in which hyperplastic vascular wall changes in the area of the anastomosis occur, this seems to be insufficient since the reconstructed lumen collapses within a short period and again leads to an obstruction (14). Until now, surgical measures have remained the only alternative in such cases. Either the bypass was reinserted or the complete new establishment of a bypass was done.

Implantation of endoprostheses as an alternative to anastomoses that are difficult to handle surgically have gained consideration. The goal of this study was to demonstrate if stent implantation in these segments was technically possible, if the vessel was kept open, and if an interaction between the anastomosis and the stent material occurred.

MATERIALS AND METHODS

If occlusion of a peripheral bypass is suspected, an antegrade puncture with a typical 0.65-mm angioneedle is made in order to perform an angiography. If there is an indication for the suspected bypass occlusion and an existing reconnection distal to the bypass, a 4 Fr lysis catheter is exchanged into the bypass and advanced until it is in the thrombus, once contraindications for a local lysis therapy with a fresh thrombosis have been ruled out. The first 4 cm of the lysis catheter are perforated so that imbibition of the thrombus with urokinase is possible. After an initial infusion of urokinase 100,000 IU, the patient is perfused with 70,000 to 100,000 IU/hour, depending on weight, along with heparin 1000 IU/hour at the same time (20,23). If, as a result of the lysis procedure or because of the case history, there is any indication that an embolus is the cause of the thrombosis, an attempt is made to suction off the embolus including the thrombotic material as an alternative (21,24). Intensive monitoring of the patient is necessary if local lysis is continued. Individual lyses in the above dosed form often still proved successful after 48 hours with somewhat older occlusions.

If a stenotic obstruction below the bypass or at the distal anastomosis results from the lysis procedure, the stenosis is dilated with a balloon catheter after a larger sheath has been substituted and the flow is then checked. It is absolutely necessary to administer an antispasmodic agent to the peripheral vascular region before the contrast medium series is done so that genuine obstructions can be distinguished from spasms. If unobstructed flow results, the same procedure as that after the PTA of an occlusion is adapted for the further peri-interventional measures. In case of a collapse of the distal or proximal anastomosis and the following slowing of flow, an endoprosthesis is implanted.

INDICATIONS

The insufficient dilatability of a distal or proximal anastomosis after recanalization and lysis, with consecutive slowing of flow above the obstruction, is accepted as an indication for stent implantation in bypass vessel anastomoses. Endoprosthesis implantation can only be done if there are no contraindications to anticoagulation treatment. Besides sufficient flow above the anastomosis segment which is to be fed with the stent, at least one patent lower leg vessel below this area is required.

PATIENT DATA

A total of five patients with bypass occlusions were treated (four male, one female; Table 1). Their mean age was 64 years (range, 56 to 74 years). There was a relatively fresh thrombosis of the bypass in all cases (2 days to 3 weeks). In one case, stent implantation was the first therapy after establishing the bypass following lysis and PTA. In four cases multiple surgical interventions had already occurred (mostly maneuvers with the Forgaty balloon after arteriotomy) with only relatively brief patency periods ranging from 3 days to 5 months. All patients had a year-long case history of advanced stage arterial occlusive disease (AOD). The ankle-arm index (AAI) before intervention was between 0.1 and 0.3 and the clinical stage according to Fontaine was between III and IV.

The first patient was 56 years old, had generalized pronounced AOD and multiple coronary bypass operations. The patient also had an iliacopopliteal bypass which had already been surgically revised after occlusion and which had rethrombosed after only a brief patency rate of 3 months despite Marcumar® therapy. The patient had an AAI of 0.2 on the right and 0.89 on the left side. The clinical stage according to Fontaine was III. Due to the cardiac case history, other surgeons were not inclined to perform a new revision. The iliacopopliteal bypass was a Goretex endoprosthesis which was placed proximally on the iliaca communis and distally on the side of the poplitea. We decided to use a transbrachial method with exposition of the left brachial artery. After the Terumo

Table 1. Implantation of Tantalum Endoprostheses in Bypass Anastomoses

Patient No.	Age/Sex	Implant Location	Stent Dimensions	Problems		Follow-up[a]
				With Implant	After Lysis and PTA	
1	56/Male	Distal iliacopoliteal bypass	5-mm wide 4-cm long	No	Yes	36 months
2	67/Male	Distal femoropopliteal bypass	5-mm wide 4-cm long	No	Yes	19 months
3	74/Female	Distal femoropopliteal bypass	5-mm wide 4-cm long	No	Yes	12 months
4	62/Male	Proximal femoropopliteal bypass	6-mm wide 4-cm long	No	Yes	4 months
5	64/Male	Distal femoropopliteal bypass	6-mm wide 8-cm long 6-mm wide 4-cm long	No	Yes	4 months

a No recurrences were noted during the follow-up period for any patient.

guidewire was advanced into the proximal branch of the bypass, the Beerenstein catheter was exchanged for a 9 Fr guide catheter, through which the spindle of a Rotacs drill with an olive-shaped tip was then advanced to the bypass. After the spindle was connected with the motor unit, it was advanced caudally during careful rotation. The drill spindle went only as far as the proximal third of the thigh because of the long distance. A second puncture was made in the area of the right groin towards the spindle which was in the Goretex bypass. It served as a "road map" if there was no pulsation of the bypass. It was possible to successfully probe this bypass. An 8 Fr Terumo sheath was exchanged, and the Rotacs spindle was then advanced caudal from the groin during motor-powered rotation. It was only possible to force a passage at the distal foot-point of the bypass under great difficulty, because the drill spindle had snagged in a pocket-formed sag. Once this

anastomosis was passed, lysis treatment using the above described technique was carried out for approximately 10 hours. After that, the bypass was patent but also demonstrated clear congestion of the contrast medium flow and thus, of blood flow. Finally, a PTA was performed in the anastomosis area with a 5-mm balloon catheter. It successfully expanded the constriction, but also led to an immediate collapse of the anastomosis with consecutive congestion because of the sag which was present at the lower end of the anastomosis. The patient was receiving the prescribed anticoagulation therapy for the duration of the procedure. We decided to implant a stent in the anastomosis which was 5 mm in diameter and 4-cm long since the distal segment of the anastomosis had collapsed.

The second patient was a 67-year-old man with known generalized AOD (Fontaine stage III) and an acute femoropopliteal bypass occlusion. The AAI on the left was only 0.1 and was 0.66 on the right side. The patient had massive pain at rest and an almost completely white lower leg. Since the patient had a long cardiac case history, he was referred to us. Angiographically, the bypass was occluded a few centimeters below its origin, so that it turned out to be possible to probe the bypass. A lysis catheter was inserted and local lysis using the above described technique was carried out. After this treatment was concluded there was a persisting constriction in the distal anastomosis which could also not be satisfactorily eliminated with PTA because of pronounced recoiling. In view of these problems, we decided to implant a 5-mm wide, 4-cm long stent.

The third patient was a 74-year-old woman with severe generalized AOD (Fontaine stage IV) and a bypass anastomosis at the distal point of a femoropopliteal bypass. It had already been revised twice and the second reocclusion occurred within 6 months. The patient had an AAI of 0.2 on the right and 0.75 on the left; she also had an ulcer on the sole of the right foot. The lower leg was lividly discolored but it wasn't white yet due to a still well-preserved profunda with the corresponding collaterals. Besides nicotine abuse, the patient also had diabetes for many years. After the bypass (Goretex) was punctured in the antegrade direction at the level of the groin, we were able to advance a wire into the thrombus and do a lysis under the above described conditions after changing in the lysis catheter. The bypass was patent after 6 hours of lysis therapy, but a stenotic area at the height of the distal anastomosis caused a persisting obstruction. Dilatation with a 5-mm balloon catheter also could not eliminate the obstruction. Implantation of a 5-mm wide, 4-cm long stent was performed.

The fourth patient was a 62-year-old-man with a completely occluded bypass. The patient suffered from generalized AOD, with an AAI of 0.3 on the right and 0.7 on the left and a clinical stage of IV according to Fontaine. The femoropoliteal bypass had al-

ready been surgically revised after an occlusion and had reoccluded after 3 weeks. Based on the case history, we did an antegrade puncture as high up as possible, since we did not know the exact location of the bypass origin due to the lack of previous radiographs. Although a stump of the superficial femoral artery as well as a rudimentary profunda were visualized, the origin of the bypass was not located. After thorough injections we were convinced that a vessel system which was fed by profunda collaterals was filled up below the bypass. After several exploratory probes were done, we finally managed to successfully probe the occluded bypass segment. Lysis with a 4 Fr catheter according to the above described technique followed. At the 12-hour follow-up, thrombotic material with flow around it was recognized, but there was no connection towards the distal part. We decided to substitute a 9 Fr sheath into the bypass and aspirate the thrombotic material. A relatively large amount of thrombotic material was removed. We managed to advance a guidewire caudally through the distal anastomosis. We continued the lysis therapy for 24 hours because thrombus material was still recognizable in the bypass and the situation in the lower leg was unclear, although we knew that no blood flow could pass into the bypass from above because of the sheath's size. Finally, severe constriction with questionably old thrombus formation at the caudal pole of the femoropopliteal anastomosis became recognizable. We decided to implant a 6-mm wide, 4-cm long stent into the distal anastomosis because of the risk of dispersing thrombotic material, which could no longer be lysed, into the caudal segment of the lower leg.

The fifth patient was a 64-year-old man who also had known generalized AOD (Fontaine stage IV) with a femoropopliteal bypass that had been surgically revised twice. He had been referred to us for visualization because of suspected reocclusion. The AAI was 0.2 on the left and 0.8 on the right. After an antegrade puncture of the femoralis communis, which was performed high up, the profunda, but not the bypass origin, could be visualized. After several probe attempts, we finally managed to insert a Terumo wire into the bypass lumen and insert a lysis catheter. Lysis therapy according to the above described conditions was carried out. A persisting anastomosis constriction, which covered a long distance and extended itself to the following vessel segment, resisted our efforts to successfully eliminate the constriction with a 6-mm balloon catheter. We decided to implant a 6-mm wide, 8-cm long stent along with a second 6-mm wide, 4-cm long stent.

Walking distance could not be determined, with two exceptions (10 and 20 m), because the patients were all confined to bed at the time of examination. All patients were subjected to a precise follow-up which provided for regular determination of the AAI and the pain-free walking distance before and after stent implantation, as well as the changes in clinical stage. AAI and the possible walking distance were determined 3, 6, 12, 18, 24, 36, and 48 months after stent implantation. Routine intravenous digital subtraction angiography (DSA) was carried out 6, 12, 24, and 48 months after stent implantation or in case of a clear reduction of the AAI.

RESULTS

All six stents at six different sites in five patients could be successfully implanted (Ta-

ble 2; Figures 1 and 2). Three 5-mm wide, 4-cm long stents; two 6-mm wide, 4-cm long stents; and one stent that was 6-mm wide and 8-cm long were implanted. Five stents were implanted in the distal anastomoses of three femoropopliteal bypasses and one iliacopopliteal bypass, and one stent was placed in the proximal anastomosis of a femoropopliteal bypass. The AAI changed from 0.1 to 0.3 before implantation to 0.8 to 1.0 after implantation. The clinical stage according to Fontaine was able to be improved from stage III or IV to stage I or IIb in all cases. All ulcerous changes healed. Until now, the patency rates in the follow-up are between 4 and 36 months and thus are clearly higher than before the last revision.

DISCUSSION

The above results showed a good success rate for the implantation of stents in anastomoses. Of course, the number of interventions carried out is still very small, and the individual cases are quite different from one another. Nevertheless, one of the most commonly used arguments, an increased risk of thrombosis because of lack of epithelialization of the Goretex bypass and thus also of the stent, can be weakened as a result of the long-term follow-up for individual anastomoses after stenting (14). The anticoagulation was also done in normal vessel stenoses as after stent implantation (25-28). It is surprising that no stenosis recurred in spite of the in-

Table 2. Implantation of Tantalum Endoprostheses in Bypass Anastomoses

Patient No.	Age/Sex	Clinical Stage (Fontaine) Before/After Stenting	AAI Before/ After Stenting	Walking Distance After Stenting
1	56/Male	III/I	0.2/0.9	Unlimited
2	67/Male	III/IIa	0.1/0.8	> 500 m
3	74/Female	IV/IIa	0.2/0.9	> 500 m
4	62/Male	IV/I	0.3/1.0	Unlimited
5	64/Male	IV/IIb	0.2/0.8	> 300 m

convenient position of the stent in the vessel, although final conclusions cannot be made due to the small number of cases. The explanation may lie in the deviating flow behavior of the blood in the bypass. Besides increasing the possibilities for implanting endoprostheses in other anastomoses, the implantation of such endoprostheses in anastomosis connections with inconvenient locations could be possible (6,10,12,16-18). A further interesting variation is the prophylactic implantation of endoprostheses in vessel anastomoses which are in considerable danger of occlusion. Among these is the relatively high rate of anastomosis occlusions between donor and recipient organ arteries as in the case of liver transplants. Naturally, further animal testing in this regard must be conducted (16,17,29).

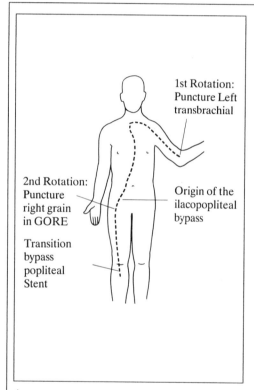
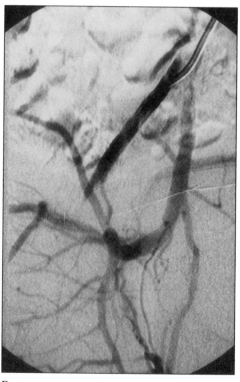

A   B

Figure 1. Recanalization of an occluded iliacopopliteal bypass transbrachial and transfemoral (GORE) using rotation, PTA, and stenting in the popliteal transition. Difficult recanalization of an occluded iliacopopliteal bypass with rotation angioplasty and implantation of a 5-mm stent into the distal anastomosis between bypass and arteria poplitea. Scheme of the access to recanalization of the bypass and for stent implantation in the distal anastomosis of the transbrachial recanalized iliacopopliteal prosthesis *(1A)*. The tip of the rotation catheter inserted transbrachially is in the origin of the occluded bypass *(1B)*. The reopened distal anastomosis collapses immediately after recanalization and PTA *(1C)*. Visualization after implantation of a 5-mm stent into the distal anastomosis *(1D)*. Complete patency of the bypass at the follow-up after 36 months *(1 E/F)*.

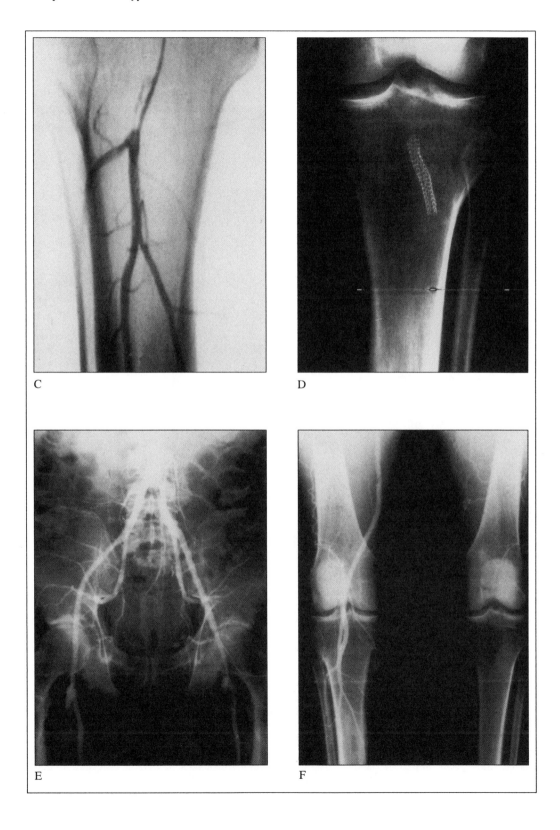

C

D

E

F

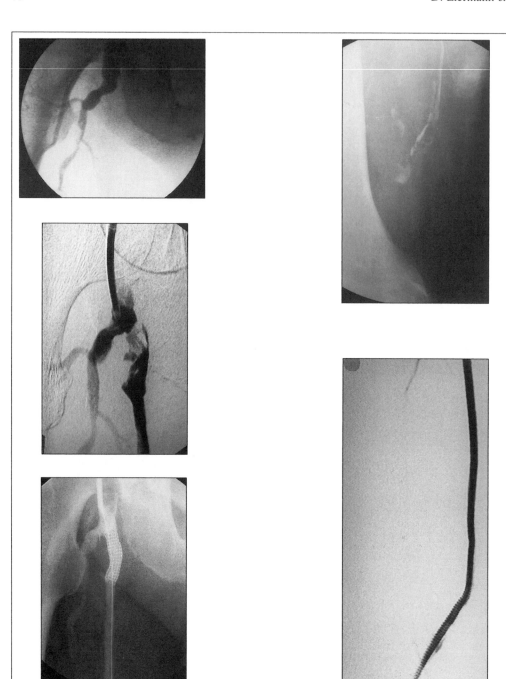

Figure 2. Recanalization and stent implantation with complete occlusion of a right femoropopliteal bypass. Angiographic visualization of the A. femoralis profunda *(top left)*; the origin of the bypass is completely occluded. The bypass origin after lysis and PTA with persistence of occluding material in the lumen *(middle left)*. PTA cannot be considered because of the danger of diffusing unlysed material into the distal vessels. Visualization of the situation in the bypass exit after lysis *(bottom left)*, PTA and stent implantation demonstrating good flow. Visualization of the distal anastomosis of the same bypass after lysis and PTA *(top right)*. The distal anastomosis also remains patent after stent implantation *(bottom right)*.

REFERENCES

1. Müller-Wiefel H. Gefäßprothesen. Chirurg 1985;57:64-71.
2. Denck H. Der akute Extremitätenverschluß. In: Heberer G and van Dongen RJAM, eds. *Gefäßchirurgie*. Berlin: Springer; 1987;373-386.
3. van Dongen RJAM, Franke F. Chronische Verschlußprozesse der Unterschenkelaterien. In: Heberer G and van Dongen RJAM, eds. *Gefäßchirurgie*. Berlin: Springer; 1987;415-430.
4. Giessler R. Gefäßrekonstruktionen. In: Heberer G and van Dongen RJAM, eds. *Gefäßchirurgie*. Berlin: Springer; 1987;73-88.
5. Holcroft JW, Conti S, Blaisdell FW. Extraanatomic bypass grafts. Surg Clin N Am 1979;59:649-658.
6. Schmitz W, Vollmar J. Komplikationen des alloplastischen Gefäßersatzes. Ursachen, Verhütung und Behandlung. Langenbecks Arch Klin Chir, Kongressbericht 1963; 304:963.
7. Trede M, Thiele HH. Aortoiliakale Verschlüsse; hohe Aortenverschlüsse. In: Heberer G and van Dongen RJAM, eds. *Gefäßchirurgie*. Berlin: Springer; 1987;387-402.
8. Vollmar J. Gefäßersatz durch synthetische Kunststoffe. Fortschr Med 1963;81:387.
9. Hamann H, Vollmar J. Expanded PTFE Gefäßprothesen — Ein neuer Weg des Arterien — und Venenersatzes? Chirurg 1979;50:249-256.
10. Paes E, Vollmar JF, Mohr W, Hamann H, Brecht-Kraus D. Biologische Unverträglichkeit von Kunststoffendoprothesen: Differential-dianostik und Therapie. In: Hepp W, Raithel D, Loeprecht H, eds. *Aktuelle Herausforderung in der Gefäßchirurgie*. Darmstadt: Steinkopff; 1991;85-91.
11. Porter J. *In situ* versus reversed vein graft: is one superior? J Vasc Surg 1987;5:779-780.
12. Schlicht L. Zur Behandlung von Verschlüssen der Beinarterien mittels Kunststofflransplantaten. In: Hess V, ed. *Die Obliterierenden Gefäßerkrankungen*. München: Urban & Schwarzenberg; 1959.
13. Blaisdell FW, Hall AD. Axillary-femoral artery bypass for lower extremity ischemia. Surgery 1963;54:563.
14. Clowes AW, Gown AM, Hanson SR, Reidy MA. Mechanisms of arterial graft failure: 1. Role of cellular proliferation in early healing of PTFE prostheses. Am J Pathol 1985;118:43-54.
15. De Weese JA. Anastomotic intimal hyperplasia in vascular grafts. In: Sawyer PN and Kaplitt MJ, eds. New York; 1978; 147-152.
16. Linton RR, Menendez CV. Arterial homgrafts: a comparison of the results with end-to-end and end-to-side vascular anastomosis. Ann Surg 1955;142:568.
17. Payr E. Zur Frage der circulären Vereinigung von Blutgefäßen mit resorbierbaren Prothesen. Arch Klin Chir 1904;72:32.
18. Upson JF. The comparative development of atherosclerosis in normal aorta, vascular grafts and endatherectomized aorta. J Surg Res 1963;3:384.
19. Blair JM, Gewertz BC, Moosa H. Percutaneous transluminal angioplasty versus surgery for limb-threatening ischemia. J Vasc Surg 1989;9:698-703.
20. Hess H. Lokale Lyse bei peripheren arteriellen Verschlüssen. Herz 1989;14: 12-21.
21. Lammer J, Ascher PW, Choy DSJ. Transfemorale Katheter-Laser Thrombendarterektomie (TEA) der arteria carotis. Dtsch Med Wochenschrift 1986;11:607-610.
22. Wolf GL, Le Veen RF, Ring EJ. Potential mechanism of angioplasty. Interv Radiol 1984;7:11-17.
23. Liermann D, Strecker EP, Peters J. The Strecker stent: indications and results in iliacal and femoropopliteal arteries. Cardiovasc Intervent Radiol 1992;15:298-305.
24. Stark E, McDermott J, Crummy A, Turnipseed W, Acher C, Burgess J. Percutaneous aspiration thromboembolectomy. Radiology 1985;156:61-66.
25. Albert JP, Regensburger D, Rudolf I, Yükseltan I, Sievers HH, Bruhn HD. Rezidivprophylaxe operativ korrigierter Arterienverschlüsse der unteren Extremitäten. Med Welt 1982;33:1829-1831.
26. Bruhn HD, Jipp P, Schellmann J, Sedlmeyer I, Müller-Wiefel H, Borm D. Zur Antikoagulantienprophylaxe bei chirurgischer undkonservativer Therapie chronischer Becken Bein-Arterienverschlüsse. Med Klin 1972;67:1514.

27. Genton E, Clagett GP, Salzman EW. Antithrombotic therapy in peripheral vascular disease. Chest 1986;2:75-81.

28. Liermann D, Strecker EP, Vallbracht C, Kollath J. Indikation und klinischer Einsatz des Strecker-Stents. In: Kollath J and Liermann D, eds. *Stents ein aktueller Überblick.* Konstanz: Schnetztor Verlag; 1990;24-37.

29. Kuhn FP, Kutkuhn B, Fürst G, Torsello G, Mödder U. Einsatz des Strecker Stents zur Therapie der Nieren — und Transplantat-nierenarterienstenose. In: Kollath J and Liermann D, eds. *Stents II.* Konstanz: Schnetztor Verlag; 1992;194-203.

The Use of Stents in Venous Vessels

Christopher L. Zollikofer, Francesco Antonucci, Gerd Stuckmann, Paul Mattias

Institute for Radiology, Cantonal Hospital, Winterthur, Switzerland

INTRODUCTION

The treatment of venous stenoses by percutaneous transluminal angioplasty (PTA) is afflicted with a high relapse rate (1,2). In addition, cicatrized fibrotic stenoses, stenoses in the outflow path of a dialysis shunt, or tumor stenoses can often not be effectively dilated in the first place. Endovascular expandable metal prostheses have been used successfully in the arterial area to treat dissections, truly dilatable stenoses, or recurrences thereof. Thus, the venous system is also a logically consistent area for further application of such endovascular stents, to prevent collapse or compression of the lumen by means of an internal mechanical support (3-9). We report our results of 15 patients in whom we treated malignant and benign stenoses in the area of the vena cava, as well as larger veins, with self-expanding endovascular stents.

PATIENTS AND METHODS

Our study was comprised of 44 patients, 26 men and 18 women, aged between 18 and 83 years (mean, 49 years). The localization and etiology of the lesions, as well as the stents used, are listed in Table 1. The patients were divided into three groups:

- Tumor-based stenoses (22 patients).
- Post-operative or post-thrombotic relapse stenoses (including a so-called venous spur) of large veins in the pelvic femoral area (12 patients, 12 stenoses).
- Stenoses of the brachiocephalous veins (vena anonyma and subclavia) in hemodialysis patients (9 patients, 9 stenoses) and one patient with a corto-clavicular compression syndrome.

The self-expanding prostheses that were used were the Wallstent™ (Medinvent, Lausanne, Switzerland) and the Gianturco™

Table 1. Lesion and Stent Characteristics

Etiology	Localization	No. of Patients	Stent Diameter (mm)	Stent Type
Tumor	superior vena cava, vena anonyma	12	14 - 30	WS (11)/GT (1)
Tumor	inferior vena cava, pelvic vein	10	10 - 30	WS (9)/GT (1)
Benign	iliac vein	7	12 - 16	WS (7)
Benign	femoral vein	5	10 - 11	WS (5)
Benign	subclavian vein	11	10	WS (1)
Hemodialysis	vena anonyma, vena subclavia	9	10 - 14	WS (9)

KEY: WS = Wallstent; GT = Gianturco

types (Cook, Bloomington, IN). They have been described in detail elsewhere (3,4). All stents were inserted using a percutaneous inguinal access. The cross-over technique was used for two patients with stents in the vena femoralis communis. An ipsilateral retrograde axis was chosen for patients with stenting of the vena femoralis superficialis; in one patient a transjugular approach was used. In addition, an introducer was always used for stent implantation and all stenoses were pre-dilated with a balloon catheter before stent implantation. The dimensions of the balloon were at least 1 mm smaller than the diameter of the fully expanded stent. With the large central veins of the vena cava, however, the chosen balloon diameter was generally much smaller. In cases in which the endoprosthesis unfolded incompletely after being detached, a balloon dilatation was additionally performed in the implanted stent. Analogous to a conventional PTA, heparin 5000 IU was intravenously administered during the operation. After completion of the operation, patients were heparinized for another 2 to 4 days and, unless there were contraindications, were anticoagulated perorally with Sintrom® in overlapping fashion for at least 6 months. If contraindications to peroral anticoagulation existed, aggregation inhibitors were ordered.

Whenever possible, follow-up examinations were scheduled 1, 3, 6, and 12 months after stent implantation and then yearly thereafter. During the last 18 months, color Doppler studies were also performed. If at all possible, a phlebography was also performed at the 6- and 12-month follow-up visits.

RESULTS

Tumor Stenoses

Seventeen of the 22 patients with an upper and lower blockage died 6 weeks to 24 months after stent implantation without any symptoms. In the case of one patient with an upper blockage, however, the vena cava was phlebographically obstructed 4 weeks after stent implantation. Three days after insertion of the prosthesis, a recanalization with thrombolysis and aspiration had to be performed because of obstruction. The blockage did not recur, however, until the patient's death 3 months later. One patient has had a well-patent vena cava inferior shunt for 17 months (Figure 1). There were two additional recurrences from tumor progression in the mediastinum which were treated with additional stents. In the 10 patients with lower leg inflow obstruction, two suffered from recurrent symptoms after 6 months secondary to tumor progression. Both patients were treated with additional stents. One patient suffered from acute thrombosis of her left pelvic stents due to lack of inflow because of extensive, pre-existing deep vein thrombosis. The overall patency rate until death or last follow-up is 86%.

Post-Operative Relapse Stenoses

All patients continue to have patent stents and have been asymptomatic over a follow-up period of 1 to 96 months. A patient with a stented stenosis after surgical removal of a venous spur shows a basically patent stented lumen without significant intima reaction, even after 96 months. With regard to the patient with a stented vena femoralis superficialis after a traumatic injury, a moderate intimal reaction was observed with a maximum lumen constriction of about 25%. This patient still remains asymptomatic, even after 4 1/2 years. Despite stenting of the hip-joint area, the five patients with stents in the vena femoralis communis (status after crossectomy with consecutive short stenoses of the vena femoralis communis or peri-interventional stenoses) show no signs of relapse after 3 and 6 months, respectively (Figure 2).

Stenoses of the Vena Anonyma and Subclavia

One female patient died after 5 months due to an underlying disease; dialysis was possible until death. The control phlebography

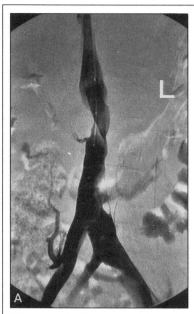 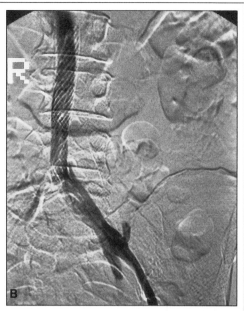

Figure 1. A 47-year-old patient with metastasized ovarian carcinoma, operated on and irradiated. *Left:* Cavography shows a severe infrarenal stenosis and eccentric lumen compression as far as the vena iliaca communis left. (Secondary finding: the right vena iliaca interna flows into the vena iliaca communis left). *Right:* Cavography 6 months after two 25-mm stents showed good patency. The patient continues to be asymptomatic after 15 months.

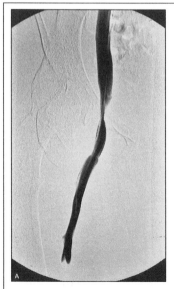 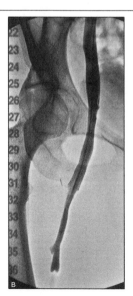 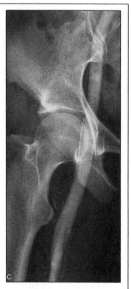

Figure 2. A 34-year-old patient with swelling of the right leg after crossectomy. Phlebography shows a high grade stenosis of the vena femoralis communis *(left, A)*. After implantation of two overlapping 12-mm stents using the cross-over technique, only a discrete residual stenosis was detected *(middle, B)*. Six-month follow-up phlebogram shows complete expansion of the stent with generally patent lumen *(right, C)*.

obtained one month before her death, however, showed a new stenosis 3 cm proximal to the wide open stented area (Figure 3). The control periods of the other seven patients range from 8 to 41 months; all seven patients remain asymptomatic, but only one patient still has a functioning distal AV-shunt. The control phlebography in two patients showed a relapse stenosis in the vena subclavia that, upon further expansion, became increasingly shortened out of the tight stenosis. In both patients, relapse stenosis was eliminated with another stent, placed centrally. A truly intimal reaction could not be detected.

In the other patients, the stented area remains wide open; a new stenosis distal to the stent appeared after 18 months, however, in the patient with the longest follow-up. This stenosis was not treated because of a lack of symptoms and because an AV-shunt was no longer needed after kidney transplantation.

COMPLICATIONS

Altogether, two acute obstructions occurred, one of which could be treated with primary success percutaneously by means of fibrinolysis and thrombus aspiration (cava stent in connection with an upper blockage). In the other patient with an upper blockage with a short stenosis of the vena cava superior, a cranial dislocation of the Gianturco stent by about 3 cm occurred and thus, two additional stents had to be placed to eliminate the tumor constriction. No other serious complications occurred. In particular, no further stent migrations, vascular ruptures, or infections occurred. In two patients with a benign subclavial stenosis, a relapse occurred because the chosen stent was too short and also because of severe secondary shortening of the stent.

DISCUSSION

The most frequent application of percutaneous angioplasty in the venous system concerns stenoses in hemodialysis patients. These stenoses are primarily found in the venous outflow tract of AV-dialysis fistulas or in the area of the brachiocephalous veins (2,10,11). Until now there have been only a few reports about the percutaneous treatment of other benign or tumor-induced venous stenoses (12,13). The application of

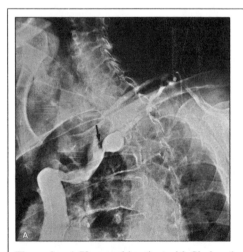 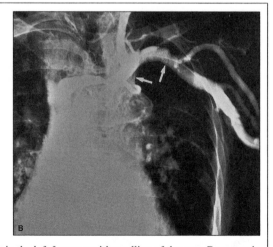

Figure 3. A 78-year-old patient with Cimino shunt in the left forearm with swelling of the arm. Retrograde phlebography shows a high grade stenosis at the place where the vena subclavia flows into the vena anonyma (arrow) *(left, A)*. Four months after a 12-mm endoprosthesis was implanted, very good patency of the stented area was seen (between the arrows) *(right, B)*. No intima reaction was detected, but a new stenosis can be seen in the vena anonyma. Since dialysis was possible, no further therapy was administered.

flexible, endovascular prostheses, however, opens up new perspectives as a supplement or alternative to the surgical treatment of venous constrictions. Tumor-induced obstructions which are refractory to chemical or radiation therapy can now be successfully treated by means of endoluminal splints. The symptoms of the upper blockage, which occur in about 3 to 4% of all patients with bronchial carcinoma, are discontinuously improved (9-14). Our own experience shows that endoluminal stenting of the vena cava superior helps to relieve obstruction by an ingrowing tumor within hours. The endoluminal vascular prostheses are also suitable for the treatment of tumor compression or fibrotic stenoses after irradiation in the area of the vena cava inferior and the pelvic veins. If a closed segment can be reopened by a guidewire, there is a good chance that the obstruction can be kept open by means of an endoprosthesis. If necessary, a cava segment can additionally be opened fibrinolytically before the stent is implanted. This has been proposed by Rösch et al (14). On the other hand, limits of this therapy have also been seen in cases of tight and rigid tumor-based stenoses which do not allow sufficient expansion despite the self-expansion force of the stent. This, among other reasons, is why we pre-dilated all tumor stenoses in order to obtain an idea of the resistive power of a tumor stenosis. As is true for PTA in general, an attempt with an endoprosthesis is always indicated for tumor patients, as long as the situation is not thereby worsened.

Stenoses after surgical reconstruction of the veins, anastomoses, or pelvic thrombosis and the so-called venous spur are further important indications for the implantation of endoprostheses in the venous system. Our two cases with long-term follow-up examinations of 90 and 96 months indicate that late complications or recurrent blockages are not to be expected in large veins. Consequently, we also believe that balloon dilatation combined with the insertion of an endoprosthesis represents the method of choice for patients with a venous spur (May-Thurner syndrome), and should replace surgical therapy. In the area of the vena femoralis, too, our results seem very promising despite joint-crossing stents. By 3 years after stent insertion, no significant intima reactions occurred.

Stenoses of the brachiocephalic vessels are unpleasant complications of hemodialysis (10,15-17). Conventional balloon dilation of these lesions has a very high recurrence rate. For this reason, we and others (18) approach these problems with endoprostheses. The stents seem to prove themselves in this area, even though new stenoses in the neighborhood of the stented area are to be expected. A direct causal connection with the stent appears improbable to us, however, because in our follow-up examinations, the stent areas themselves were completely free of signs of intimal hyperplasia or significant thrombotic deposits.

As the recent publications of Rösch et al and Irving et al (14,18) have shown, no significant differences were found between the results of lesions in the area of the vena cava, the vena subclavia, and the pelvic veins that were stented with Wallstents or Gianturco stents. As was the case in two of our patients, the tendency of the Wallstent to shorten if the chosen prosthesis was too short, can prove to be a problem, since the prosthesis extends further into the area of the normal lumen and thus shortens out of the stenosis. On the other hand, problems can occur with the Gianturco prosthesis in connection with very high-grade stenoses, because of its relative stiffness along the longitudinal axis. Because of this, the prosthesis may slide out of the stenosis under the worst possible case. This risk is reduced by using so-called double stents. If one or possibly several further stents are placed, the above mentioned problem associated with the use of both types of stents can be eliminated immediately, however.

In our opinion, the choice of stent type for large veins should be based primarily on the required diameter and on availability. At this time, vascular Wallstents are only commercially available at diameters up to 16 mm;

20 to 25 mm diameters exist only for esophageal stenoses and should soon be available for vascular use.

CONCLUSIONS

The palliative treatment of tumor-based venous obstruction by means of endoprostheses represents an important indication for the treatment of venous blockage. The vascular endoprosthesis also seems to be an outstanding alternative to surgical intervention in the case of benign stenoses which cannot be readily dilated or which tend to relapse.

REFERENCES

1. Wilms G, Baert AL, Nevelsteen A, et al. Balloon angioplasty of venous structure. JBR-PTR 1989;72:273-277.
2. Hunter DW, Castenada-Zuniga WR, Coleman CC, et al. Failing arteriovenous dialysis fistulas: evaluation and treatment. Radiology 1984;152:631-635.
3. Zollikofer CL, Largiader I, Bruehlmann WF, Uhlschmid GK, Marty AH. Endovascular stenting of veins and grafts: preliminary clinical experiences. Radiology 1988;167:707-712.
4. Charnsangavej CH, Carrasco CH, Wallace SZ, et al. Stenosis of vena cava. Preliminary assessment of treatment with expandable metallic stents. Radiology 1985;161:295-298.
5. Günther RW, Vorwerk D, Bohndorf K, et al. Venous stenoses in dialysis shunts: treatments with self-expanding metal stents. Radiology 1989;170:401-405.
6. Moradian GP, Hunter DW, Castenada F, et al. Clinical experience with placement of Gianturco vascular stents in the venous system. Presented at the 75th Annual Meeting of the RSNA, Chicago; 1989.
7. Antonucci F, Zollikofer CL, Salomonowitz E, Hugentobler M, Stuckmann G. Stenotic veins, grafts, and dialysis shunts: treatment with self-expanding prostheses. Presented at the 76th Annual Meeting of the RSNA, Chicago; 1990.
8. Rousseau H, Morfaux V, Joffre F, et al. Treatment of hemodialysis arteriovenous fistula stenosis by percutaneous implantation of a new intravascular stent. Intervent Radiol 1989;4:161-169.
9. Putman JS, Uchida BT, Antonovic R, Rösch J. Superior vena cava syndrome associated with massive thrombosis: treatment with expandable wire stents. Radiology 1988;167:727-728.
10. Canherwegher JL, Cabolet P, Dhaene M, et al. Complications related to subclavian catheters for hemodialysis. Am J Nephrol 1986;6:339-345.
11. Schwab SJ, Quarles LD, Middleton JP, Cohan RH, Saeed M, Dennis VW. Hemodialysis associated subclavian vein stenosis. Kidney Int 1988;33:1156-1159.
12. Werner WR, Sievers KW, Serdarevic M. Concerning a percutaneous transluminal angioplasty (PTA) of the vena brachiocephalica in the case of a sarcoidosis with upper blockage. Radiologe 1988;28:429-432.
13. Capek P, Cope C. Percutaneous treatment of superior vena cava syndrome. AJR 1989;152:183-184.
14. Rösch J, Uchida BT, Hall LD, et al. Gianturco-Rösch expandable Z-stents in the treatment of superior vena cava syndrome. Cardiovasc Intervent Radiol 1992;15:319-327.
15. Glanz D, Gordon DH, Lipkowitz GS, Butt KMH, Hong J, Sclafani SJ. Axillary and subclavian vein stenosis: percutaneous angioplasty. Radiology 1988;168:371-373.
16. Ingram TL, Reid SH, Tisnado J, Cho SR, Posner MP. Percutaneous transluminal angioplasty of brachiocephalic vein stenoses in patients with dialysis shunts. Radiology 1988;166:45-47.
17. Barrett N, Spencer S, McIvor J, Brown EA. Subclavian stenosis: a major complication of subclavian dialysis catheters. Nephrol Dial Transplant 1988;3:423-425.
18. Irving JD, Dondelinger RF, Reidy JF, et al. Gianturco self-expanding stents: clincial experience in the vena cava and large veins. Cardiovasc Intervent Radiol 1992;15:328-323.

Endoprostheses in the Therapy of Stenoses and Occlusions in Hemodialysis Fistulas

D. Liermann[1], J. Berkefeld[1], E. P. Scheuermann[2]

Departments of [1]Radiology and [2]Nephrology, J.W. Goethe University Hospital
Frankfurt am Main, Germany

INTRODUCTION

Treatment methods for renal failure often allow patients to have a normal life expectancy. Besides transperitoneal dialysis, the most successful method for systemic lavage is hemodialysis through filter systems and machines. A high pressure vessel like the brachial artery has to be punctured for hemodialysis in order to be able to obtain a sufficient amount of blood to pass through the high-volume needle. At the same time a large vessel is needed for retransfusion of the hemofiltrated blood. Thus, arteriovenous shunts have to be set, mostly between a lower arm artery and a large vein.

The first shunts had glass tubes with valves or little faucets. Over time, however, an accessible direct anastomosis between an artery and vein or an artificial interposition prosthesis like a Gore-prosthesis between an artery and vein became the method of choice (1-4). The useful life of these shunts varies greatly between only some hours after its first use up to 23 years (own patient population) without significant problems (4). Changes in the set-up of the shunt caused by the pressures exerted to the anastomosis itself and to secondary venous flow areas, as well as by the frequent punctures, consist primarily of stenoses with frequent pre-stenotic vascular dilatations. In addition to the unpleasant optics of these changes we have to deal with a gradually deteriorating dialytic function accompanied by difficulties in the puncture of the post-stenotic vascular section of the shunt. There is the possibility, in appropriate cases, of a shunt revision by percutaneous transluminal angioplasty (PTA) or surgery (4-8).

Shunt stenoses frequently exhibit extreme rigidity caused by scar tissue formation and this differs from the classic arterial vessel stenosis related to intimal hyperplasia. These stenoses can often be burst open by applying pressures above 18 atm (7,9,10). Thus a suitable catheter material, along with sensitivity, are required for opening the shunt stenosis without risk of rupture. However, outflow obstructions often persist if the stenosis collapses in spite of the pressure. In these cases the implantation of a supporting tissue such as an endoprosthesis for maintaining lumen patency can be a solution (11,12). A problem with this procedure thus far has been the fact that a stented puncture segment could no longer be used for dialysis because the stent was damaged by the consequences of clot formation. In consideration of these problems, and due to skepticism from nephrologists, we refrained from implanting the common types of stents with which we had already had success in arterial vessels. It was not until the development of a nitinol prototype whose thrombogenic and possibly allergy-resistant properties were established in animal studies and which had been successfully implanted, punctured, and extracted in human cadaver arteries that we ventured to apply this type of endoprosthesis in therapy-resistant stenoses and dialysis shunts.

EXPERIMENTAL PUNCTURE OF NITINOL ENDOPROSTHESES AFTER IMPLANTATION IN ARTERIAL VESSELS

Vessel Material and Preparation of Experimental Set-Up

We chose vascular specimens from patients whose case history indicated severe pelvic arterial occlusive disease (AOD) combined with Fontaine stage IIb to IV. In addition we accepted specimens for the experimental series where incidental findings during autopsy revealed severe visible and palpatable pathologic AOD changes (Table 1). In cooperation with the Department of Pathology, the following specimens were removed in one piece and exposed: distal abdominal aorta including bifurcation, both iliac arteries including 2 cm of both internal iliac arteries, and both femoral arteries until 4 cm below the subdivision in the superficial femoral and deep femoral arteries. Specimens were probed and flushed in a saline solution and then occluded by clamping or suturing at the dissections on the distal aorta, both sides of the internal iliac arteries and other exits, and on the superficial femoral or both sides of the profound femoral arteries. The specimen was mounted and extended on a block of wood. After an incision in the common femoral artery and a purse-string suture, a sheath (10 Fr) was introduced via a guidewire. Through the introducer set we were able to obtain an x-ray of the entire vascular lumen by injecting a saline-radiopaque medium with a volume of 50 to 100 mL. When the radiopaque medium gave too intensive coloring, the mixture was aspirated and only a saline solution was injected because the wall coating from the radiopaque medium was often sufficient after the first filling. This procedure allowed us to radiologically identify vascular stenoses and to document them with a 100-mm camera.

After positioning the mounted specimen on the x-ray table, a contrast medium was injected through the sheath using the technique described above in order to exactly locate the site of the stenosis in the vascular section. A 0.035-inch curved tip guidewire and a 7 Fr plain survey catheter were then introduced via the sheath in order to safely pass the stenosis under x-ray control. When the guidewire was in the correct position, the plain survey catheter was replaced by a balloon catheter and the vessel was expanded to the balloon diameter by a manometer-controlled pressure tip. The pressures applied ranged mostly between 6 and 10 atm. The balloon remained inflated for about 1 minute and was then deflated and extracted. Subsequently, the type of endoprosthesis under examination was introduced and deployed in the stenosis.

Methodology

We implanted prototypes of the nitinol stent. The experiment was set up according to the conditions described above. The study objective was to examine the metal properties of the nitinol stent for its application in the treatment of hemodialysis fistulas. A total of six nitinol stents were implanted using the technique described above. Subsequently, these stents were punctured up to 100 times from the outside through the vessel. The experiments were controlled for stent deformation or migration during puncture by an

Table 1. Experimental Puncture After Implantation of Nitinol Endoprostheses in Human Cadaver Iliac Arteries[a]

Sex	Age	Location	Arterio-sclerosis	Punctur-ability	Filament Damage	Elasticity Post-Puncture
Male	78	I. ext.	Mild	Good	None	Good
Male	81	I. com.	Mild	Good	None	Good
Female	62	I. ext.	Severe	Good	None	Good
Female	56	I. com.	Mild	Good	None	Good
Male	78	I. com.	Severe	Good	None	Good

[a] Each stented artery was punctured in the stent region about 100 times.
Key: I. ext. = external iliac; I. com. = common iliac.

angioscope inserted into the vessel. The punctures were made by the usual hemodialysis needles. A new needle was employed after 10 consecutive punctures in order to imitate normal conditions as closely as possible. Next, we made a longitudinal section of the vessel and removed the endoprostheses for examination of evidence of deformation and filament damage.

Results and Discussion

In none of the cases did the puncture of the implanted stents pose any problem. It is felt that a little more physical strength is required to puncture stented sites as compared to the puncture of an unstented artery. No crepitation or bothersome noises were noticed. Examination of the angioscope-transmitted monitor picture indicated a slight compression of the stent with a protrusion of the network into the stent lumen. However, due to the known material properties of the prosthesis, this protrusion was immediately compensated after releasing the needle pushed into the lumen. During needle extraction, the endoprosthesis assumed a tent-like configuration but thereafter the stent filaments resumed their initial shape. Even after more than 100 punctures this mechanism was not changed, and under magnification after explantation, the stent filaments showed no evidence of puncture. The endoprosthesis was easily compressed by hand and then resumed its initial configuration (Table 1). Based on these experimental findings, we can say that the endoprosthesis showed 100% stress resistance and conformed to the expectations in all experiments. There were no complications. These results allowed us to consider this endoprosthesis for puncture sites.

CLINICAL CONDITION

Material and Methods

The nitinol-type endoprostheses were implanted as described above. According to the peri-interventional and post-interventional anticoagulation protocol, follow-up included intravenous digital subtraction angiography (DSA) after 3, 6, and 12 months as well as every 12 months thereafter to avoid recurrent stenoses in the stent. Unlike patient follow-up after stent placement in peripheral arterial vessels due to AOD, additional follow-up parameters have not been determined as all patients are subject to continuous monitoring during dialysis and even insignificant deteriorations are reported and checked.

Indications

The only indication accepted for nitinol stent implantation in dialysis shunts was multiple recidivism of stenoses at the same site following PTA or surgical revision. In general, the patients should be above 60 years of age and peri-interventional, high-dose anticoagulation must be possible. No contraindication for long-term aspirin or Marcumar® therapy should exist before therapy. A nickel allergy has to be excluded because the stent is made of a nickel-titanium alloy.

Patient Population

To date, the conditions for nitinol stent implantation have been met by 13 patients (9 men, 4 women). All have undergone dialysis for several years and their age was between 60 and 78 years (mean, 71 years). Seven patients suffered from the third relapse at the same site, another patient had the second relapse after PTA within a period of 8 months. In all cases recidivism was so severe that continuation of dialysis was jeopardized. A surgical shunt revision was the alternative therapy. We present three case histories as examples.

A 74-year-old patient had a third relapse after PTA with a 3-cm stenosis in the venous part of the shunt. A small, sacculated aneurysm was found in the stenosed area. There was a pre-stenotic saccular, partly sclerosed dilatation of the venous segment; the arterial segment was unstenosed. No obstructions were found in the post-stenotic outflow to the central and caval vein. The general condition of the patient was relatively poor. After normal puncture of the artery to visualize vascular conditions, the vein was punctured behind the stenosis and a 9 Fr sheath introduced. The stenosis was dilated in an ascending direction up to 7 mm with a pressure of up to 16 atm, without success. Due to persistent stenosis, the need for stent implantation was diagnosed.

The second case was a 62-year-old female patient who had already had her third post-PTA relapse in the venous shunt segment. The stenosed vascular section was about 2-cm long. The vein could not be palpated sufficiently in the post-stenotic segment. The venous segment available for puncture was only about 4-cm long. The patient was in a good general condition. After visualization by arterial puncture, the post-stenotic vein was punctured in a retrograde direction and a 9 Fr sheath was inserted. Subsequent PTA to a diameter of 8 mm at a pressure of 18 atm was not able to satisfactorily remove the stenosis. Stent implantation was indicated.

The third case was a 69-year-old patient with a short-distance stenosis in the venous shunt segment that had occurred within 8 months of PTA. The segment was about 3-cm long. After puncture in the arterial section to visualize outflow conditions, the post-stenotic section of the venous segment was punctured, and the stenosis was expanded up to 7 mm at pressures of 16 mm Hg by balloon catheters introduced through a sheath. Stent implantation was indicated due to persistent stenosis and the short recurrence-free intervals.

Results

Nitinol endoprosthesis implantation was successful in all shunts. The follow-up was from 6 to 18 months (mean, 12.5 months). In the first of the three cases mentioned above the stent could only be deployed through a 10

Fr Cook sheath. The reason for this was an iatrogenous kinking of the shaft of the prototype deployment set which made it impossible to insert the catheter through the guidewire. No replacement set for the prototype was at hand. After the deployment system was slightly deformed through the manipulations during insertion of the guidewire, we saw no possibility to introduce the set via the 9 Fr sheath without crepitation. In order to avoid future detachment problems we decided to use the 10 Fr sheath which could be fed over the stenosis without any problems. We were then able to coaxially advance the prototype to the stenosed section without a guidewire. The sheath shaft was retracted and the stent was deployed as described above. Unlike the first experimental procedure, subsequent detachment was successful and did not pose any problems. The stent was sufficiently visible under radiopaque control. After compression of the puncture sites, application of a pressure bandage, and initial heparinization, the patients were controlled by long-term therapy with aspirin 300 mg. Punctures in the stent region were unproblematic due to the metal properties of the stent and no thrombosis occurred in this region (Figure 1). In the case of the 62-year-old patient, the stent could be placed via the guidewire through the 9 Fr sheath. Also in this case, the stent was sufficiently visible under x-ray control. No stent dislocation occurred. During deployment set retraction, no interaction occurred between the stent filaments and the deployment set due to the now tapered shape of the backside of the guide rod. Puncture of the stented region by the dialysis needle was no problem. In the third case, stent implantation after PTA through the inserted 9 Fr sheath was also unproblematic and the stent could virtually be deployed under x-ray control.

So far no problems have occurred in the stented region. Stents were not dislocated or misplaced despite known contraction during deployment. Patients did not report any bothersome sensations in the stented region, nor

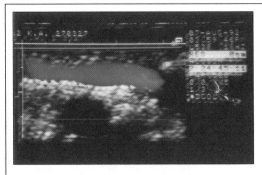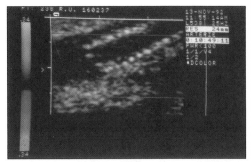

Figure 1. The color ultrasound Doppler shows a good flow in the shunt after implantation of a puncturable nitinol stent. The figures *(left* and *right)* clearly show the filaments as white dots to the sides of the flow lumen.

did the stent puncture cause any unpleasant sensations different from those of normal puncture. The physician or nurse had no problem with puncture of the stented region (Figure 2). The relatively high recidivism rate as compared to other stent types was certainly a negative result that became obvious during follow-up. Eight months post-stenting, for example, 60% of all patients had restenoses in the stent or in another shunt section. No correlation between restenosis and the impossibility or difficulty to puncture the stent area was seen. So far there have been only five cases with an indicated re-PTA in the stented area or a secondary stenosis which, in addition to routine angiography, resulted in a clinically important flow reduction and finally made it impossible to proceed with routine dialysis. In one case with two relapses, we had to place a new shunt after 13 months. In all cases of diagnostic atherectomy, the histologic examination showed a hyperplastic reaction with mesenchymal cells and myxoid degenerations, but also classical cicatrized changes.

DISCUSSION

Stent implantation for treatment of stenoses in dialysis shunts is certainly an interesting alternative to surgical revision. Günther et al (11,12) reported good immediate results but mentioned a considerable number of relapses in the mid- and long-term

follow-up of the Wallstent. We know from our own experiments that the stent significantly contracts after deployment, thus making it difficult to determine the exact position. At the same time, this type of stent cannot be extracted after deployment. In the case of restenosis in the stent a repeated PTA in the stent lumen which led to longer patency of the shunt lumen (12) was the therapy of choice. As a result of the difficulties described above, and due to the problems arising from the shortened puncture site for dialysis after placement of all the stent models known so far, we decided after consultation with our nephrologists to refrain from stent implantation for the time being and to limit our treatment of restenoses to repeated PTA. The further development of the nitinol stent with its outstanding material properties, together with the adoption of the tantalum stent design, led to a prosthesis which, contrary to other models, allows puncture of the shunt volume after implantation in the dialysis shunt without damage to the stent design (Figure 3).

Prior to our clinical study, we performed a series of experiments to verify the repositioning of initial stent filament formation. After finishing these experiments we decided to implant this stent type into the stenosed shunt. One of our primary considerations was to maintain puncturability over as long a period of time as possible. The low number of nitinol stents implanted into the vascular system or the shunt is explained by the relatively

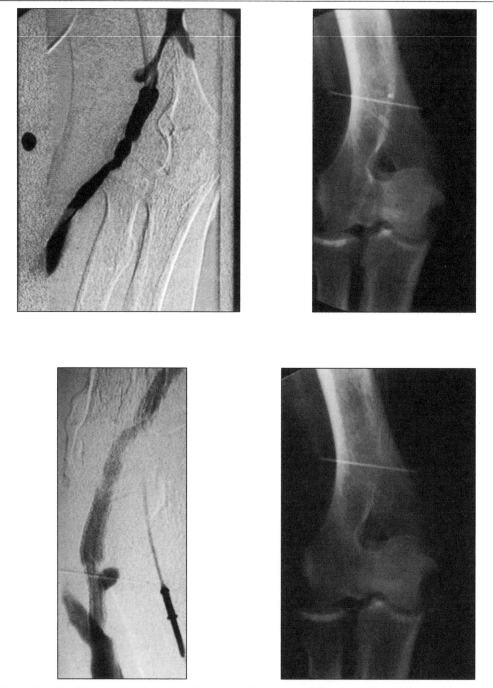

Figure 2. Arteriogram of implantation of a puncturable nitinol stent in a hemodialysis fistula with therapy-resistent restenoses. Intraarterial image of shunt stenoses *(top left)*. The introducer set of the nitinol stent deployment system is visible under the marking *(top right)*. The DSA shows a good flow in the shunt after stent implantation *(bottom left)*. An incomplete thrombosed aneurysm and the not yet completely expanded stent can be seen. The stent, still slightly wasted, can hardly be recognized in the plain picture *(bottom right)*.

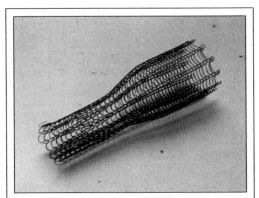

Figure 3. Prototype of a self-expandable nitinol stent with Strecker stent design.

late development of this type of stent which was available to us as a prototype. We were the first worldwide to successfully implant a nitinol stent into the vascular system and dialysis shunt without resulting problems. The problems encountered during experimental applications, such as entanglement of the stent and the backside of the guide rod, were no longer evident due to the new conical design of the reverse side. X-ray representation was surprisingly improved compared to pre-tests. The expansion properties of the stent seem to match very well with the mostly cicatrized, very rigid stenoses which frequently can only be revised under pressures of 18 atm and in many cases result in recidivism when unsplinted.

The fact that the stent, due to the nickel content in the nickel-titanium alloy, should not be applied in patients with a known nickel allergy constitutes a disadvantage (5,13). If a nickel allergy should become evident after implantation, the stent can be extracted using a polyp forceps until about 3 months afterwards. Later, however, a surgical intervention would be required. Unreliable patients who do not comply with their prescribed anticoagulation drugs should not receive an endoprosthesis for risk of thrombosis caused by the thrombogenic material. Furthermore, we have to wait for results concerning mid- and long-term patency rates of the stented shunt sections, as well as for the reaction of the vessel walls in the stented region to the repeated punctures. Based on the results available at this moment, a stenosed shunt section after repeated PTA seems to constitute an indication for stent implantation if a nitinol stent is used that can be percutaneously punctured for dialysis.

REFERENCES

1. Dardik H. Graft materials in vascular surgery. Symp Spec Inc, Miami; 1978.
2. Giessler R. Gefäßrekonstrukitonen. In: Heberer G and van Dongen RJAM, eds. *Gefäßchirurgie*. Berlin: Springer; 1987;73-88.
3. Müller-Wiefel H. Gefäßprothesen. Chirurg 1985;57:64-71.
4. Rühland D, Husemann F. Hämodialyseshunts. In: Heberer G and van Dongen RJAM, eds. *Gefäßchirurgie*. Berlin: Springer; 1987;661-687.
5. Bensmann G, Baumgart F, Haasters J. Osteosyntheseklammern aus Nickel-Titan. Herstellung, Vorversuche und klinisher Einsatz. Techn Mitt Krupp Forsch Ber 1982;40:23-134.
6. Glanz S, Bashist B, Gordon DH, Butt K, Adamsons R. Angiography of upper extremity access fistuale for dialysis. Radiology 1982;143:45-52.
7. Hunter DW, Sos KS, Castaneda-Zuniga WR, Coleman CE, Sutherland DE, Amplatz K. Failing or thrombosed Brescia-Cimino arteriovenous dialysis fistulas: angiographic evaluation and percutaneous transluminal angioplasty. Radiology 1983;149:105-109.
8. Zollikofer CL, Largiader I, Bruhlmann WF, Uhlschmid GK, Marty AH. Endovascular stenting of veins and grafts: preliminary clinical experiences. Radiology 1988;167:701-712.
9. Imparato AM, Bracco A, Kim GE, Zeff R. Intimal and neointimal fibrous proliferation causing failure of arterial reconstructions. Surgery 1972;172:1007-1017.
10. Rittgers SE, Karayannacos PE, Guy JF, et al. Velocity distribution and intimal proliferation in autologous vein grafts in dogs. Circ Res 1978;42:792-801.

11. Günther RW, Vorwerk D, Bohndorf K. Venous stenosis in dialysis shunts: treatment with self-expanding metallic stents. Radiology 1989;170:401-405.

12. Vorwerk D, Günther RW. Perkutane vaskuläre Endoprothesen bei Verschlüssen oder Stenosen von Hämodialyse-Shunts. DMW 1990;115:43-47.

13. Castleman LS, Motzkin SM, Bonawit VL. Biocompatible nitinol alloy as an implant material. J Biomed Mater Res 1976;10:695-731.

Stent Placement in Supraaortic Artery Disease

K. Mathias

Department of Diagnostic Radiology, Teaching Hospital, Dortmund, Germany

Stent placement in supraaortic artery disease has broadened the types of indications for PTA. In addition, it has improved the immediate and probably long-term results and has reduced the complication rate of PTA. Wallstents were implanted in 33 of 410 subclavian, 9 of 34 innominate, and 42 of 305 internal carotid artery obstructions. The PTA result was improved in all 84 stent applications. Two patients developed transient ischemic attacks during carotid stenting. No further complications occurred, although two stents could not be placed in the exact desired position and one end of the stent protruded several millimeters into the aortic arch. No hemodynamically-significant restenosis was seen during the mean follow-up period of 27 months.

MATERIALS AND METHODS

From October 1984 to March 1994, 759 narrowed or occluded supraaortic arteries in 688 patients were treated by percutaneous transluminal angioplasty (PTA). Of these 688 patients, 245 (35.6%) were female and their mean age was 57 years (range, 12 to 86 years).

Six hundred fifty-one (94.6%) patients suffered from atherosclerosis and 18 had recurrent stenosis after carotid desobliteration, 3 of which were at the anastomosis of a bypass graft. Eleven females presented with fibromuscular dysplasia and another three had Takayasu's disease. Post-irradiation stenosis were treated in five patients (Table 1).

Table 1. Etiology of Supraaortic Artery Obstruction

Indication	No. of Patients (%)	
Atherosclerosis	651	(94.6%)
Postoperative Restenosis	18	(2.7%)
Fibromuscular Dysplasia	11	(1.5%)
Post-Irradiation	5	(0.7%)
Takayasu's Disease	3	(0.5%)
TOTAL	688	(100.0%)

After it became commercially available in 1989, we began using the self-expandable Wallstent™ (Medinvent, Lausanne, Switzerland) in selected patients. The diameter of the stents we inserted varied from 6 to 10 mm and the length varied from 3.2 to 5.7 cm. A total of 84 stents were placed in 79 patients. The mean age of these patients did not differ from that of the other patients who were referred to us for supraaortic PTA.

The Wallstent was chosen because of its special properties, including flexibility, which allows for its use in curved or moving artery segments. In addition, its self-expanding capability produces a force against the recoil of the dilated artery that would normally create a larger vessel diameter than with simple balloon dilatation. Ruptured intima and loosened material of the atheroma are pressed to the vessel wall and kept in place. The meshwork of the Wallstent is narrow enough to prevent protrusion of the material between the struts of the stent, thus reducing the risk of embolization.

Placement of the stent was performed using the road mapping technique of digital subtraction angiography. The ostium of the vertebral artery can be exactly located using this technique, thus avoiding an extension of the stent across its offspring. Crossing of the external carotid artery while placing a stent in the internal carotid artery is sometimes necessary. All patients tolerated the crossing of the origin of the external carotid artery without clinical signs.

All patients received at least heparin 5000 IU as well as aspirin 100 mg before, during, and after PTA. A drip infusion of Haes 6%® 1000 mL (dextran) was given within 24 hours of starting the procedure. We recommended an adjuvant treatment with platelet aggregation inhibitors for at least 6 months; 55 of 72 patients (76.4%) complied with this regimen. The other patients stopped taking the medication for various reasons.

INDICATIONS

When sufficient arterial dilatation can be achieved by PTA alone, any additional technique is superfluous, expensive, and accompanied by its own risk. In our opinion, stent placement is useful or necessary under the following conditions:

* Primary stenting, i.e., stenting before PTA, for subclavian and innominate artery occlusion or complex internal carotid artery lesion.
* Secondary stenting, i.e., stenting after PTA, for residual stenosis > 30% after PTA, severe intimal cracking with intimal flaps, or thrombotic material.

Stents are implanted to improve the treatment results when intimal dissection, flaps, or hemodynamically-significant residual stenosis is revealed by angiography after PTA. Stenting is also helpful in overcoming elastic recoil of the arterial wall which might endanger the final treatment results. In the supraaortic territory, stents are especially useful in preventing possible complications of PTA such as embolization or early reocclusion.

RESULTS

The distribution of our 84 implanted stents in the different locations is shown in Table 2. Nineteen stents were implanted in

patients with subclavian artery stenosis in whom we found a residual stenosis of more than 30% after PTA. In all cases the treatment results were improved and even in calcified arteries, a greater diameter of the vessel could be achieved, sometimes with repeated PTA within the stent.

Table 2. Distribution of the Stents in Supraaortic Arteries

Placement Site	No. of Patients (%)
Subclavian Stenosis	19 (22.6%)
Subclavian Occlusion	14 (16.7%)
Innominate Stenosis	3 (3.6%)
Innominate Occlusion	6 (7.1%)
Internal Carotid Stenosis	42 (50.0%)
TOTAL	84 (100.0%)

The necessity to use a stent is much more frequently seen in recanalization of occluded subclavian or innominate arteries (Figure 1). The occluded artery is filled with additional atherosclerotic or thrombotic material which cannot be redistributed by simple balloon angioplasty to create an arterial lumen with sufficient diameter. The risk of embolization in treating these occlusions is not known, but seems to be higher than in simple stenosis. This is another reason why we generously place stents (Figure 2).

Using the road mapping technique, 82 of 84 stents were placed in the planned position. One stent projected from the recanalized innominate artery while another projected from the subclavian artery into the aortic arch. This stent location might be unfavorable concerning the late outcome of the procedure because the free part of the stent will not be covered by endothelium and has to be considered as a possible source of thromboembolism (Figure 3).

Of the 79 patients, 71 returned for regular follow-up examinations and had control procedures performed for an average of 25 months. None of the patients reported neurological events or showed recurrent stenosis

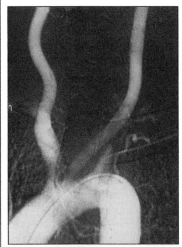

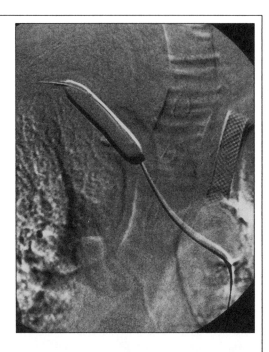

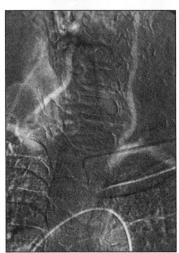

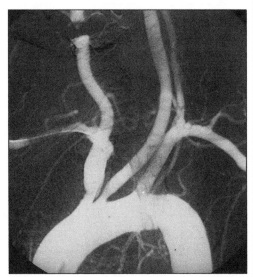

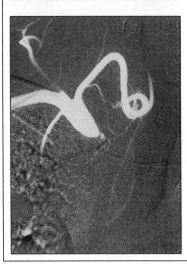

Figure 1. Bilateral subclavian artery occlusion *(top left)*. Retrograde blood flow in both vertebral arteries *(middle left)*. Recanalization and stent placement (arrow heads) of the left subclavian artery *(bottom left)*. Recanalization of the right subclavian artery *(top right)*. Patent subclavian arteries: smooth vessel contour after stenting of the left subclavian artery and good opacification of the left vertebral artery *(bottom right)*.

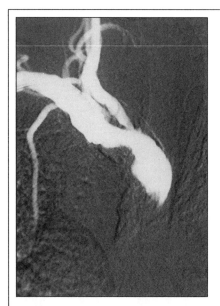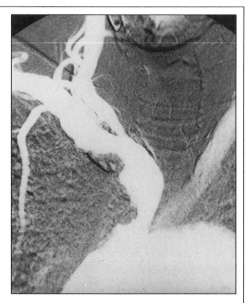

Figure 2. Calcified innominate artery occlusion and ostial stenosis of common carotid artery *(left)*. After stent placement and dilatation within the stent, patent artery with residual stenosis: no pressure gradient at rest *(right)*.

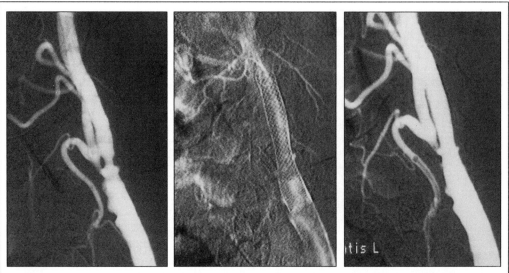

Figure 3. Ulcerative atherosclerosis of the common and internal carotid artery. Ostial stenosis of the external carotid artery *(left)*. Stent placed across the origin of the external carotid artery *(middle)*. Ulceration can still be seen, but the stenosis is removed *(right)*. Thrombus formation in the superior laryngeal artery is apparent.

during that period. Two patients died due to myocardial infarction 9 and 26 months after the procedure, respectively. Duplex ultrasound showed some vessel wall thickening in 23 patients with carotid stents, but no flow pattern typical for recurrent stenoses was registered.

DISCUSSION

Stenting is one of the newer options of percutaneous treatment for occlusive arterial disease and has won broad acceptance in coronary, renal, iliac, and femoropopliteal arteries (1-8). We could only find one report in the literature, however, of stents in the supraaortic territory dealing with subclavian occlusion (9). Normally, stenting is used to repair damage to the arterial wall inflicted by PTA or to prevent immediate restenosis or even reocclusion. In supraaortic arteries, prevention of embolism during PTA is another important argument for stenting. With primary stenting in complex lesions involving 42 carotid arteries, we observed two transient ischemic attacks; no brain infarctions were noted, however.

In general, three stent types are regularly used: the balloon-expandable Palmaz and Strecker stents, and the self-expandable Wallstent. Our experiences with 84 stents in the supraaortic arteries are based solely on the placement of Wallstents which have the advantage that the bloodstream is not interrupted during the grafting procedure. Thus, blood flows through the meshes of the net during stent release. Stenting in the carotid artery is safer with this stent compared to the balloon-expandable stents which require blocking of the artery. The Wallstent does not tend to change its position after grafting. In contrast, the Strecker stent needs overdilatation at its ends for safe anchorage or it might move and even embolize. Its compressibility is a disadvantage because accidental neck compression might lead to a collapse of the stent with acute arterial occlusion. The Palmaz stent is stiffer and does not

have this problem. It may even support the dilatation result in severely calcified lesions better than the Wallstent. Shortening of the Wallstent during expansion makes it necessary to gain experience with this tool to warrant precise positioning of the stent. In addition, better visualization during fluoroscopy is desirable.

The vessel wall reacts to the dilatation injury and the implanted foreign body by the development of intimal hyperplasia (10). In small diameter arteries such as the coronaries, this process will deteriorate the primary treatment result within months requiring additional interventions. In supraaortic arteries which are characterized by a constantly high flow rate and larger diameters of 6 to 10 mm, we have not seen as high a recurrence rate as in the coronary, iliac, and femoropopliteal arteries. Wall thickening as shown by digital subtraction angiography, Duplex scanning, and computed tomography did not exceed 1 to 2 mm. Therefore, intimal hyperplasia does not have the same clinical consequences in the supraaortic arteries as it does in other vascular regions. It is currently unknown, however, how the stented arteries will react to the progression of atherosclerosis.

REFERENCES

1. Haude M, Erbel R, Hafner G, et al. Multicenter Ergebnisse der koroanaren Implantation balloon-expandierbarer Palmaz-Schatz Gefäßstents. Z Kardiol 1993;82:77-86.
2. Hausegger KA, Lammer J, Hagen B, et al. Iliac artery stenting — clinical experience with the Palmaz stent, Wallstent, and Strecker stent. Acta Radiol 1992;33:292-296.
3. Joffre F, Rousseau H, Bernadet P, et al. Midterm results of renal artery stenting. Cardiovasc Intervent Radiol 1992;15:313-318.
4. Liermann D, Strecker EP, Peters J. The Strecker stent: indications and results in iliac and femoropopliteal arteries. Cardiovasc Intervent Radiol 1992;15:298-305.
5. Palmaz JC, Laborde JC, Rivera FJ, Encarnacion CE, Lutz JD, Moss JG. Stenting of the iliac arteries with Palmaz stent: experi-

ence from a multicenter trial. Cardiovasc
Intervent Radiol 1993;15:291-297.

6. Sapoval MR, Long AL, Raynaud AC, Beyssen
    BM, Fiessinger JN, Gaux JC. Femoro-
    popliteal stent placement: long-term results.
    Radiology 1992;184:833-839.

7. Scott NA, Weintraub WS, Carlin SF, et al.
    Recent changes in the management and out-
    come of acute closure after percutaneous
    transluminal coronary angioplasty. Am J
    Cardiol 1993;71:1159-1163.

8. Vorwerk D, Günther RW. Stent placement
    in iliac arterial lesions: three years of clinical

experiences with the Wallstent. Cardiovasc
Intervent Radiol 1992;15:285-290.

9. Mathias KD, Lüth I, Haarmann P.
    Percutaneous transluminal angioplasty of
    proximal subclavian artery occlusions.
    Cardiovasc Intervent Radiol 1993;16:214-218.

10. Carrozza JP, Kuntz RE, Fishman RF, Baim
    DS. Restenosis after arterial injury caused
    by coronary stenting in patients with diabe-
    tes mellitus. Ann Intern Med 1993;118:344-
    349.

Bail-Out Stenting Following Percutaneous Transluminal Coronary Angioplasty

N. Reifart, T. Massa, A. Langer, H. Störger, F. Schwarz, W. Preusler, M. Hofmann

Red Cross Hospital and Heart Center, Frankfurt am Main, Germany

In our practice, stents are implanted mainly as bail-out devices after percutaneous transluminal coronary angioplasty (PTCA) if prolonged inflations fail to seal the dissection. In 164/10,000 consecutive patients (1.6%), a dissection could not be sealed with prolonged balloon inflations (77% with perfusion balloon) and resulted in total (28%) or subtotal occlusion prior to stent implantation. A total of 185 stents (88 Palmaz-Schatz, 97 Strecker) were implanted. All patients were pretreated orally with aspirin and intravenously with heparin 20,000 IU. Before stent implantation patients also received intracoronary aspirin 500 mg, heparin 5000 IU, and dextran 500 cc. After implantation they received between 1000 and 2200 units/hour of heparin which overlapped a 3-month treatment regimen with coumadin, aspirin, and dipyridamole. The results following implantation are shown below.

Outcome	Strecker (N=84)	Palmaz-Schatz (N=80)
Technical Success	97%	95%
Acute Thrombosis (< 24 hours)	11%	12%
Subacute Thrombosis (2-18 days)	8%	14%
Severe Bleeding	15%	9%
Myocardial Infarction	7%	4%
Emergency CABG	8%	4%
Death in Hospital	11%	6%
Restenosis	34%	34%
Reocclusion	13%	7%
Late Death (6-12 months)	5%	3%

Bleeding complications with subsequent stent thrombosis prompted us to surgically repair the puncture site in 39 patients. Severe bleeding, stent thrombosis, and death occurred less often in patients who had elective surgical repair of the puncture site (6%, 3%, 0%) compared to those who received mechanical compression in the groin region (9%, 26%, 6%). In bail-out situations after failed prolonged balloon inflations, there is a high incidence of early thrombotic occlusion. We recommend elective surgical repair of the groin in these patients to facilitate aggressive anticoagulation.

INTRODUCTION

Dissections are frequent after percutaneous transluminal coronary angioplasty (PTCA) (20 to 40%) and are the main cause of severe complications. The availability of perfusion balloons and stents allow for the effective treatment of dissections and abrupt closures. The indication for stenting as a bail-out device varies from early in the course of dissection (10 to 20% of the total PTCA population) to implantation only after prolonged balloon inflations fail to achieve a satisfactory result (less than 2% of the total case load). There is no doubt that restrictive use of stents means negative patient selection. We believe that total complications and costs are less with this latter approach compared to a more liberal therapeutic approach.

MATERIALS AND METHODS

Patients

From January 1990 to December 1992, we performed 10,000 PTCA procedures. Dissections requiring treatment with prolonged balloon inflations occurred in 26% of the patients. In 164/10,000 (1.6%) patients, it was obvious that the abrupt or threatening closure could only be treated by emergency bypass grafting or stenting. Eighty patients received a Palmaz-Schatz™ stent (Johnson & Johnson Interventional Systems Co., Warren NJ) while 84 patients received a Strecker™ stent (Boston Scientific Corp., Denmark) (Table 1).

Methods

In this patient population stents were used as a bail-out device to treat occlusive dissection after repeated prolonged inflations failed. In 77% of patients the use of perfusion balloons did not result in a residual narrowing of less than 75%.

Both the Strecker and Palmaz-Schatz stent were used. The Strecker stent (Figure 1) was preferred for vessels with acute take-off, severe tortuosity, dissection in a bend (Figure 2), or long dissections (> 15 mm); the Palmaz-Schatz stent was preferred in smaller vessels. In contrast to the Palmaz-Schatz stent, the Strecker stent has considerable recoil (10 to 15%) and, therefore, it was necessary to choose catheters with a balloon size 0.5-mm larger than the vessel size and to deploy the stent with at least two inflations of 8 to 10 bar. Two or more stents were implanted when long dissections could not be fully covered with one stent.

Table 1. Clinical Characteristics

	Strecker	Palmaz-Schatz
No. of Patients/Stents	84/97	80/88
Male/Female	65/19	61/19
Mean (± SD) Age (years)	58.9 ± 8	59.4 ± 6
Placement		
Left Anterior Descending	44	50
Circumflex	9	6
Right Coronary Artery	26	24
Graft	13	8
Stent Size		
3.0 mm	18	69
3.5 mm	34	16
4.0 mm	45	3
Indication for Stent Implantation		
Abrupt closure	28%	
Occlusive dissection	62%	
Saphenous vein graft with a residual stenosis > 75% after PTCA	10%	

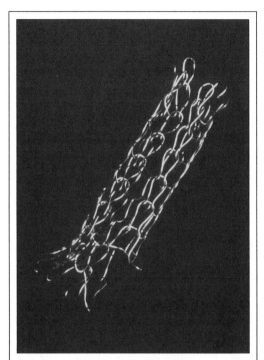

Figure 1. Strecker Stent: Balloon-mounted flexible endoprosthesis of knitted tantalum wires (vertical position).

Our patients were closely watched for 10 to 15 days to guarantee an optimal anticoagulation and to be able to immediately react upon stent thrombosis. To reduce bleeding complications and secondary stent thrombosis due to counter reaction, the last 39 patients with bail-out stenting have had immediate elective surgical repair of the puncture site.

Medication

All PTCA patients received oral aspirin (1000 mg) and heparin 2000 IU via a guiding catheter prior to balloon dilatation. Before stent implantation they further received heparin 5000 IU, intracoronary aspirin 500 mg, and dextran 500 cc (Haes). This medication was followed by intravenous heparin infusion to maintain partial thromboplastin time (PTT) to 3 times normal and activated coagu-

lation time (ACT) at 180-220 seconds, aspirin 1000 mg, and dipyridamole 200 mg daily as well as coumadin. Heparin was reduced by 500 IU/hour daily when the prothrombin time (PT) reached therapeutic levels. Coumadin, aspirin, and dipyridamole were continued for 3 to 4 months.

Management of Acute Stent Thrombosis

Angina at rest or ischemia after stent implantation resulted in immediate recatheterization. In a stent setting thrombosis reopening was tried with a Magnum wire (Schneider, Minneapolis MN) and balloon dilatation. Residual thrombi, if angiographically visible, were lysed with intracoronary infusion of urokinase (250-500,000 units).

Follow-Up

Patients remained hospitalized for 8 to 14 days. A stress test with maximal workload was performed on Day 10. After 4 months all patients were recatheterized except those who died or had doubtless stent thrombosis or coronary artery bypass grafting (CABG).

RESULTS

Results and inhospital complications are summarized in Table 2. Both types of stents were implanted with a high success rate. Some vessels receiving a Strecker stent were obviously not suitable for the Palmaz-Schatz stent because of marked tortuosity, acute take-off, or sharp bends. In one patient with failure to place a Palmaz-Schatz stent, a Strecker stent could be deployed successfully. Acute thrombosis (symptomatic stent occlusion within 24 hours) and subacute thrombosis (stent occlusion after 24 hours during hospital stay) occurred in 19 and 26% of the patients in the Strecker and Palmaz-Schatz stent groups, respectively. In all patients with acute occlusions, the anticoagulation was within the therapeutic range. In five patients with subacute occlusion, the event could have been caused by insufficient levels of anticoagulation. One

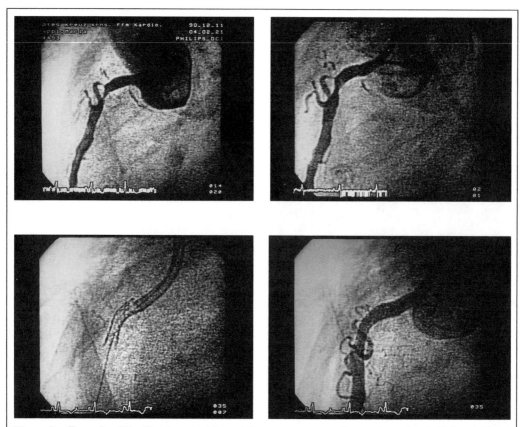

Figure 2. Example of the Strecker stent in a right coronary artery dissected at a bend. Before balloon angioplasty *(top left)*. After balloon angioplasty *(top right)*. Strecker stent *(bottom left)*. Final result with 20% recoil at the stent site *(bottom right)*.

Table 2. Inhospital Results

Outcome	Strecker (N=84)	Palmaz-Schatz (N=80)
Technical Success	97%	95%
Acute Thrombosis (< 24 hours)	11%	12%
Subacute Thrombosis (Day 2 to 12)	8%	14%
Reopened	14/16	17/21
Emergency CABG	8%	4%
Myocardial Infarction	7%	4%
Severe Bleeding	15%	9%
Early Death	11%	6%

patient received blood transfusions because of severe gastrointestinal bleeding, while four patients received transfusions and were operated on because of severe inguinal bleeding.

Reopening with a Magnum wire and balloon catheterization was successfully attempted in 31/37 patients with acute or subacute occlusion. In 10 of these patients, intracoronary urokinase infusion (250-500,000 units) was administered to desolve residual thrombus. Two patients in the Strecker group and four patients in the Palmaz-Schatz group died before re-PTCA could be attempted. One patient in each group died because of recurrent stent thrombosis (Figure 3).

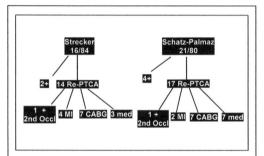

Figure 3.   Outcome of acute and subacute stent thrombosis.

Severe bleeding at the puncture site was a result of the aggressive anticoagulation regimen: eight patients in the Strecker group and seven in the Palmaz-Schatz group needed surgical repair of the groin. The rigorous anticoagulation regimen is substantiated by six deaths (all in the Strecker group). Three patients died because of gastrointestinal bleeding with eventual stent thrombosis: one due to cerebral bleeding, and the other two because of hemopericardium, despite therapeutic levels of PTT and PT. Bleeding complications with subsequent stent thrombosis resulted in our switching from groin compression to surgical repair of the puncture site immediately after stenting in the final 39 patients in this series. Table 3 shows a comparison of the patients with conventional protocol (sheath removal after 6 to 8 hours when ACT reached 200-220 seconds, manual groin compression followed by mechanical compression with a C-clamp or Femostop) and of the patients who had surgical closure of the puncture site. This more recent strategy dramatically decreased the incidence of stent thrombosis and death, most likely because the anticoagulation regimen was not interrupted (for sheath removal) and facilitated during the first days.

Table 3.	Comparison of Results in Patients with Conventional Groin Management and Those with Elective Surgical Closure of Puncture Site after Sheath Removal	
Outcome	Compression (N=80)	Surgical Repair (N=39)
Acute Thrombosis	12%	0%
Subacute Thrombosis	14%	3%
Q-Myocardial Infarction	4%	3%
Emergency CABG	4%	9%
Elective CABG	20%	18%
Inhospital Death	6%	0%
Severe Bleeding	9%	6%
Mean Hospital Stay (days)	13 ± 5	11 ± 4

Follow-Up

Four months of follow-up data were available for all 164 patients. Four patients with a Strecker stent and two patients with a Palmaz-Schatz stent died during this time (Table 4). The cause of late deaths were: ventricular fibrillation (N=1), cardiogenic shock (Strecker) (N=2), reinfarction (Palmaz-Schatz) (N=1), bypass thrombosis (N=1) and low output syndrome (N=1). Forty-seven patients in the Strecker group and 44 in the Palmaz-Schatz group were angiographically restudied after 4 months. Of the 73 patients who were not recatheterized, 22 had previously documented stent thrombosis, and/or CABG (N=42) and/or died (N=20). Angiographically documented recurrence occurred in 47% of the Strecker patients and in 41% of the Palmaz-Schatz patients (Table 4).

Table 4. Four-Month Follow-Up Results

Outcome	Strecker (N=84)	Palmaz-Schatz (N=80)
Death	5%	3%
Restenosis	34%	34%
Reocclusion	13%	7%

DISCUSSION

Stents are widely used to prevent restenosis, to improve an unsatisfactory PTCA result, and for bail-out situations. Elective stent implantation is associated with a favorable outcome with less than 5% of the patients experiencing stent thrombosis (1,2). The same results may be achieved with liberal stenting of unfavorable PTCA results, such as dissections which have not been treated with prolonged balloon inflations.

If bail-out stenting is only restricted to patients with failed prolonged inflations, however, high complication rates as compared with elective implantation are a consistent observation (3-5) and appear to be independent of the stent model used. Our strategy in occlusive dissections is to apply prolonged inflations before stenting. This is successful in 75% of the patients (residual stenosis ≤50%, no major complications during hospital course) (6). The patients in whom prolonged inflations fail have a severely damaged vessel wall which may represent an unfavorable situation for coronary stenting. This might be a major reason that acute and subacute stent thrombosis occurs in 20 to 30% of the cases (3). On the other hand, earlier use of stents in patients with unfavorable PTCA results would increase the implantation rate from 1.6% to approximately 15%. This would considerably increase procedural costs without a significant change in the overall complication rate, i.e., out of 1,000 PTCA cases and 1.6% bail-out stent procedures, four patients (25%) might experience stent thrombosis. With a more liberal implantation rate of 10% (100 patients), a subacute stent thrombosis of 4% indicates four patients as well.

Elective surgical closure of the puncture site enabled us to anticoagulate patients more aggressively and thus, consecutively reduce stent thrombosis and mortality, even in this high risk subgroup. Therefore, we recommend this strategy after bail-out stenting, especially following prolonged inflations. This appears to obviate the need for preventive bypass surgery after bail-out stenting.

CONCLUSIONS

Stent thrombosis occurs more often in bail-out situations than after elective stenting with both the Strecker and Palmaz-Schatz stents. Both stent thrombosis and mortality can be reduced if the puncture site is surgically closed at the time of sheath removal. Randomized trials are necessary to compare the different strategies for bail-out situations (i.e., perfusion balloon versus stenting).

REFERENCES

1. Schatz RA, Baim DS, Leon M, et al. Clinical experience with the Palmaz-Schatz coronary stent. Circulation 1991;83:148-161.

2. Kimura T, Nosaka H, Yokoi H, Hamasaki N, Nobuyoshi M. Initial clinical experience with Strecker coronary stent (abstr). J Am Coll Cardiol 1992;19:198A.
3. Fajadet J, Jenny D, Guabliumi G, et al. Immediate and late outcome of bail-out coronary stenting (abstr). J Am Coll Cardiol 1992;19:109A.
4. Herrmann HC, Hirshfeld JW, Buchbinder M, et al. Emergent coronary stenting for failed PTCA (abstr). Circulation 1991;84:II-590.
5. Carrozzo JP, Kuntz RE, Levine MJ, et al. Angiographic and clinical outcome of intracoronary stenting: immediate and long-term results from a large single-center experience. J Am Coll Cardiol 1992;20:328-337.
6. Reifart N, Langer A, Preusler W, Hofmann M, Störger H, Schwarz F: Drohender Verschluß nach PTCA: perfusionsballon oder Stent? Z Kardiol 1992;81:108.

RECOMMENDED READING

Hamm CW, Beythien C, Sievert H, et al. Management of acute coronary occlusions after angioplasty with the Strecker tantalum stent. Submitted for publication.

Rabenseifner I, Küsswetter W, Wünsch PH, Schwab M. 1st die Knochenbruchheilung bei den gewebeverträglichen Implantatwerkstoffen Tantal und Niob gegenüber Stahlimplantaten verändert? Z Orthop 1984;122:349-355.

Reifart N, Kupka J, Störger H, Preusler W, Schwarz F. Akuter Gefäßverschluß durch perkutane transluminale Koronarangioplastie: früh- und Spätergebnisse der Re-PTCA. Z Kardiol 1991;80:317-321.

Reifart N, Langer A, Störger H, Schwarz F, Preusler W, Hofmann M. Strecker stent as a bail-out device following percutaneous transluminal coronary angioplasty. J Intervent Cardiol 1992;5:79-83.

Sawyer PN, Stanczewski B, Srinivasan S, Stempak JG, Kammlott GW. Electron microscopy and physical chemistry of healing in prosthetic heart valves, skirts and struts. J Thorac Cardiovasc Surg 1974;67:25-43.

Strecker EP, Liermann D, Barth KH, et al. Expandable tubular stents for treatment of arterial occlusive diseases: experimental and clinical results. Radiology 1990;175:97-102.

von Holst H, Collins P, Steiner L. Titanium, silver, and tantalum clips in brain tissue. Acta Neurochir 1981;56:239-242.

Current Clinical and Technical Status
of the Gianturco-Roubin Flex Stent

Michael Parks and Gary S. Roubin

Departments of Medicine and Radiology, University of Alabama,
Birmingham, AL USA

Recent developments in the field of interventional cardiology have resulted in a variety of newer devices, allowing the cardiologist to approach much more difficult lesions than previously possible. Despite this explosion in technology, the incidence of acute and threatened closure remains fixed at approximately 10 to 15%. For this reason, the Gianturco-Roubin Flex stent was developed. A multicenter trial concluded in September, 1992 demonstrated a significant reduction in the incidences of myocardial infarction, CABG, and death among patients stented for acute and threatened closure. As our experience has grown, the incidences of stent-related complications have dramatically decreased such that stent thrombosis currently occurs in only about 1 to 2% of patients, and a bleeding rate of less than 5% is expected.

INTRODUCTION

Since its introduction by Andreas Gruentzig, percutaneous transluminal coronary angioplasty (PTCA) has become the predominant method of coronary revascularization in the world today. It is estimated that in 1992, 350,000 procedures were performed in the United States alone. Despite this wide acceptance, PTCA remains limited by the occurrence of restenosis and acute closure. The incidence of restenosis (30 to 40%) has remained essentially unchanged despite the development of second generation devices (DVI, rotobladder, TEC, eximer laser). However, the incidence of acute closure and the need for emergent bypass surgery have been significantly reduced by the recent approval of the Gianturco-Roubin™ Flex stent (Cook, Bloomington IN). This stent, initially designed by Cesare Gianturco and modified in collaboration with Gary Roubin, was first placed in human subjects in 1987. In the Fall of 1988, the multicenter trial investigating the use of the Flex stent was begun. In the Spring of 1992, data were presented to a Food and Drug Administration (FDA) Scientific Advisory Board and the product was approved for marketing in the United States in May, 1993. Since its introduction, approximately 10,000 Gianturco-Roubin Flex stents have been placed worldwide (personal communication). Over the same period, one would expect approximately 13,500 episodes of acute closure in the United States (5% incidence of closure x 30,000 PTCA's per month). This report will update the technical and clinical data currently available on the Gianturco-Roubin Flex stent and will outline future trends in the rapidly expanding use of this endoprosthesis.

MATERIALS AND METHODS

The Gianturco-Roubin Flex stent is composed of a single continuous strand of six-thousandths-of-an-inch surgical grade stainless steel. The wire is folded back and forth to form a series of loops, which are then wrapped around a compliant balloon catheter to form a cylinder or tube of interdigitating loops. To simplify deployment, there is no covering sheath. The compliant balloon upon which the stent is mounted behaves in a rather unique way when deployed within atherosclerotic coronary arteries. At low pressures, it is essentially constrained by the diameter of the artery and/or those geometric dimensions determined by the prior dilatations with the standard angioplasty balloon. High pressures are inappropriate with this compliant balloon because, at higher pressures, it may expand over time and result in distal dissection. This balloon, however, is ideal for ensuring the stability of the stent during its passage into position in the coronary artery.

Stent Compatible Equipment

The placement of the Gianturco-Roubin Flex stent is straightforward. There are general guidelines, however, which during the multicenter trial resulted in a marked improvement in successful deployment. Primary among these is the choice of stent compatible equipment. Both the guide catheter and guidewire should allow for maximal "backup" support. In addition, the inner diameter of the guide catheters have to be sufficiently large to allow for passage of the stent and enough dye to visualize the coronary (Table 1). The large lumen 8 Fr Cook Lumax guide (ID = 0.086-inch) will permit the passage of all stent sizes (2 to 4 mm). The 9 Fr guides listed also provide excellent support and permit the placement of all stent sizes. A variety of extra-support wires are available (Table 2) and, in 0.016- and 0.018-inch diameters, provide excellent support.

Stent Sizing

The correct use of the Gianturco-Roubin Flex stent involves choosing a stent of a nominal size that is slightly larger than the reference diameter of the vessel to be stented. The stent should then be deployed at the lowest possible pressure at which it is completely expanded (usually between 3 and 4 atm). It is important to realize that it takes somewhat longer to deploy at pressures of 3 to 4 atm. This means that in vessels of 2.6 to 3.0 mm in diameter, a 3.0 mm stent should be

utilized. Similarly, for vessels 3.1 to 3.5 mm in diameter or 3.6 to 4.0 mm in diameter, 3.5 and 4.0 mm stents are appropriate, respectively. Intracoronary ultrasound has demonstrated that following successful deployment, dilation within the stent at high pressures (14 to 20 atm) with a non-compliant balloon results in optimal apposition of the stent struts against the vessel wall (1) (Figures 1 and 2). For this reason, we feel that optimal sizing of the balloon is best done after ultrasound interrogation of the artery. We recommend the sheath CVIS 2.9 Fr device. Care should be taken not to over-inflate the vessel immediately distal to the stent.

Adjunctive Pharmacology

All patients undergoing PTCA and who are a candidate for stent placement must receive soluble aspirin 325 mg and persantine 75 mg. When the decision to proceed with stenting occurs, the patient should be given intravenous Solu-Medrol® (125 mg) followed

Table 1. Stent Compatible Guide Catheters[a]

Manufacturer	French	ID
Cook (Lumax)	8	0.086-inch
USCI (Super 9)	9	0.089-inch
Schneider (Soft Tip)	9	0.089-inch
Medtronic (Giant Lumen)	9	0.089-inch

[a] All allow for the passage of 2.0- to 4.0-mm stents.

Table 2. Extra-Support Guidewires

Product Name	Manufacturer	Diameter
Roadrunner	Cook	0.018-inch
Hi-Torque Floppy II	ACS	0.018-inch
Hi-per Flex	USCI	0.016-inch
Flex	USCI	0.017-inch
Ultra Select Nitinol	Microvena	0.016-inch
Reflex	Cordis	0.018-inch
Entre	Scimed	0.018-inch

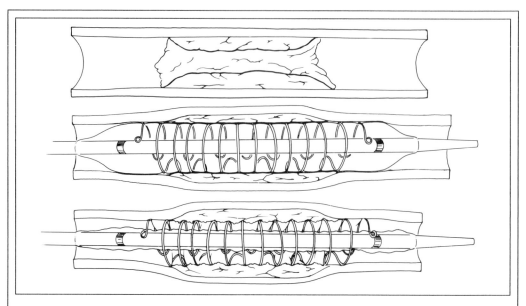

Figure 1. Atherosclerotic lesion following balloon dilation demonstrating a suboptimal result (*top*). Deployment of Gianturco-Roubin Flex stent at a low pressure (3 to 4 atm) (*middle*). Following successful deployment, the balloon is deflated and removed slowly (*bottom*).

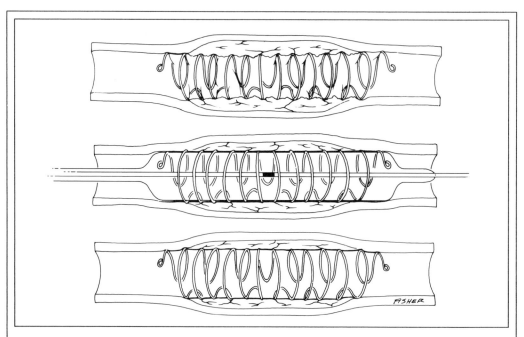

Figure 2. Following deployment, incomplete expansion of the stent coils with significant residual stenosis (*top*). A non-compliant balloon is placed within the stent and the stent dilated to high pressures (14 to 20 atm) (*middle*). Final result demonstrating complete stent coil expansion and no residual stenosis (*bottom*).

by dextran (10%). Dextran should be bolused (about 250 cc), then the infusion should be reduced to 50 cc/hour. Routine intravenous heparin is given and activated coagulation time (ACT) measured every 30 minutes to assure that it remains above 300 seconds. Following successful placement, the sheaths are pulled when the ACT drops below 150 seconds; the dextran infusion continues during this period. Two hours after achieving hemostasis, heparin 1000 IU/hour is begun (without a bolus) and dextran is continued until the partial thromboplastin time (PTT) is > 55 seconds. Coumadin is begun on the day of the procedure and heparin is continued until the INR is between 3 and 4. Patients should not be allowed to get out of bed until the second post-stenting day to minimize the incidence of groin bleeding. Recently, protocols using 48 hours of heparin followed by subcutaneous heparin (PTT 45 to 55 seconds) or a low-molecular weight heparin (Lovenox, 30 mg SQ bid) have begun. In addition, protocols utilizing antiplatelet therapy alone (aspirin and Ticlid®) in patients undergoing IVUS-guided stent placement are beginning.

RESULTS

Multicenter Trial in Acute or Threatened Closure

This study occurred from September, 1988 to September, 1992 and included 973 pa-

tients. Indications for stent placement were acute closure (32%) and threatened closure (68%). A total of 1099 stents were placed, with successful deployment occurring in 94.3%. Of particular note, the most common stent size was the 3.0 mm stent. Using our current sizing strategy, the most common stent sizes are 3.5 and 4.0 mm. When compared to historic controls (NHLBI registry) for outcomes in patients with acute closure (Table 3), the stent resulted in a significant decrease in myocardial infarction, coronary artery bypass grafting (CABG), and death.

Clinical Experience in Treating Acute Closure

The initial University of Alabama (UAB) experience (2) included 115 patients undergoing intracoronary stents for acute or threatened closure (8.8% of total patients undergoing PTCA). For the purposes of this study, threatened closure was defined as the presence of two or more of the following four criteria: a residual stenosis of $\geq$ 50%; TIMI grade 2 flow; a significant dissection (> 15 mm); and evidence of clinical ischemia (either typical angina or ECG changes). Twelve patients (10%) met the criteria for acute closure, 87 vessels (73%) satisfied the criteria for threatened closure, and 20 vessels (17%) had only one criteria for threatened closure. The Gianturco-Roubin Flex stent was successfully deployed in 97% of patients. Overall, in-hospital mortality was 1.7% and

Table 3. Incidence of MI, CABG, and Death in Multicenter Registry Following Stent Implantation Compared to 1985-1986 NHLBI Registry

| | Multicenter Registry Results | | 1985-1986 NHLBI Registry | |
	In-hospital	After 6 months	In-hospital	After 6 months
MI	6.7%	1.6%	42.0%	0.0%
CABG	8.4%	7.6%	40.2%	5.8%
Death	2.6%	1.2%	5.0%	2.0%

[a] The difference was significant with respect to MI and CABG. The difference in the incidence of death was not statistically significant between the two groups.

KEY: MI = myocardial infarction; CABG = coronary artery bypass grafting

CABG was required in 4.2% of patients. Q-wave myocardial infarction occurred in 7% and non-Q myocardial infarction was evident in 9%. Stent thrombosis occurred in nine patients (7.6%).

A more recent review of the UAB experience included 240 consecutive stenting procedures (44 for acute closure; 196 for threatened closure) (3). Patients were divided into three groups based on the presence of 0, 1, or 2 to 3 predictors of stent thrombosis (stent diameter < 3.0 mm; presence of residual dissection; presence of residual filling defect). In 92 patients who had none of the three predictors, stent thrombosis occurred in 1% compared to 8% of those who had one of the predictive factors and 28% of those who had two or three predictors present. The group having no predictors of stent thrombosis also had a lower rate of late myocardial infarction and repeat PTCA.

Prevention of Restenosis

The first prospective randomized trial to examine the ability of the Gianturco-Roubin Flex stent to reduce restenosis in PTCA has demonstrated that the stent is extremely effective in improving late results in selected patients (4). The patient population selected in this study included 69 patients who, on angiography 24 hours after routine PTCA, demonstrated a 10% or greater increase in diameter narrowing and/or a 0.3-mm loss in the minimum lumen diameter. These parameters have been shown in previous studies to be associated with a restenosis rate of 60 to 79%. Of the 69 patients, three were excluded because the vessels were not suitable for stenting. The remaining 66 patients were randomized to receive either a Gianturco-Roubin Flex stent or continued standard medical therapy. The two groups were well-matched with respect to age, gender, and the presence of coronary risk factors. All patients in the study were classified as having unstable angina and 15% had a prior myocardial infarction. There were no complications in the medically-treated group, but three patients had subacute closure in the stent group and one patient experienced Q-wave myocardial infarction. At the follow-up angiography, the mean diameter in the control group was 63% compared to 23% in the stented group (p < 0.0001). Using a binary definition of restenosis (> 50% diameter narrowing), the restenosis rate was 21% in the stent group and 76% in the control group (p < 0.01).

DISCUSSION

In its brief history, the Gianturco-Roubin Flex stent appears to favorably alter the natural history of acute and threatened closure as demonstrated by the multicenter registry. The data presented in this registry represents the earliest experience with this device and incorporates the learning curves of all participating centers. The incidence of complications following stent placement decreased dramatically during the course of the registry and was inversely related to the number of cases performed at the institution. The more recent UAB experience demonstrates that the learning curve is continuing. We now expect, with proper stent placement and care, an approximate 1% subacute thrombosis rate and a less than 5% significant bleeding rate.

During these earlier studies, restenosis appeared to be reduced in a subset of patients. These preliminary observations led to the Rodriguez trial (4) which is the first prospective, randomized trial comparing conventional therapy to elective stenting. In this selected group of patients, the incidence of restenosis was markedly reduced by the elective placement of a Gianturco-Roubin Flex stent. As impressive as these data are, many of the stents during this trial would be considered to be undersized by our current stent sizing strategy. It is our hope that this newer strategy will not only decrease the complications of stent thrombosis but will result in a "bigger" lumen and perhaps even a lower restenosis rate.

Finally, the current approved stent represents 1985 technology (as mandated by the FDA). Newer stents made of tantalum which may be less thrombogenic, and newer prototypes, lower in profile and capable of being deployed up to 6 mm, are currently under study. In addition, a unique polymer coating has been developed, allowing for the coupling of drugs to this stent. Studies involving methotrexate demonstrated significant local concentration of drug 3 weeks after stent deployment (5). While no effective drug has been identified, the ability to use a stent as a method of drug delivery, allowing for inhibition of both elastic recoil and smooth muscle cell proliferation, is an exciting possibility.

CONCLUSION

Since its introduction, the Gianturco-Roubin Flex stent has established itself as the mainstay in the treatment of threatened and acute closure complicating PTCA. Recent randomized trials also have demonstrated that, in a subset of patients, elective placement of the Gianturco-Roubin Flex stent markedly reduces restenosis. With these data available, the need for a large multicenter, randomized trial using the elective placement of the Gianturco-Roubin Flex stent to reduce the incidence of restenosis is planned.

REFERENCES

1. Ho D, Roubin GS. Sizing of the Gianturco-Roubin coronary Flex stent. Submitted.
2. Roubin GS, Cannon AD, Agrawal SK, et al. Intracoronary stenting for acute and threatened closure complicating percutaneous transluminal coronary angioplasty. Circulation 1992;85:916-927.
3. Liu MW, Agrawal SK, Cannon AD, et al. Is coronary stenting for acute or threatened closure a temporary bail-out device or definitive therapy (abstr.). J Am Coll Cardiol 1993;21:177A.
4. Rodriguez A, Santaera O, Larribau M, et al. Rational use of coronary stenting to prevent restenosis: A randomized study in lesions with early minimal luminal diameter loss after PTCA (abstr.). J Am Coll Cardiol 1994;22:118A.
5. Cox DA, Anderson PG, Roubin GS, Chou CY, Agrawal SK, Cavender JB. Effect of local delivery of heparin and methotrexate on neointimal proliferation in stented porcine coronary arteries. Coronary Artery Dis 1992;3:237-248.

Clinical Results and Long-Term Patency of Renal Artery Stenting with the Wallstent Endoprosthesis

Hervé P. Rousseau[1], Laurent M. Hennequin[2], Francis G. Joffre[1]

[1]Department of Radiology, C.H.U. Toulouse Rangueil, Toulouse, France
[2]Department of Radiology, C.H.U. Nancy-Hôpital Central, France

To evaluate the long-term patency and clinical success of renal artery stenting, 27 Wallstent endoprostheses were placed in 22 patients during 25 procedures to treat inadequate immediate post-angioplasty response (N=8) or delayed restenosis after previous balloon angioplasty (N=14). All patients had hypertension. The stenosis was atheromatous in 16 patients, involving the ostium in 8 cases. The kidney was solitary in five patients. Due to misplacement of the first stent, five patients had two stents; technical success was achieved in all patients (correct stent implantation, covering the lesion without residual stenosis). Early benign complications occurred in four patients. At the end of the angiographic follow-up period (12 to 60 months), four patients (20%) had restenosis within the stent. The cumulative patency rate (Kaplan-Meier) was 95% at 7 months, 86% at 9 months, and 78% at 15 months. The secondary patency rate was 92% at 15 months. At the clinical follow-up (12 to 60 months), hypertension was cured in 3 patients and improved in the other 19. Renal artery stenting has good clinical results and a high patency rate in long-term follow-up. It is beneficial in many patients with poor results from conventional renal angioplasty, especially in ostial lesions.

INTRODUCTION

Technical and clinical success rates of percutaneous transluminal renal angioplasty (PTRA) are similar to those of surgery (1,2). PTRA is a well-accepted alternative method for treating renal artery stenosis as an initial therapy, both for management of renovascular hypertension and for improvement or stabilization of renal function (3). Limitations of PTRA include initial failure, occluding dissection, and short- or mid-term restenosis. Poor results are especially expected in atheromatous ostial lesions (4-7).

Endovascular stenting has been proposed and tested as an endovascular mechanical support that can be introduced percutaneously to compensate or to prevent the limitations of PTA. A stent is an effective means of providing non-operative management of flow-compromising PTA-induced dissection (8) and vessel reclosure during PTA. Stent placement has been proposed for treating delaying post-PTA restenosis (9,10) and for reducing the likelihood of a second restenosis. The long-term patency of the stents in the renal artery, however, is not yet known. We report our experience with the placement of 27 stents in 22 patients, with a mean angiographic follow-up period of 28 ± 15 months.

MATERIALS AND METHODS

Study Group

Stenoses were located in 20 renal arteries (11 on the right, 9 on the left), in one renal transplant artery, and in one aortorenal by-pass graft in 22 patients (11 male, 11 female) aged 27 to 74 years (mean, 55 ± 11 years).

The clinical indication for PTRA was hypertension for all patients and was presumedly of renovascular origin in 16 patients. In seven patients, preservation of the renal vasculature and nephronic protection was also indicated. Six patients had renal failure. No patient had diabetes mellitus.

The lesions were on the main renal artery in all patients, with no accessory renal artery on the same side. In five patients, the lesions were located on a solitary kidney. The cause of renal artery stenosis was atheromatosis in 16 patients (including the ostium in 8 patients), fibromuscular dysplasia in 3 patients, and Takayasu arteritis, renal transplant stenosis, and aortorenal bypass stenosis in 1 patient each.

The indication for stent placement was an immediate inadequate post-angioplasty response (N=8) or delayed restenosis after previous angioplasty (N=14). Among the 14 patients with restenosis, the stent was implanted in six despite an immediate positive result from a redilation, because of a supposed risk of a second restenosis.

Stent Placement Technique

A Wallstent™ endoprosthesis (Medinvent, Lausanne, Switzerland) was used in all patients. The stent diameter was 7 mm (N=7), 6 mm (N=12), or 5 mm (N=8) and was 10 to 15% greater than that of the balloon used for the preceding dilation of the lesion. Stent length was 20 to 30 mm.

All procedures were performed under local anaesthesia through a 7 Fr sheath via the femoral artery (N=21) or the left axillary artery (N=1). A 0.020-inch, 4-cm long soft tipped guidewire was used. Conventional balloon dilation was first performed in every case after injection of heparin 5000 IU and calcium channel blockers. Manometric and angiographic controls were performed in order to quantify the efficacy of the dilation.

The Wallstent delivery catheter was deployed over the guidewire in the renal artery by retraction of the doubled-over rolling membrane as previously described (11). In cases of ostial stenosis a catheter introduced via the contralateral femoral artery was used for control of the exact position of the ostium. Angiography of the final stent placement and

manometric control were then performed with the guidewire in the renal artery, allowing for additional dilation or a second stent if necessary.

Heparinization was maintained for 24 hours. Aspirin (250 mg/day) was prescribed the day before the procedure and for a minimum of 6 months. Additional oral anticoagulation therapy was given in the first 12 patients for 2 months.

Follow-Up Examinations

All patients underwent continual follow-up examinations. Clinical and angiographic follow-ups included general status; 24-hour monitoring of arterial blood pressure, drug regimen, and serum creatinine levels; and renal angiography. Follow-up angiograms were planned at 1, 6, and 12 months, and yearly thereafter. Intraarterial angiography at 1 year was performed in all but one patient.

The criteria used to determine cure or improvement of hypertension were those used by the Society of Cardiovascular and Interventional Radiology (12). Survival curves were generated according to the Kaplan-Meier method. Cumulative patency rates were indicated using product-limit estimation analysis, and graphically presented following recommendations of the Ad Hoc Committee on Reporting Standards from the Society for Vascular Surgery (13).

RESULTS

General clinical and angiographical data are presented in Table 1.

Technical Results

Twenty-seven stents were implanted in 22 patients during 25 procedures. Immediate correct placement without residual stenosis was obtained in 17 patients, with a slight protrusion into the aorta of about 2 mm in 2 patients.

Table 1. Clinical Data and General Results

Pt No./ Age/Sex	Renal Failure	Solitary Kidney	Nature of Stenosis	Indication	No. Stents	Stent Diameter (mm)	Clinical Follow-up (Months)	Angiographic Follow-up (Months)	Restenosis/ Redilatation	Late Anastomotic Result	Clinical Hypertensive Result	Renal Failure Result
1/46/M	No	No	ARB	IMM	1	5	15	14	+	+	I	
2/41/F	Yes	No	ATH OST	RESTEN -	2	5	60	12	+	+	I	F
3/87/F	Yes	Yes	ATH	RESTEN -	1	6	50	48	+	+	I	U
4/39/F	No	No	FMD	RESTEN +	1	5	48	46	+	+	C	
5/30/F	No	No	FMD	IMM	2	6	60	60	+	+	C	
6/47/F	No	No	TAKA	RESTEN -	1	6	48	48	+	+	I	
7/59/M	No	No	ATH	RESTEN +	1	7	37	36	+7M/+29M	+	I	
8/51/M	Yes	Yes	ATH	IMM	1	6	13	13	+	+	I	I
9/12/F	No	No	ATH	RESTEN -	1	5	14	14	+	+	I	
10/83/F	No	No	ATH OST	RESTEN +	2	6	39	14	+	+	I	
11/74/M	Yes	Yes	ATH OST	IMM	1	5	45	45	+	+	I	U
12/51/M	No	No	ATH	RESTEN +	1	7	32	32	+	+	C	
13/31/M	No	No	ATH	RESTEN -	1	7	25	23	+	+	I	
14/50/F	No	No	ATH OST	RESTEN +	1	6	30	30	+9 & 15M/ +12 & 22M	+	I	
15/46/M	No	No	ATH	IMM	1	6	40	40	+	+	I	
16/27/M	Yes	Yes	RT	RESTEN +	1	5	39	39	+	+	I	U
17/67/M	No	No	ATH OST	RESTEN -	1	6	20	28	+	+	I	
18/61/F	No	No	ATH OST	IMM	1	6	19	19	+15M/-	-	I	
19/50/M	No	No	ATH OST	RESTEN -	1	6	16	16	+9M/+16M	+	I	

Table 1 (Cont). Clinical Data and General Results

Pt No./ Age/Sex	Renal Failure	Solitary Kidney	Nature of Stenosis	Indication	No. Stents	Stent Diameter (mm)	Clinical Follow-up (Months)	Angiographic Follow-up (Months)	Restenosis/ Redilation	Late Anastomotic Result	Clinical Hypertensive Result	Renal Failure Result
20/56/F	No	Yes	FMD	IMM	1	6	12	12	+	+	I	
21/67/M	Yes	No	ATH	IMM	2	7	12	0	+	+	I	F
22/56/F	No	No	ATH	RESTEN -	2	7	12	12	+	+	I	

KEY:

Nature of Stenosis: ARB = aortorenal bypass graft; ATH = atheromatous lesion; OST = ostial lesion; FMD = fibromuscular dysplasia; TAKA = Takayasu arteries; RT = renal transplant.

Indication for Stenting: IMM = immediate post-PTRA poor result; RESTEN = delayed restenosis after previous PTRA; RESTEN + = good result obtained from redilatation; RESTEN - = poor result obtained from redilatation.

Restenosis: + = delay in months (M); if redilatation within the stent, date in months (M)

Late Anatomic Result: Final angiographic aspect; + = no stenosis; - = stenosis within the stent and the renal artery.

Clinical Hypertensive Result: C = cured; I = improved.

The stent was placed too distally and did not cover the lesion in five latter patients with ostial or very proximal stenosis which required placement of a second stent during the same procedure (N=2) or respectively at 2, 3, and 3 months (N=3).

Complications

No acute stent occlusion occurred. The following early complications occurred in four patients:

- Distal cruoric embolism, treated by local infusion of streptokinase.
- Renal hilar hemorrhage, requiring no specific treatment or transfusion.
- Acute deterioration of renal status, supposedly due to cholesterol embolization downstream from a misplaced stent, improving after correct placement of a second stent.
- Occlusion of a polar branch of the renal transplant artery distal to the stent.

Clinical and Angiographic Results

No migration of the stent occurred. After a mean angiographic follow-up of 28 ± 14.9 months (range, 12 to 60 months) (N=21), 17 patients showed a patent stent. The mean angiographic follow-up for these 17 patients was 30 ± 16 months (range, 12 to 60 months). The cumulative primary patency rate was 95% at 7 months, 86% at 9 months, and 78% at 15 months (Figure 1).

Restenosis within the stent occurred respectively at 7, 9, 9, and 15 months in four patients (20%). Successful PTRA was performed in two patients with an excellent immediate result at 29 and 16 months, respectively. In the third patient, balloon angioplasty was successfully performed at 12 months. Restenosis occurred at 15 months and required a second PTA at 22 months; a good angiographical result was ascertained at 30 months. For the fourth patient, restenosis proximal in the stent was diagnosed at 15 months, but no PTRA was performed because the patient's hypertension was controlled with medication. The cumulative secondary patency rate was 92% at 15 months (Figure 2).

During a mean clinical follow-up period of 31.2 ± 15.9 months (range, 12 to 60 months), one patient died after 15 months due to a myocardial infarction.

Blood pressure immediately improved within 24 hours of stent placement in 16 patients. At the end of the clinical follow-up period, hypertension was cured in 3 patients and improved in the other 19 patients. None of the three cured patients had a restenosis. Among the four patients with restenosis, three had had a relapse of hypertension. Blood pressure at the end of the clinical follow-up period was significantly reduced compared to that prior to renal artery stenting (p < 0.01) (Table 2).

Serum creatinine levels remained normal at the end of follow-up in the patients with normal renal function before stenting; one patient showed a slight deterioration of renal function due to restenosis in the stent, since serum creatinine levels became normal after PTA in the stent. Of the six patients with renal failure before stenting, two showed a deterioration of their renal function due to the evolution of underlying nephropathy, since neither had restenosis. Renal status was stabilized in three patients and improved in one; none of these patients had restenosis.

DISCUSSION

Our series described the 1- to 5-year long-term follow-up of renal artery stenting in 22 patients. In eight, the indication for stenting was an immediate poor result from PTRA. An unsatisfactory immediate post-dilation appearance is susceptible to improve within several months (14,15). Because of a high risk of restenosis, however, this now represents a well-accepted indication for stenting, especially in ostial lesions (2,4,16,17).

In the case of restenosis after PTRA, there is a potential controversy concerning the use of a stent, despite a positive result

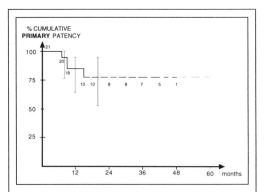

Figure 1. Primary patency rates of stents in the renal artery. Numbers below line indicate number of patent stents at start of interval, i.e., the number remaining at risk at beginning of each period. The 95% confidence interval is indicated for each step as a vertical segment.

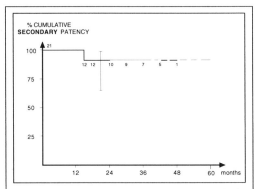

Figure 2. Secondary patency rates of stents in the renal artery. Numbers below line indicate number of patent stents at start of interval, i.e., the number remaining at risk at beginning of each period. The 95% confidence interval is indicated for each step as a vertical segment.

after a second dilation, and requires further experience.

Selection of the correct stent size is a major determinant of Wallstent endoprosthesis patency in small arteries (9,18). The mild overexpansion of the stent, by imbedding the metal stent struts away from the circumference of the lumen, allows rapid reendothelialization by multicentric growth from the tissue mounds protruding between the troughs (19).

The positioning step is particularly important in ostial lesions (20). Our experience shows the importance of completely covering the lesion, even with a slight protrusion of the proximal extremity of the stent into the aortic lumen. The placement of a second stent does not seem to be a problem since five of our patients had two stents with an immediate excellent result after the second stent and without late restenosis.

Complications of renal artery stenting are not specific and are mainly due to balloon angioplasty (1). Wilms et al have described cholesterol embolization as a complication of stenting (21); this is a well-known complication of both aortography and previous renal angioplasty (22).

Our drug regimen was similar to that used by others: heparinization during the procedure and for 24 hours after, and long-term antiplatelet therapy with aspirin. No acute or late occlusion occurred in our first 12 patients with oral anticoagulation, nor in the nine latter without this medication, according to low thrombogenicity of the device and high flow rate in the renal arteries.

Table 2. Evolution of Arterial Blood Pressure at the End of Follow-Up in 22 Patients

Systolic Arterial Blood Pressure		Diastolic Arterial Blood Pressure	
Before Stenting	After Follow-Up	Before Stenting	After Follow-up
183 ± 22 mm Hg (150 to 240)	137 ± 15 mm Hg (100 to 170)[a]	108 ± 9 mm Hg (100 to 130)	78 ± 8 mm Hg (65 to 90)[a]

[a] p < 0.01 by T-test as compared to arterial blood pressure before stenting.

The Wallstent endoprosthesis provides a limited intimal proliferation and low occlusion rate, which are closely related to the small wire size, its self expansion, inherent pliability, and longitudinal flexibility (23). The smooth transition from the stented segment to the adjacent native vessel limits blood flow turbulence and abrupt changes in the diameter, reducing the likelihood of restenosis or thrombosis (23,24).

Restenosis in renal arteries is often silent and does not necessarily lead to relapse of hypertension or renal function deterioration (15). An angiographic follow-up is thus required, since angiographic restenosis exists in some patients with ongoing clinical benefit, i.e., improvement in hypertension (20) and because relapse of hypertension may be associated with a patent stent. Restenosis in the stent is amenable to redilation using a conventional balloon (20,21,25) without particular difficulty and with normal inflation pressures.

Our angiographic follow-up period (mean, 28 months; range, 12 to 60 months) is longer than that reported for other series of renal artery stenting using the Palmaz stent (20,26,27), the Strecker stent (25,28), and the Wallstent (21). Correct placement (i.e., immediate technical success) is generally achieved in more than 75% of the cases. Although stent misplacement can occur with the Palmaz stent (20), it seems to be more frequent with the Wallstent (about 20%) because of retractability and lower radiopacity, especially in ostial lesions. The Wallstent endoprosthesis is flexible, however, and can be retrieved in cases of bad placement if complete expansion has not been achieved.

Clinical results are comparable, both in terms of improvement in hypertension and renal failure, with beneficial rates for hypertension of greater than 60%. Restenosis rates at mid-term follow-ups are also comparable: 20 to 30% (21,29) with the Wallstent, 18% with the Strecker stent (25,28), and 6 to 38% with the Palmaz stent (20,26,27).

CONCLUSIONS

In conclusion, long-term results in renal arteries are similar with the three major metallic stents undergoing active clinical investigation. Renal stenting is an important adjunct to renal angioplasty. The long-term patency rates are quite acceptable, clinical efficacy is good, and the complication rate is low.

Renal stenting is now a widely accepted method and should be proposed as an adjunct to renal arterial angioplasty. Its indications are usually poor results after first angioplasty or after redilation of a restenosis. This unfavorable evaluation is amenable, however, to a second PTA within the stent without any significant difficulties. Further experience is needed in order to know if endoprostheses may be proposed as a first-line treatment of ostial stenosis, even with a good result from a first angioplasty.

REFERENCES

1. Tegtmeyer CJ, Selby JB, Hartwell GD, Ayers C, Tegtmeyer V. Results and complications of angioplasty in fibromuscular disease. Circulation 1991;83(Suppl. I):I155-I161.
2. Sos TA. Angioplasty for the treatment of azotemia and renovascular hypertension in atherosclerotic renal artery disease. Circulation 1991;83(Suppl. I):I162-I166.
3. Canzanello VJ, Millan VG, Spiegel JE, Ponce SP, Kopelman RI, Madias E. Percutaneous transluminal renal angioplasty in management of atherosclerotic renovascular hypertension: results in 100 patients. Hypertension 1989;13:163-172.
4. Sos TA, Pickering TG, Phil MB, et al. Percutaneous transluminal renal angioplasty in renovascular hypertension due to atheroma or fibromuscular dysplasia. N Engl J Med 1983;309:274-279.
5. Tegtmeyer CJ, Kellum CD, Ayers C. Percutaneous transluminal angioplasty of the renal artery: results and long-term follow-up. Radiology 1984;153:77-84.
6. Cicuto KP, McLean GK, Oleaga JA, Freiman DB, Grossman RA, Ring EJ. Renal artery

stenosis: anatomic classification for percutaneous transluminal angioplasty. AJR 1981;137:599-601.

7. Dean RH, Callis JT, Smith BM, Meacham PW. Failed percutaneous transluminal renal angioplasty: experience with lesions requiring operative intervention. J Vasc Surg 1987;6:301-307.

8. Becker GJ. Intravascular stents. General principles and status of lower-extremity arterial applications. Circulation 1991;83(Suppl I):I122-I136.

9. Duprat G, Wright KC, Charnsangavej C, Wallace S, Gianturco C. Self-expanding metallic stents for small vessels: an experimental evaluation. Radiology 1987;162:469-472.

10. Sigwart U, Puel J, Mirkovitch V, Joffre F, Kappenberger L. Intravascular stents to prevent occlusion and restenosis after transluminal angioplasty. N Engl J Med 1987;316:701-706.

11. Joffre F, Rousseau H, Bernadet P, et al. Midterm results of renal artery stenting. Cardiovasc Intervent Radiol 1992;15:313-318.

12. Standards of Practice Committee of the Society of Cardiovascular and Interventional Radiology. Guidelines for percutaneous transluminal angioplasty. Radiology 1990;177:619-626.

13. Rutherford RB and the Ad Hoc Committee on Reporting Standards, Society for Vascular Surgery. Suggested standards for reports dealing with lower extremity ischemia. J Vasc Surg 1986;4:80-94.

14. Srur MF, Sos TA, Saddekni S, Cohn DJ, Rozenblit G, Wetter EB. Intimal fibromuscular dysplasia and Takayasu arteritis: delayed response to percutaneous transluminal renal angioplasty. Radiology 1985;157:657-660.

15. Wilms GE, Baert AL, Amery AK, Staessen JA, Vermylen JG. Short-term morphologic results of percutaneous transluminal renal angioplasty as determined by angiography. Radiology 1989;170:1019-1021.

16. Park JH, Han JH, Kim SH, Oh BH, Park YB, Seo JD. Takayasu arteritis: angiographic findings and results of angioplasty. AJR 1989;53:1069-1074.

17. Sharma S, Saxena A, Talwar KK, Kaul U, Mehta SN, Rajani M. Renal artery stenosis caused by nonspecific arteritis (Takayasu disease): results of treatment with percutaneous transluminal angioplasty. AJR 1992;158:417-422.

18. Rousseau H, Raillat CR, Joffre FG, Knight CJ, Ginestet MC. Treatment of femoropopliteal stenosis by means of self-expandable endoprostheses: midterm results. Radiology 1989;172:961-964.

19. Palmaz JC. Intravascular stents: tissue-stent interactions and design considerations. AJR 1993;160:613-618.

20. Rees CR. Palmaz stent in atherosclerotic stenoses involving the ostia of the renal arteries: preliminary report of a multicenter study. Radiology 1991;181:507-514.

21. Wilms GE, Peene P, Baert AL, et al. Renal artery stent placement with use of the Wallstent endoprosthesis. Radiology 1991;179:457-462.

22. Baert A, Wilms G, Amery A, Vermylen J, Suy R. Percutaneous transluminal renal angioplasty: initial results and long-term follow-up in 202 patients. Cardiovasc Intervent Radiol 1990;13:22-28.

23. Zollikofer CL, Largiader I, Bruhlman WF, Uhlschmid GK, Marty AH. Endovascular stenting of veins and grafts: preliminary clinical experience. Radiology 1988;167:707-712.

24. Rousseau H, Puel J, Joffre F, et al. Self-expanding endovascular prosthesis: an experimental study. Radiology 1987;164:709-714.

25. Kuhn FP, Kutkuhn B, Torsello G, Mödder U. Renal artery stenosis: preliminary results of treatment with the Strecker stent. Radiology 1991;180:367-372.

26. Henry M, Amor M, Ethevenot G, et al. Renal artery stenting with the renal Palmaz-Schatz balloon-expandable endoprosthesis. A single center experience. 65th Scientific Session of American Heart Association, November 16-20, 1992, New Orleans. Circulation 1992;86(4, Suppl I):635.

27. Henry M, Amor M, Ethevenot G, Henry I, Allaoui M, Beron R. Palmaz-Schatz stent in the treatment of peripheral vascular diseases: 2-year follow-up — a single center experience. 78th Scientific Assembly and Annual Meeting, Radiological Society of North America, December 2, 1992, Chicago. Radiology 1992;185(Suppl P):259.

28. Kuhn FP, Malms J, Kutkuhn B, Torsello G, Mödder U. Three-year experience with

renal artery stents. 78th Scientific Assembly and Annual Meeting, Radiological Society of North America, December 1, 1992, Chicago. Radiology 1992;185(Suppl P):209.

29. Hennequin LH, Joffre FG, Rousseau HP et al. Long-term results of renal artery stenting with the Wallstent endoprosthesis. Radiology 1994, in press.

Five Years' Experience with Strecker Stent Implantation in Renal Arteries: An Epicritical Summary

J. Malms[1] and F.-P. Kuhn[2]

[1]Institute of Diagnostic Radiology, Heinrich Heine University, Düsseldorf, Germany
[2]Institute of Diagnostic and Interventional Radiology, Städtische Kliniken Kassel, Germany

In 27 of 137 patients (19.7%) who underwent percutaneous transluminal renal angioplasty, renal stent implantation was indicated due to insufficient success of the angioplasty. In seven cases (26%), primary stent implantation failed. In all other cases stent implantation led to full recanalization of the vascular segment treated. After a mean angiographic follow-up period of 16.8 months we recorded a 50, 55, and 80% restenosis within the vascular segment treated in three cases. In two patients, single or multiple PTRA was successfully repeated. The third patient showed spontaneous regression of the neointimal cover.

INTRODUCTION

Percutaneous endovascular implantation of metal mesh prostheses can now look back on 7 years of clinical experience. Endoprostheses are used in virtually all vascular regions: supraaortic, coronary, abdominal, and in the sector of extremity arteries and deep veins, as well as extraanatomically in cases of TIPS intervention. Compared with these indications, stent implantation in renal arteries is still a relatively new field of application.

Reliable 5-year results are not yet available so that at present, acute obstructing intimal dissection after percutaneous transluminal renal angioplasty (PTRA) is the only absolute indication for renal stent implantation. We should like to contribute our experience with renal stent implantation by reporting on our 5 years of experience with Strecker™ stents (Boston Scientific Corp., Denmark).

INDICATIONS

From February, 1989 to December, 1993, a total of 144 PTRA procedures were performed at our institute on 137 patients. Renal stent implantation was indicated for 27 patients (11 women, 16 men) (18.8% of all angioplasty procedures). Indications for stenting in these patients were:

- Residual stenosis of >30% after the primary PTRA in 17 patients. The extent of residual stenosis ranged from 40 to 85% (mean, 58% ± 7).
- Intimal dissection after primary PTRA in one patient. Stent implantation in this case was performed because of the danger of acute obstruction.
- Residual stenosis of >30% after primary PTRA of a transplanted renal artery in two patients. The extent of the residual stenosis was 50% in one case and >60% in the other.
- Restenosis after primary PTRA in three patients.
- 80% restenosis of transplanted renal artery 5 months after primary PTRA in one patient.
- PTRA with consecutive stent implantation after acute obstructing intimal dissection following transaortic renal artery desobliteration in two patients. Stent implantation was necessary as the intimal flaps could not be reconnected to the vascular wall by balloon angioplasty and led to a 75% and 95% vascular obstruction, respectively.

• 60% restenosis 6 months after transaortic renal artery desobliteration in one patient. Practically no lumen expansion was achieved by the prior PTRA and stent implantation was subsequently performed.

RESULTS AND COMPLICATIONS OF STENT IMPLANTATION

In 20 patients, stent implantation resulted in an exact and desired complete vascular recanalization; tandem stent implantation was necessary in two cases due to a lengthy dissected flap. In seven cases (26%), primary stent implantation was unsuccessful. In one of these cases, surgical desobliteration of the renal artery was necessary due to stent compression and consequent vascular occlusion. In all other cases the stent which was misplaced (1 case), dislocated into the artery (2 cases), or which failed to separate from the delivery balloon (3 cases) could be recovered percutaneously without any complications. No attempt was made to implant a second stent in the same session because of the strain on the patient (high overall dose of contrast medium, new transfemoral access, lengthy examination period). The technique of Strecker stent implantation in renal arteries, analysis of our patient population according to clini-

cal aspects of renal function and blood pressure behavior, and the possibility of percutaneous recovery of the tantalum vascular prosthesis have already been described in detail elsewhere (1-4).

Long-Term Follow-Up Observations

For 17 of the 20 patients successfully treated with stent implantation, the average angiographic follow-up observation period was 16.8 months, with the shortest interval between stent implantation and angiographic examination being 5 months and the longest, 31 months (Figure 1). In 3 of the 17 (17.6%) patients, a 50, 55, or 80% restenosis, respectively, occurred within the vascular implant during the course of that follow-up period. The stenosis was observed 6 months after stent implantation in two cases and after 12 months in one case. In two cases of restenosis, PTRA was again performed immediately; in one of these patients PTRA was again necessary 6 months later. In all cases, PTRA led to complete recanalization of the vascular implants. In one of the three cases of restenosis, PTRA was not repeated at the patient's request. This patient had originally had two overlapping stents implanted due to acute obstructing intimal dissection following transaortic renal artery desobliteration.

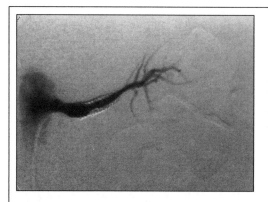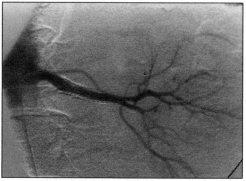

Figure 1. Angiogram of the left renal artery of a female patient 6 months *(left)* and 31 months *(right)* after tandem Strecker stent implantation. A noticeable feature is the spontaneous regression of neointimal tissue overlap which had led to 50% stenosis within the treated segment of the artery 6 months after stenting.

Angiographic examination after 6 months showed clear intimal hyperplasia (>50% stenosis, Figure 1, *left*) in the middle third of the vessel segment treated. Thirty-one months after tandem stent implantation, the follow-up angiography surprisingly revealed a complete regression of the intimal restenosis with a non-stenotic, smoothly-defined vascular lumen (Figure 1, *right*).

DISCUSSION

In PTRA treatment of renovascular hypertension and/or renal insufficiency, an indication for renal artery stent implantation was observed in 18.8% of our cases due to inadequate angioplasty success. Study groups under Rabbia (5; personal communication) and Blum (personal communication) showed a higher percentage indication for stenting, 89 stents in 351 PTRA procedures (25.4%) and 90 stents in 357 PTRA procedures (25.2%), respectively. The literature does not contain corresponding data for other study groups (6-8). The higher proportion of stent implantations can perhaps be explained in view of the inclusion of stenoses involving the ostia of the renal arteries in PTRA (5-7). Our patient population included only one case in which ostium stenosis was treated by PTRA. Ostial stenosis of renal arteries must be considered separately and the importance of stent implantation will first have to be determined from the long-term results of a multicenter study (7), especially in comparison with surgical procedures.

We achieved a lower primary success rate for stent implantation than study groups working with Palmaz stents or Wallstents. In three of our seven cases where primary stent implantation was unsuccessful, the release mechanism failed. One stent protruding into the aortic lumen and two stents dislocated into the aorta could be successfully recovered percutaneously without any adverse consequences for the patient. The possibility of a traumatic percutaneous stent recovery has previously been described for the Strecker stent only (2,4,9).

High elastic recoil strength led to complete stent compression in one of our first patients whose renal artery stenosis was due to peri-adventitial fibromuscular dysplasia. As the recoil factor can be evaluated (3,4) prior to intervention by assessing the degree of calcification of a stenosis, preference should be given to a stent type with good pressure stability in such cases (10).

In three patients we observed a 50 to 80% restenosis within the stent. While PTRA was again performed on the two more severe cases, spontaneous regression of the neointimal tissue cover was observed in the third case. This characteristic early and late form of tissue response to implantation of a metal endoprosthesis has previously been observed clinically and in animal experiments (summarized in 11,12).

The two cases of substantial neointimal thickening involved previously damaged kidneys with reduced organ size and in which the respective overall clearance was reduced to 30%. On the basis of this observation, we assume that restricted kidney function with reduced blood supply to the organ constitutes a prognostically unfavorable factor for stent implantation.

CONCLUSION

In keeping with recent publications (5-8), our experience implies that stent implantation may improve the long-term efficiency of PTRA in the treatment of renovascular hypertension and kidney insufficiency. This, however, has yet to be verified by the long-term results of ongoing studies. Empirical values are available for Wallstents (8) as well as for Palmaz (5-7) and Strecker stents. In addition to the differences in manipulation, the pressure stability of the endoprosthesis is presumably decisive for selection of the stent type (9). Multicenter studies have not yet shown whether the satisfactory results seen to date can also be achieved in the treatment of stenoses involving the ostia of renal arteries, particularly when compared with the results of surgical procedures.

A focal point of current research is the development of wrapped vascular endoprostheses. The aim of wrapping stents is to reduce intimal hyperplasia during the early stage in particular. Stents are wrapped with biocompatible membranes which do not reduce the pressure stability of the stent, do not themselves have a thrombogenic effect, and offer the possibility of favorably influencing the trigger mechanisms of tissue reaction by means of drug impregnation.

REFERENCES

1. Kuhn F-P, Kutkuhn B, Torsello G, Mödder U. Renal artery stenosis: preliminary results of treatment with the Strecker stent. Radiology 1991;180:367-372.
2. Kuhn F-P, Kutkuhn B, Fürst G, Torsello G, Strecker EP, Mödder U. Einsatz des Strecker-Stents zur Therapie der Nieren- und Transplantatnierenarterienstenose. In: Kollath J and Liermann D, eds. *Stents II.* Konstanz: Schnetztor-Verlag; 1992.
3. Kuhn F-P, Malms J, Kutkuhn B, Fürst G, Torsello G, Mödder U. Renale stent-implantation. Fortschr Röntgenstr 1992; 157: 65-71.
4. Malms J, Kuhn F-P, Torsello G, Kutkuhn B, Joerss Ch. Indikationen, Technik, Nachsorge und Langzeitbeobachtungen der Nierenarterien-Stentimplantation. Radiologia Diagnostica 1994; (in press).
5. Rabbia C, Savio D, Rossato D, Margarita G. Stenting of renal artery stenosis: preliminary results. Stent Forum (Johnson & Johnson Nr. 6; June 1993).
6. Joffrey F, Rousseau H, Chemali R, Meites G. Long-term results with artery stenting. In: Kollath J and Liermann D, eds. *Stents II.* Konstanz: Schnetztor-Verlag; 1992.
7. Rees RC, Palmaz CJ, Becker GJ, et al. Palmaz stent in atherosclerotic stenoses involving the ostia of the renal arteries: preliminary report of a multicenter study. Radiology 1991;181:507-514.
8. Wilms GE, Peene TP, Baert LA, et al. Renal artery stent placement with use of the Wallstent endoprosthesis. Radiology 1991;179:457-462.
9. Liermann D, Zegelman M, Kuhn F, Herrmann G, Satter P, Kollath J. Experimentelle Untersuchungen zur Entfernbarkeit unterschiedlicher implantierter. Stenttypen Radiologe 1993;33:525-562.
10. Wehrmeyer B, Kuhn F-P. Experimentelle Untersuchungen zur Druckstabilität vaskulärer Endoprothesen. Fortschr Röntgenstr 1993;158:242-246.
11. Palmaz CJ. Intravascular stents: tissue interaction and design considerations. AJR 1993;160:613-618.
12. Richter GM, Nöldge G, Palmaz JC, Tio F. Generalisierte Arteriosklerose und Stentimplantation. Radiologe 1991;31:114-119.

Therapy of Ostium Stenoses in Renal Arteries

D. Liermann[1] and E.H. Scheuermann[2]

Departments of [1]Radiology and [2]Nephrology, J.W. Goethe University Hospital, Frankfurt am Main, Germany

INTRODUCTION

Arterial hypertension poses a serious threat, particularly the secondary sequelae related to chronic elevated blood pressure, such as cerebral hemorrhaging and arteriosclerosis. For most forms of hypertension, the only treatment is lifelong conservative drug-based or dietetic therapy to reduce blood pressure (1). For some patients, it is possible to detect a renal genesis for the elevated pressure using laboratory and renal function tests. Further methods succeed in differentiating between parenthymatous disease such as glomerulonephritis and vascular stenotic diseases, including renal artery exit stenosis, isolated arteriosclerotic renal artery stenosis, stenoses as part of fibromuscular dysplasia, and cicatrized stenosis following or as part of inflammatory vascular diseases such as Takayasu's disease (1-5). Depending on the cause of the stenosis and its localization, a strategy can be developed for eliminating the stenosis and thus treating the elevated blood pressure.

Since the introduction of percutaneous transluminal angioplasty (PTA) as an alternative to surgery for renal artery stenosis, PTA has been used more or less successfully for different types of stenosis. It has become the established therapy for inflammatory and fibromuscular stenoses (2,5-7). Good long-term results have been achieved for several types of stenoses along the renal arteries with long recurrence-free intervals (6,8). Results for artery exit stenoses, however, have been generally unsatisfactory because of the stenosis genesis and corresponding immediate recurrence of restenosis after PTA. Thus, stenosis in the renal artery exit has remained a case for the vascular surgeon (9,10).

Vascular endoprostheses have recently joined the discussion as an alternative for avoiding restenosis in the renal artery. The endoprostheses were initially used and tested for stenoses in occlusive disease of the iliac artery, but the range of possible applications was soon extended to the peripheral arteries. On the basis of our own experimental studies, we decided to use only one specific stent (tantalum stent) for implantation in renal arteries. Because of its good visibility upon x-ray, this stent was the only one which could be reliably positioned; it also remained sufficiently flexible to cope with several bends, and could be removed from the renal artery in the event of malpositioning. The purpose of this clinical study was to ascertain whether the stent, which had been convincing in experimental trials and intraoperative applications, would also produce the same positive results *in situ*.

EXPERIMENTAL EXPLANTATION OF TANTALUM STENTS FROM RENAL ARTERIES

The entire distal abdominal artery was prepared out of its site up to just above the renal artery exit. In addition, both kidneys were removed together with the prepared blood vessels, and the entire preparation was fixed onto a wooden board. In this way it was possible to probe and stent both the left and right renal arteries from the right and left common femoral arteries.

In this series of tests through the positioned Terumo sheath, a renal catheter (7 Fr; Angiomed, Karlsruhe, Germany) was introduced by wire and one of the two renal artery exits probed. A guidewire was inserted into the kidney through the positioned catheter according to the contrast medium image. Under the experimental conditions, the renal artery was not dilatated since the preparations were free of stenoses. A tantalum stent was then inserted through the sheath and positioned guidewire, and placed and deployed in the normal way just behind the renal artery exit. Care was required to ensure that the guidewire created a good curve from its tip in the caudal kidney pole area through the renal artery into the distal aorta so that the dilatation catheter could be removed without problems caused by snaring of the stent.

Deviating from normal stenting techniques, a curved catheter such as those used in cardiology was inserted and positioned with its nose in the exit area of the renal artery. After the guidewire had been withdrawn, it was then possible to push the catheter described above with polypus forceps through the 5 Fr inner lumen of the cardiology catheter and around the nearly 90° bend of the renal artery exit to the aorta to reach the positioned stent. Under the conditions described above, the recovery forceps catheter snared with the stent mesh and the catheter was withdrawn together with the stent through the guidewire.

Results

Altogether, six stents were implanted and then explanted in three cadaver preparations using the techniques described above. None of the preparations had any notable constriction in the renal artery area and thus we managed without the normal PTA prior to stent implantation. Apart from minor problems in withdrawing the implant set following stent deployment, no serious problems were encountered during implantation or explantation of the endoprosthesis. The problems encountered were caused essentially by crepitation of the balloon catheters on the stent filaments, with a risk of dislocation; these were mastered easily.

For the explantation procedure, it did not matter whether the stent was to be removed from the left or right side of the left or right renal artery. Although it was possible to introduce and expand the recovery forceps into the guide catheter through the 90° bend, in only some cases was it possible to pull the recovered stent into the catheter but not beyond the 90° bend. In spite of this incomplete withdrawal, the guide catheter and recovery forceps/stent tandem were removed through the positioned sheath without difficulty. Apart from the already typical damage to the valve following the distal end of the sheath, no further material damage was detected. Subsequent inspection of the preparations revealed no evidence of damage to the vascular walls (Table 1).

Table 1. Explantation of Tantulum Endoprothesis in Renal Arteries From Human Cadavers

| Age/Sex | Localization | Atherosclerosis | Difficulty During: | | Damage to Vessel Wall? |
			Implantation	Explantation	
72/Male	LH renal artery	No	None	None	No
	RH renal artery	No	None	None	No
53/Male	LH renal artery	No	None	None	No
	RH renal artery	No	Slight	None	No
64/Female	LH renal artery	Slight	Slight	None	No
	RH renal artery	Slight	None	None	No

CLINICAL EXPERIENCE

Methods

In contrast to the techniques used in other organs, after scanning the renal artery but before angiography to localize the stenosis, a single dose of heparin 20,000 IU was applied directly into the renal artery through a catheter in order to avoid any thrombosis during the following manipulations. The tantalum endoprosthesis was then implanted using normal techniques.

In the renal artery, pressures of more than 6 atm are rarely required to overcome an existing stenosis. After two-fold dilatation of the same renal artery stenosis for a period of 2 minutes in each case, the corresponding PTA catheter was removed via the inserted wire, and the pressure was again measured by an inserted 4 Fr catheter. Before introducing the stent catheter, another set of x-rays were obtained using contrast medium in order to recognize any change in the vessel walls such as dissections after the PTA. Following another scan and introduction of a 0.035-inch Terumo wire, a ballon catheter carrying the stent was inserted. Care was taken to ensure that the guidewire was inserted beyond the stenosis into the caudal pole of the kidney to guarantee a better hold when implanting the stent. The tantalum stent which was then introduced should have had at least the same final diameter as the last PTA balloon used before stent implantation to avoid dislocation of the endoprosthesis on withdrawing the insertion set. The stent was inserted through the sheath and positioned guidewire and deployed in the normal way just behind the renal artery exit.

After stent release, the balloon catheter was carefully removed with pushing, pulling, and rotating movements from or through the lying stent after being deflated and with the patient breathing out to achieve a better angle. It was essential to avoid crepitation of the distal catheter section with the rolled back silicone sleeve, or of the catheter tip itself with the stent filaments, as under certain circumstances this could result in stent dislocation. When the angle of the renal artery exit caused problems, it was often possible to straighten this angle by pushing the wire further or by assuming a certain breathing-out position, so that the implant set could be removed without dislocating the stent.

After the implant set had been removed, a further x-ray was taken using contrast medium, and pressure measured using a 4 Fr catheter introduced through the wire behind the stent. Post-treatment of the renal artery treated with the stent included a strict peri-interventional regime, as for all other stent implantations. A long-term course of Marcumar® therapy was gradually introduced for at least 6 months, with a decision regarding the need for continued therapy to be taken after this time. Follow-up examinations were conducted after 3, 6, and 12 months and then at 6-month intervals checking normal laboratory parameters such as creatinine, kidney function tests such as the Mac 3 clearance or the captopril test, blood pressure, intravenous digital subtraction angiography (DSA), magnetic resonance, and color Doppler. Any signs of deteriorating kidney functions or increasing blood pressure required immediate control to rule out any restenosis and permit immediate intervention where necessary.

The use of stent implants for transplanted kidney stenosis was subject to basically the same prerequisites as for renal artery stenosis. It was important to know whether the transplanted kidney was from a relative or from a human cadaver. In the case of the former, the kidney could not be removed with part of an aortal vessel. It was therefore directly anastomosed with the internal iliac vessel, and not attached directly to the common iliac artery with the aortal patch containing the human cadaver kidney. As far as interventional access was concerned, a human cadaver kidney transplant indicated an ipsilateral approach for arterial stenosis, while a transplant involving a relative's organ indicated a contralateral approach in the cross-over technique.

Indications

The following prerequisites were accepted as indications for stent implantation to treat stenosis in the kidney or transplanted kidney:

- Restenosis of a vessel within a 6-month period following PTA or restenosis during PTA.
- Stenosis following an iatrogenic vessel dissection during the PTA.
- More than three recurrences in the renal artery following PTA in within 6 to 8 months.

Unsatisfactory results after PTA were only accepted in so far as recoiling of the stenosis could be expected to result in restricted flow with probable restenosis. There were also relatively reserved indications for renal artery exit stenosis which could not be surgically treated because of the patient's condition, and for transplanted kidneys with restenosis after a recurrence-free interval of less than 5 months.

Patient Data

Thirty patients with 30 renal artery stenoses were treated. All patients were referred to us from the hospital's nephrology clinic or from the outpatient departments of neighboring clinics. There were 18 female and 12 male patients with a mean age of 64 years (range, 48 to 74 years). All patients had between one and four stenosis recurrences following PTA before they were recommended for stent implantation amd all had hypertension with systolic blood pressure values between 200 and 240 mm Hg prior to stent implantation.

The localization of the renal artery stenosis was in the left renal artery in eight patients and in the right renal artery in six. Ten patients had renal artery exit stenoses in the right renal artery, four had renal artery exit stenoses in the left renal artery, and two

had kidney stenosis in a kidney transplant from a relative involving the right renal artery.

The stenoses in all patients were short, ranging from 1 to 1.5 cm and could be adequately treated by implanting a 2- or 3-cm long stent. In all cases, a clear pressure gradient was obtained before the re-PTA, ranging from 190 mm Hg with an occlusion to 80 mm Hg with the third restenosis. Three cases are described below as examples.

One case involved a 48-year-old woman with a kidney transplant who had suffered from four restenoses in the 6-month period following transplantation, with consecutive deterioration of the creatinine and near cessation of diuresis. Systolic and diastolic blood pressure in this patient increased to approximately 210 and 120 mm Hg, respectively, despite medication. A 4-mm stent was implanted in this woman using a cross-over technique from the other side.

The second case concerned a 53-year-old male patient who had suffered an acute hypertension crisis 5 weeks previously which could not be brought below levels of 200 mm Hg systolic and 110 mm Hg diastolic with medication. Examination revealed occlusion of the left renal artery with evidence of a smaller pole vessel on the left side. This pole vessel had apparently given poor service to the kidney and was thought to be responsible for the arterial hypertension. Following several futile recanalization attempts, we finally succeeded in recanalizing the vessel and dilatating it to 6 mm using the Sidewinder technique (7 Fr) with insertion under massive resistance. Although necessary in this case, we normally reject this technique. The final check revealed no more pressure gradient, and the DSA revealed minor dissections. Blood pressure fell to within the normal range and the patient could be discharged home.

Three months after this treatment, this patient returned with a reocclusion and excessive blood pressure of about 240 mm Hg systolic and 120 mm Hg diastolic. The occlusion was recanalized again, dilated, and treated with a 6-mm stent. During the general angiography, evidence of a previously undetected stenosis was found near the exit of the right renal artery which was dilated to 6 mm at a pressure gradient of 100 mm Hg during the same session. The patient was discharged with normal blood pressure levels. Six months later he returned with a blood pressure of 210 mm Hg systolic and 110 mm Hg diastolic. The general angiography revealed free passage on the left with a subtotal stenosis of the right kidney with a pressure gradient of 160 mm Hg, which could be treated during another PTA by insertion of a 6-mm stent.

A third case consisted of a 70-year-old male patient with severe arterial occlusive disease, coronary bypasses, bilateral carotid stenosis, and hypertension with systolic levels around 240 mm Hg and diastolic levels around 120 mm Hg which could not be controlled by medication. Two PTAs had already been performed on a right-hand renal artery exit stenosis with only short recurrence-free intervals of just 6 months. The position of the stenosis would have indicated a purely surgical solution, but surgery was not possible because of the patient's generally poor health. After being referred to us, the patient was treated with a 6-mm stent extending from the right-hand renal artery exit into the lumen of the aorta, following a prior PTA. The pressure gradient was 90 mm Hg.

Results

Stent implantation was successful in nearly all of the 30 patients referred to us, with one patient receiving two stents, one in the right and one in the left renal artery. In one case referred to us with a positioned sheath and dissection of the left renal artery, we managed to introduce the catheter with a stent into the left renal artery and to insufflate the balloon; however, it was not possible to separate the stent from the balloon at its distal fixing point. Following several futile attempts to expand the balloon sufficiently, we finally succeeded in releasing the stent from its implant set by rotation and manipulation. The stent which had been dislocated in the vessel exit during the disconnection attempt was eventually recovered using a 5 Fr polypus forceps via a pre-bent catheter with an inner lumen of 5 Fr. The patient was then treated a few days later with a renal artery angioplasty. In the other cases, there were no problems during implantation but occasionally problems occurred during withdrawal of the PTA balloon after release of the stent in the renal artery stenosis.

Frequently the catheter could only be removed following exceedingly careful manipulation and rotation out of the positioned stent without crepitation, with the risk of stent dislocation. We found that it was helpful if the patient held his breath in the expired position.

In the patient with the kidney transplant, inappropriate dosing in the transition from heparin 1000 IU/hour for 3 days to adjust to Marcumar resulted in a corresponding anticoagulation gap with consecutive occlusion of the vessel in the transplanted kidney in which the stent had been implanted. Although this occurred in the early hours of the morning, the patient was not referred to us until 12 hours later. We used the cross-over method to find and recanalize the thrombosis in the renal artery exit. In spite of an initially high-dosed lysis with urokinase 200,000 IU and a further 100,000 IU/hour for 12 hours via perfusion through a 4 Fr catheter in the renal artery, it was not possible to save the renal parenchyma. Although a complete, free vascular tree was found after the lysis with a freely passable stent region, there was no parenchyma phase. The kidney was removed 7 days later.

In the other cases, follow-up revealed free passage of the renal arteries treated with stents in 6 to 42 months (mean, 18 months). Blood pressure levels and the creatinine parameters both remained in a range that did not require treatment. DSA, MR, and color Doppler evaluations provided no evidence of restenosis after stent implantation. Even the stents in the renal artery exit with stent sections protruding into the aorta lumen were also clear and showed no signs of restenosis, external thrombosis, or deformation (Figures 1 and 2). Over the course of time, there was a 20% restenosis rate in the renal artery stents, which could be successfully dilated. There was practically no restenosis during a subsequent observation period of up to 3 years following implantation of stents in ostium stenoses, with long-term Marcumar therapy in order to avoid delayed or lacking epithelialization of the normally thrombogenic stent filaments. Apart from the complications described above, we detected no further restenosis or migrations following stent implantation.

DISCUSSION

Consideration of the above stent implantations under clinical conditions with this relatively small number of cases already shows that exact testing of the stent under initial experimental conditions was vital. In attempts to recover malpositioned stents, only the tantalum stent showed any success.

These satisfactory results with stent implantation for renal artery exit stenosis are very encouraging. Previous to these findings, surgical treatment of the stenosis was seen as the only possible therapy. Our initial results suggest that stent implantation in renal artery exits are an interesting, viable alternative to surgery, particularly when the patient's general health condition poses an operative risk (3,4,10,11). One possible explanation for the better results obtained with renal artery stents compared to arteries of a similar width in the superfical femoral artery and popliteal region could be the greater flow velocity in these arteries and perhaps, the lower turbulences.

As far as the other renal artery stenoses are concerned, the results obtained to date show that there are no true contraindications, provided the indications outlined earlier are observed and there are no contraindications

to anticoagulation treatment. The enormous significance of peri-interventional anticoagulation is revealed by the tragic loss of one related transplanted kidney. Although the development of thrombosis following even only a small gap in the anticoagulation management certainly depends on the constitution of the individual concerned, this case

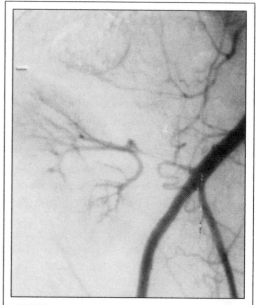

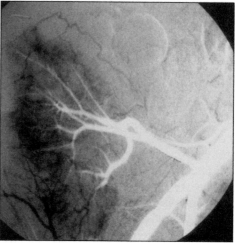

Figure 1. Renal artery stenosis in a transplanted kidney. Recurrent stenosis in a transplant renal artery anastomosed with the RH common iliac artery *(top)*. After implantation of a 5-mm stent in the renal artery *(bottom)*.

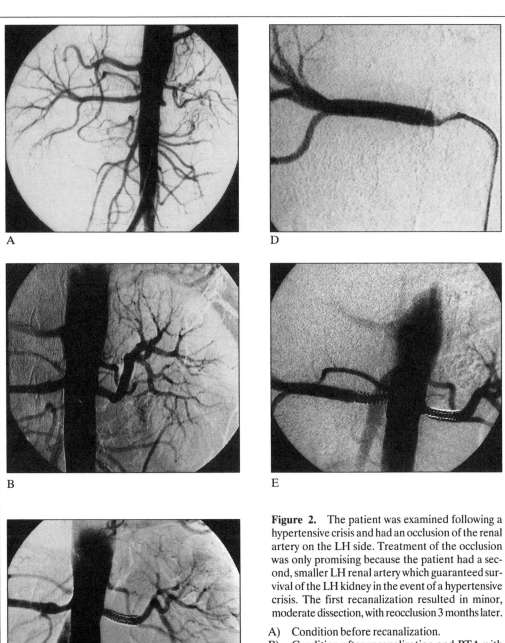

Figure 2. The patient was examined following a hypertensive crisis and had an occlusion of the renal artery on the LH side. Treatment of the occlusion was only promising because the patient had a second, smaller LH renal artery which guaranteed survival of the LH kidney in the event of a hypertensive crisis. The first recanalization resulted in minor, moderate dissection, with reocclusion 3 months later.

A) Condition before recanalization.
B) Condition after recanalization and PTA with dissection in the vessel.
C) On reocclusion, repeated recanalization and stent implantation. The stent has been open for 6 months.
D) After one year, RR increased again because of stenosis in the exit of the RH renal artery. The LH artery still has clear passage.
E) Six months after repeated PTA on the right, here too a stent is implanted.

shows very clearly that in spite of all attempts to design the stent to be as thromboresistant as possible, the development of severe thrombosis must be expected in the face of inadequate anticoagulation.

REFERENCES

1. Breslin DJ. Pathophysiology of renovascular hypertension: an overview. In: Breslin DJ, Swinton NW, Libertino JA, Zinman L, eds. *Renovascular Hypertension*. Baltimore: Williams & Wilkins; 1982;36.

2. Archibald GR, Beckmann CF, Libertino JA. Focal renal artery stenosis caused by fibromuscular dysplasia: treatment by percutaneous transluminal angioplasty. AJR 1988;151:593-596.

3. Eigler FW, Dostal G, Bock KD, Löcr E. Die Nierenarterienstenose arteriosklerotischer Genese. Dtsch Ärztebl 1984;81:271.

4. Eigler FW, Jakubowski HD. Verschlußprozesse der Nierenarterien. In: Heberer G and van Dongen RJAM, eds. *Gefäßchirurgie*. Berlin: Springer; 1987;23:628-644.

5. Srur MF, Sos TA, Saddekni S, Cohn DJ, Rozenblit G, Wetter EB. Intimal fibromuscular dysplasia and Takayasu arteritis: delayed response to percutaneous transluminal renal angioplasty. Radiology 1985;157:657-660.

6. Tegtmeyer CJ, Kofler TJ, Ayers CA. Renal angioplasty: current status. AJR 1984;142:20.

7. Zong Jun Dong, Shihua LU, Xuncheng LU. Percutaneous transluminal angioplasty for renovascular hypertension in arteritis: experience in China. Radiologie 1987;162: 477-479.

8. Powers TA, Lorenz CH, Holburn GE, Price RR. Renal artery stenosis: *in vivo* perfusion MR imaging. Radiology 1991;178:543-548.

9. Kuhn FP, Kutkuhn B, Fürst G, Torsello G, Mödder U. Einsatz des Strecker Stents zur Therapie der Nieren- und Transplantatnieren-arterienstenose. In: Kollath J and Liermann D, eds. *Stents II*. Konstanz: Schnetztor Verlag; 1992;194-203.

10. Pichlmayr R, Knitsch W, Bode U. Prophylaktische Operationen in der Transplantatchirurgie. Langenbecks Arch Chir Suppl, Kongressbericht 1991;219-255.

11. Kuhn FP, Kutkuhn B, Fürst G, Torsello G, Mödder U. Renal artery stenosis. Preliminary results of treatment with the Strecker stent. Radiology 1991;180:367.

Tantalum Stents in the Treatment of Stenotic and Occlusive Diseases of Abdominal Vessels

D. Liermann[1] and E.P. Strecker[2]

[1]Department of Radiology, J.W. Goethe University Hospital, Frankfurt am Main, Germany
[2]Department of Radiology, Diakonissen Hospital Rüppurr, Karlsruhe, Germany

INTRODUCTION

The proportion of patients with acute generalized arterial occlusive disease (AOD) is increasing as longevity is enhanced and because the opportunities for causal therapy are as yet non-existent (1-5). If conservative therapy, percutaneous transluminal angioplasty (PTA), surgical recanalization, or bypass surgery fail, amputation of the affected limb remains the last resort. If recanalization or reconstructive surgical measures fail in the area of the abdominal vessels, no further therapy is possible. The lethality of an acute arterial occlusion is between 70 and 90% (6). Post-operative lethality ranges from 3 to 20% (7), and an emergency intervention with these patients is connected with a marked increase in the operative risk and peri-operative mortality. This restricts the indications for surgery, and makes it necessary to search for alternative treatment methods. Except for cases of intestinal necrosis, carrying out a PTA of a recognizable stenosis or occlusion, even under acute conditions, seems to be the first measure which is worth trying because of the low risk involved (8-12). Compared to iliac or peripheral vessels, PTA is usually more difficult in vessels which have suffered considerable atherosclerotic change, and are partially ectatic, stenotic, and curved. In spite of this, a primary success rate of 90%, with a recurrence rate necessitating redilatation of 50%, is achieved (13).

Since 1985, there has been the possibility of stent implantation in case of insufficient results. Due to the usually severe degenerative changes, and the numerous curves in the course of the vessel encountered with the transbrachial as well as the femoral access, only a highly flexible stent that can be removed in case of detachment difficulties or misplacement is suited for this task. Experimental investigations showed that only the tantalum stent was sufficiently flexible and removable with a flexible three- or four-armed forceps (14-16).

MATERIALS AND METHODS

Besides appropriate stent selection, a prerequisite for successful intervention is a strict peri-interventional anticoagulation protocol. Beyond the initial heparinization with transbrachial access, a heparinization of 100 to 150 IU/kg body weight should be attempted and corrected upwards according to the corresponding duration of the intervention. Highly flexible tantalum stents with diameters between 5 and 7 mm and a length of 4 to 8 cm are suitable for implantation. If a diameter of up to 6 mm at the end is sufficient, transbrachial exposure can usually be done without, and the 8 Fr sheath can be inserted percutaneously to the incision. No relevant complications have been observed to date in our own patients that were initially given heparin 5000 IU and an antispasmodic agent.

If stents with a larger diameter are applied, either the brachial artery must be exposed transbrachially in order to avoid complications or the transfemoral path must be selected. As a rule, the transbrachial path should be selected for interventions in the area of the abdominal vessels because of better leverage. After properly examining the radiographs, the vessel origin of the celiac artery or the superior mesenteric artery is probed after an angiocatheter is positioned through a Terumo wire, the tip of which should either be slightly bent or straight depending on the degree of the stenosis. After the angiocatheter is advanced beyond the stenosis, a more stable wire should be substituted. The dilatation catheter, and in cases of insufficient results, the stent catheter, can be positioned through this wire. The implantation procedure for stent deployment is done with the usual technique. In case of stent deformation by pressure from the outside, it should be expanded through redilatation.

A 72-hour long heparinization with heparin 1000 IU/hour through a perfusor follows stent implantation. Marcumar® therapy for 6 months, or for an unlimited period in difficult cases, is recommended. In the other cases, long-term therapy with aspirin should follow the 6-month Marcumar treatment. Beyond the evaluation of the clinical symptoms (reduction of diarrhea and weight gain), digital subtraction angiography (DSA) is required after 6 and 12 months in order to rule out restenosing at an early stage when it is still revisable. This is repeated at 6-month intervals or when symptoms occur.

INDICATIONS

The indication for implanting a highly flexible vessel stent is the treatment of occlusive vascular disease of the abdominal vessels when PTA fails. Successful PTA with signs of restenosis does not justify the use of stents. There are no age or sex-specific restrictions, and clinical signs must be decisive. Increased operative risk or inoperability with severe abdominal angina is also a clear indication. There must be sufficient transbrachial or femoral access, and an arteriogram in which the degree of stenosis can be recognized is necessary before and after PTA. It is not possible to use stents in the event of a contraindication to anticoagulation treatment.

PATIENTS

A total of 12 patients (8 female, 4 male) with severe abdominal angina after insufficient PTA were treated with stent implantation (Table 1). All patients had varying intense symptoms of abdominal angina accompanied by weight loss, diarrhea, and colicky pain symptoms, especially after meals or physical strain. All patients had generalized AOD. Ages ranged from 63 to 86 years (mean, 79 years). Among the risk factors were nine cases of extended nicotine abuse, five cases of diabetes, and six cases of hypertonia. Symptoms occurred over a period of a few hours to 4 months (mean, 14 days before the beginning of the therapy). They consisted of intense acute process with recurring attacks and hospitalization. In three cases there was an occlusion of the superior mesenteric artery with simultaneous stenosis of the celiac artery, with perfusion of the superior mesenteric artery's supply area via the pancreas arciform arteries. In the nine other cases, there were severe constrictions of the proximal superior mesenteric artery. The extent of the stenoses varied from 65 to 95%. The constricted segments varied from 1.5 to 2.5 cm in the case of the trunk, and from 1.0 to 3.5 cm in the case of the superior mesenteric artery. All patients were being treated in a hospital at the time of diagnosis. Besides the above described stenosis, seven cases of pronounced rarefaction and peripheral severed vessels in the superior mesenteric artery's supply area were found upon angiographic evaluation.

RESULTS

It was possible to revise an insufficient result after PTA using stent implantations in all 12 patients. In 11 cases, stent release via the transbrachial path, and in one case via a transfemoral path, was selected. Stents with a diameter of 5 mm and 6 mm, respectively, and having a length of 4 cm were applied. In three cases, an obvious deformation of the stent from the outside occurred after the

Table 1. Stents in the Treatment of Abdominal Anginas

Age	Sex	Size	Access	Complications	Free of Symptoms	Survival Time Patency
82	Female	Celiac	Brachial	Hemorrhage at puncture site	Yes	48 months
64	Male	Superior Mesenteric	Femoral	None	Yes	46 months
63	Female	Superior Mesenteric	Brachial	Re-PTA after 24 months	(Yes)	35 months
57	Female	Superior Mesenteric	Brachial	Re-PTA after 24 months	(Yes)	34 months
82	Female	Superior Mesenteric	Brachial	Re-PTA after 24 months	(Yes)	32 months
71	Male	Celiac	Brachial	None	Yes	28 months
86	Male	Celiac	Brachial	Lethal myocardial infarction after 17 months	—	17 months
77	Female	Superior Mesenteric	Brachial	re-PTA after 6 months	(Yes)	21 months
79	Male	Superior Mesenteric	Brachial	Lethal apoplexy after 13 months	—	13 months
78	Female	Superior Mesenteric	Brachial	None	Yes	6 months
81	Female	Superior Mesenteric	Brachial	Lethal apoplexy after 5 months	—	5 months
71	Female	Superior Mesenteric	Brachial	None	Yes	6 months

balloon catheter had been removed. A slowing of the flow could not be observed. Nine stents were implanted in the superior mesenteric artery. Three were implanted in the constricted origin of the celiac artery upon occlusion of the superior mesenteric artery in order to achieve better filling of the supply area of the superior mesenterica via the collateral circulation from the celiac artery through the pancreas arciform arteries.

In all cases, freedom from symptoms after stent implantation was achieved. With a mean follow-up of 28 months, four restenoses that could be eliminated with PTA have occurred to date. The follow-up period ranged from 6 to 48 months. After heparinization for 72 hours, all patients received Marcumar for 6 months. Seven patients continued to receive Marcumar for an unlimited period. Three other patients were switched from Marcumar to aspirin after 6 months.

Restenosing was diagnosed based on presentation of clinical symptoms. In four cases, a restenosis of approximately 70% could be observed on the angiographic control in a ready-to-dilate state. In one case, the restenosis occurred after 6 months and in the three other cases, it did not become symptomatic until after 24 months. There was one complication in which a post-interventional hemorrhage occurred at the location where the brachial artery was exposed within the 72-hour heparinization period; this was able to be controlled conservatively. The same 82-

year-old female patient was admitted to a local hospital approximately 4 months after stent implantation because of sedimentation of tarry stool within the framework of a questionable gastrointestinal hemorrhage. Marcumar was discontinued for approximately 2 weeks with no acute thrombosis. Clinically, the patient has been free of symptoms for more than 36 months. Angiographic findings for this patient were uneventful, and there was good flow after 30 months of follow-up in spite of the stent deformation (Figures 1-2). Three patients have died of other AOD complications (myocardial infarction, cerebrovascular insult). No signs of restenosis were found at autopsy.

DISCUSSION

The phenomenon of abdominal angina has been known, described, and studied for a long time (17,18), with experimental work dating back to 1875 (19). As simple as the phenomenon may appear to be at first, its correct assessment and evaluation of the symptoms are difficult due to diagnostic differentiation from non-vascular causes of abdominal complaints (17,19,20). Besides anatomic clinical studies on asymptomatic patients with a relatively high rate of atherosclerotic changes in the visceral arteries (21), pathologic anatomical findings of the occlusive vascular disease often do not result in any symptoms (22,23). The only explanation for these phenomena is the very slow progression of the disease with the development of collaterals over time. Women appear to be affected by the disease more often than men (ratio, 2:1 to 4:1) (20). Atheromatous occlusive disease is the primary cause of abdominal angina (24). The prognosis for the condition is relatively unsatisfactory (21,25-27), with a post-operative mortality rate of 3 to 20%, a patency rate of 70 to 90%, a 5-year survival rate of 83%, and a 10-year survival rate of 62% (28,29).

An additional expansion of the non-surgical treatment of abdominal anginas is stent implantation in abdominal vessels (30). This application of endovascular stents, which appears to be especially risky in comparison to other stent indications, was only considered because of the experience gained from the use of stents in other vessel segments and in experimental investigations (14-16, 31-33). Implantation of endovascular stents provides an additional, possible form of therapy that can be used even when patients are not operable or are rated as a high operative risk because of generalized arteriosclerosis and a poor general condition. Prior to stenting, these latter patients could expect either eventual death due to mesenteric artery thrombosis with complete ischemia in the following intestinal segment, or the risk of high perioperative mortality in the event of an attempted emergency revision. The obvious discrepancy between radiologic findings of a deformed stent and the absolute freedom from symptoms in two patients in our series point to the importance of the clinical findings within the framework of the follow-up (34). The weakness of the stent design was a too low rigidity which made the prosthesis susceptible to denting from the outside (30,34). A higher rigidity was achieved by selecting a thicker tantalum wire; however, the ability to remove the stent must still be demonstrated.

REFERENCES

1. Glatzel H. Fettverzehr-Plasmacholesterin-Coronarsklerose. Die Ergebnisse der Epidemiologie. Z Kreil Forsch 1964;53:416.
2. Gresham GA. Atherosklerose: Ihre Ursachen und ihre potentielle Reversibilität. Triangel 1976;15:39-43.
3. Hess H, Marschall M. Rauchen und arterielle Gefäßerkrankung. Med Welt 1976;27:697.
4. Ratschow M. Das Altern als ätiologischer Faktor arterieller Verschlußkrankheiten. Med Welt 1963;717.
5. Völker D. Die bedeutung der Risikofaktoren für die Entwicklung der arteriellen Verschlußkrankheit. In: Trübestein G, ed. *Arterielle Verschlußkrankheit und tiefe Beinvenenthrombose.* Stuttgart: Thieme Verlag; 1984.

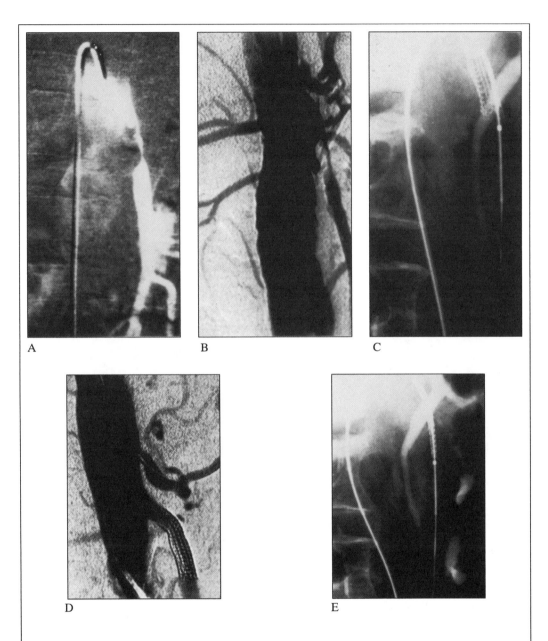

Figure 1. Among the typical symptoms of abdominal angina is severe stenosis of the superior mesenteric artery which does not demonstrate sufficient results even after PTA. It was possible to implant a tantalum stent in spite of the transfemoral access to the superior mesenteric artery. The stent is still patent 30 months after the implantation.

A) Stenosis in typical position shortly after the exit of the abdominal aorta.
B) Collapsed wall after dilation of the constricted vessel segment.
C) Inserting the tantalum stent from a transfemoral access.
D) The stent in its correct position in expanded condition.
E) Follow-up examination with patency of the superior mesenteric artery segment that is supplied with a stent.

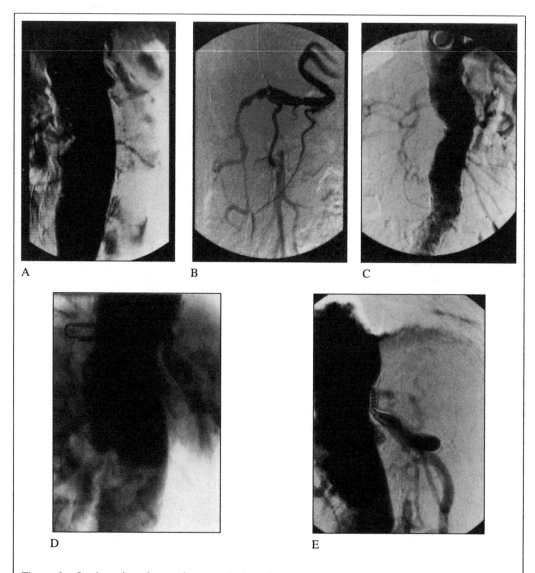

Figure 2. Implantation of a tantalum stent in the celiac artery.

A) An occlusion of the superior mesenteric artery and a severe constriction of the celiac artery in the exit area are found in an 83-year-old female patient with an abdominal angina. In the survey there was almost no visualization of the mesenteric vessels, although the abdominal aorta was already clearly filled.

B) After futile recanalization attempts of the superior mesenteric artery, the catheter was advanced beyond the exit stenosis to the area of the celiac artery. The angiographic visualization made it possible to recognize a longer occlusion of the proximal superior mesenteric artery segment. The caudal supply area of the superior mesenteric artery was also supplied via a pancreas arciform artery from the trunk.

C) The follow-up examination after attempted PTA and stent insertion demonstrated an early filling of the superior mesenteric artery's flow area, that was not filled before the distal aorta, through the supplied pancreas arciform arteries.

D) After the stent is cast off, a clear compression of the stent from the outside occurs, which prevents complete expansion but does not lead to a greater risk of thrombosis.

E) Follow-up showed patency as well as uneventful clinical signs, with good flow in spite of the stent compression.

6. Jenson CB, Smith GA. A clinical study of 51 cases of mesenteric infarction. Surgery 1956;40:930.

7. Rapp JH, Reily LM, Quarford PG. Durability of endarterectomy and antegrade grafts in the treatment of chronic visceral ischemia. J Vasc Surg 1986;4:338-344.

8. Castaneda-Zuniga WR, Gomes A, Weens C, Ketchum D, Amplatz K. Transluminal angioplasty in the treatment of abdominal angina. Röfo 1982;137:330-332.

9. van Denise WH, Zawacki JK, Phillips D. Treatment of acute mesenteric ischemia by percutaneous transluminal angioplasty. Gastroenterology 1986;91:475-478.

10. Furrer J, Gruentzig A, Kugelmeier J, Goebel N. Treatment of abdominal angina with percutaneous dilatation of an arterio-mesenteric superior stenosis. Cardiovasc Intervent Radiol 1980;5:367-369.

11. Golden DA, Ring EJ, McLean GK, Freimann DB. Percutaneous transluminal angioplasty in the treatment of abdominal angina. AJR 1982;139:247-249.

12. Saddenkni S, Sniderman KW, Hilton S, Sos TA. Percutaneous transluminal angioplasty of nonatherosclerotic lesions. AJR 1980;135:975-982.

13. Odurny A, Sniderman KW, Colapinto RF. Intestinal angina: percutaneous transluminal angioplasty of celiac and superior mesenteric arteries. Radiology 1988;165-167.

14. Liermann D, Strecker EP, Vallbracht C, Kollath J. Indikation und klinischer einsatz des Strecker-stents. In: Kollath J and Liermann D, eds. *Stents ein aktueller Überblick*. Konstanz: Schnetztor Verlag; 1990;24-37.

15. Liermann, D, Zegelman M, Kollath J, Satter P, Strecker EP. Is there a surgical contraindication against stents and is it possible to rescue a misplaced stent? Eur Radiol 1991;1:76.

16. Liermann D, Zegelman M, Jacobi V, et al. Ist ein plazierter Gefäßstent nach Fehlpazierung wieder entfernbar und stellt ein fehlplazierter Stent eine Kontraindikation zur TEA dar? Der Radiologe 1991;10,31:517-519.

17. Heberer G, Dostal G, Hoffmann K. Zur Erkennung und Behandlung der chronischen Mesenterialarterieninsuffizienz. Dtsch Med Wschr 1972;97:750.

18. Kümmel R. Über die Sklerose der Eingeweidearterien in der bauchhöhle. Zbl Allg Path Anat 1906;17:129.

19. Litten M. Über die Folgen des Verschlusses der Arteria mesenterica superior. Virchows Arch Path Anat 1875;63:289.

20. Stanton Jr PE, Hollier PA, Seidel TW, Rosenthal D, Clark M, Lamis PA. Chronic intestinal ischemia: diagnosis and therapy. J Vasc Surg 1986;4:338-344.

21. Beebe HG, McFarlane S, Raker IJ. Supraceliac aortomesenteric bypass for intestinal ischemia. J Vasc Surg 1987;5:749-754.

22. Cen M, Kämmerer K, Neef H. Verschluß der drei unpaaren Eingeweidearterien ohne klinische Symptomatik. Dtsch Med Wschr 1972;97:197.

23. Chiene J. Complete obliteration of the celiac and the mesenteric arteries, the visceral receiving their blood supply through the extraperitoneal system of vessels. J Anat Physiol 1868/69;3:65.

24. Derrick JR, Pollard HS, Moore RM. The pattern of atherosclerotic narrowing of the celiac and the superior mesenteric arteries. Ann Surg 1959;149:685.

25. Hollier LH, Bernatz PE, Pairolero PC, Payne WS. Surgical management of chronic intestinal ischemia: a reassessment. J Cardiovasc Surg 1981;22:601-602.

26. Rieferscheid M, Phillip R. Zur Problematik des rezidivierenden Adhäsionsileus. Zbl Chir 1967;92:370-374.

27. Todd IA, Pearson FG. Mesenteric vascular occlusion. Analysis of a series of cases and report of a successful embolectomy. Canad J Surg 1963;6:33.

28. Becker GJ, Katzen BT, Drake MD. Noncoronary angioplasty. Radiology 1989;170:921-940.

29. McCollum CH, Graham JM, DeBakey ME. Chronic mesenteric arterial insufficiency: results of revascularization in 33 cases. South Med J 1976;69:1266-1268.

30. Liermann, D, Strecker EP, Jacobi V, Peters J, Lörcher U, Kirchner J. Severe angina abdominalis treated by implantation of a highly flexible tantalum endoprosthesis. Angiology 1992;43:275.

31. Kollath J and Liermann D, eds. *Stents ein aktueller Überblick*. Konstanz: Schnetztor Verlag; 1990;24-37.

32. Kuhn FP, Kutkuhn B, Fürst G, Torsello G, Mödder U. Einsatz des Strecker Stents zur Therapie der nieren- und Transplantatnierenarterienstenose. In: Kollath J and Liermann D, eds. *Stents II*. Konstanz: Schnetztor Verlag; 1992;194-203.

33. Liermann D, Strecker EP, Peters J. The Strecker stent: indications and results in iliac and femoropopliteal arteries. Cardiovasc Intervent Radiol 1992;15:298-305.

34. Liermann D, Lörcher U, Rauber K, et al. Stents in the tracheobronchial system - first results. Eur Radiol 1991;1:55.

State of the Art Surgical Treatment of Portal Hypertension

V. Paolucci, B. Schaeff, K. Heller

J.W. Goethe University Hospital, Frankfurt am Main, Germany

INTRODUCTION

Since the mid-1940's surgery has played a leading role in the emergency and elective treatment of portal hypertension. However, in the last few years it has lost much of its importance due to the development of new endoscopic and interventional radiologic techniques. These latter techniques seem to produce similar results with regards to survival rate and the risk of recurrent bleeding, and at the same time cause fewer complications and side effects. The intent this paper is to give a short description of state of the art procedures and to define the present position of surgical treatment of portal hypertension.

The main objective of portal surgery is to stop esophageal variceal bleeding and to prevent recurrent bleeding. This is achieved by decreasing the portal pressure by means of a portosystemic shunt (shunt surgery) or by interrupting the spontaneous portosystemic gastroesophageal circulation (staple transsection).

SHUNT OPERATIONS

Elective or emergency shunt operations are only discussed after failed sclerotherapy (1,2). This is the case if esophageal hemorrhage occurs after two consecutive emergency interventions (3,4). We differentiate between complete shunts recanalizing the total portal blood flow, and selective shunts that bypass the esophageal region and maintain the portal hepatic blood circulation.

Common complete shunts consist of the following.

- Portacaval terminolateral anastomosis (Figure 1). The portal vein is completely ligated towards the liver and a vascular anastomosis is established end-to-side between the proximal trunk of the portal vein and the vena cava at the level of the hepatoduodenal ligament. The portal hepatic circulation is blocked completely.

- Portacaval terminolateral anastomosis with hepatic arterialization. The central portal vein stump is arterialized subsequent to portacaval anastomosis in order to compensate for the portal blood flow. For this purpose, a segment of the vena saphena is positioned between the right gastroepiploic artery (according to Adams) or the right common iliac artery (according to Matzander) and the portal vein stump. The objective is to avoid encephalopathy. The procedure requires much technique and bears the danger of over arterialization damaging the liver and causing ascites.

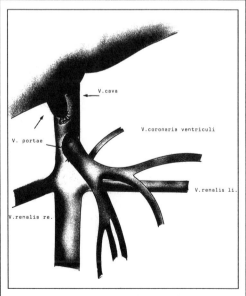

Figure 1. Portacaval terminolateral anastomosis (von Eck, 1877, Vidal 1903).

• Portacaval laterolateral anastomosis (Figure 2). A side-to-side anastomosis of about 2 cm is established between the portal vein and the vena cava. The technique of this shunt is more difficult than in the case of the terminolateral procedure. The portal vein stump remains open towards the liver which, however, does not produce a better hepatic perfusion but bears the danger of hepatofugal portal flow. For this reason the technique is hardly used anymore.

A broad shunt between the portal vein stump and the vena cava is best suited for a durable reduction of portal hypertension and thus constitutes the best treatment of esophageal bleeding (1). A disadvantage of any emergency portacaval anastomosis is the reduction in hepatic perfusion in patients with already reduced liver function prior to surgery. Mortality rates are between 10% for elective and 30% for emergency portacaval shunts. Encephalopathy rates average 30% or a little below following arterialization of the intrahepatic portal vein system. The 5-year survival rate is about 50% (5,6). Due to

these results the portacaval shunt was progressively abandoned in favor of selective anastomosis and emergency staple transsections.

• The proximal splenorenal anastomosis (Lintonshunt, Figure 3) numbers among the complete shunts. The procedure consists of splenectomy and an end-to-side anastomosis between the splenic vein and left renal vein. With a sufficient shunt volume, this anastomosis results in a massive pressure drop in the whole portal vein region with the danger of hepatofugal reflux. Experienced surgeons achieve a mortality rate during surgery of 12%, a 5-year survival rate of 41%, and an encephalopathy rate of 19% (7).

• The mesentericocaval anastomosis (H-shunt, Figure 4) consists of a shunt between the superior mesenteric vein and the vena cava. It is achieved by interposition of an 8 to 10-mm, polytetrafluoroethylene (PTFE) prosthesis. One indication is the pre-hepatic blockage of portal circulation. The encephalopathy rate corresponds to the portacaval anastomoses. In comparison, mortality during surgery is lower and the 5-year survival rate

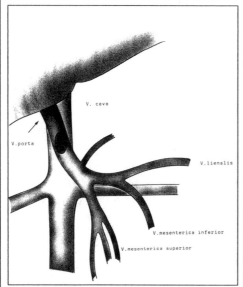

Figure 2. Portacaval laterolateral anastomosis (Rosenstein, 1912); not in use today.

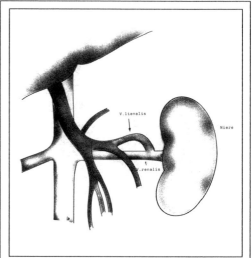

Figure 3. Proximal splenorenal shunt (Linton, 1956).

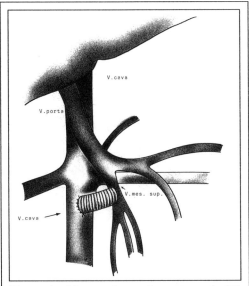

Figure 4. Mesentericocaval anastomosis (H-shunt; Drepanas, 1972).

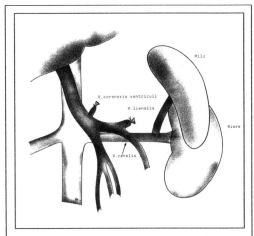

Figure 5. Distal spenorenal anastomosis (Warren, 1967).

amounts to 50% (8). The technique for this procedure is more difficult. The shunts show a thrombosis rate of about 30%.

Today, two kinds of selective shunt operations are primarily used. The best known is the distal splenorenal anastomosis (Warren shunt, Figure 5). An end-to-side anastomosis between the distal stump of the central splenic vein and the left renal vein is established (9). The spleen has to be conserved. The portal hepatic circulation is maintained through the superior mesenteric vein with the shunt leading to a selective transsplenic decompression of the gastroesophageal varices. Ligature of the coronary ventricular vein is part of this operation. Intraoperative mortality is below 10%, and a post-operative encephalopathy is observed in up to 30% of the patients (10). The main problems associated with this procedure (which has been favored in the last few years), are frequent thrombotic occlusions and an often insufficient pressure drop (11).

The coronariocaval anastomosis (Meursing-Shunt) is a rare kind of shunt between the coronary ventricular vein and the vena cava. The small size and the thin walls of the ventricular coronary vein explain why this selective shunt has little efficacy and is rarely applied.

STAPLE TRANSSECTIONS

In most cases, closure operations are a last resort for interrupting the collateral circulation. They do not result in a decrease of the portal vein pressure. The most common procedure for this is a combination of splenectomy, transsection of the ventricular coronary vein, and interruption of the blood supply to the distal esophagus by a clip suture anastomosis through the stomach (Figure 6). About 100 different modifications of this procedure have been described. Mortality during elective procedures is at about 12% and rises to 28.5 to 80% for emergency operations in Child stage C liver disease. A study under controlled conditions shows the best results for closure operations during emergency treatment of acute variceal bleeding. For this reason the authors recommend using the staple transsection in bleeding patients where sclerotherapy has not resulted in sufficient bleeding control (4,12).

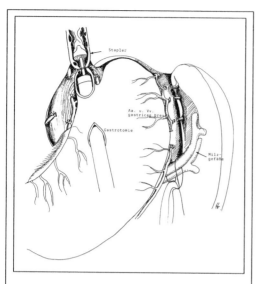

Figure 6. Typical staple transsection.

REFERENCES

1. Terblanche J. Portal hypertension management. Surg Endosc 1993;7:472-478.
2. Vogt DP, Hermann RE. End-to-side, side-to-side and interposition portacaval shunts. In: Nyhus LM and Baker RJ, eds. *Mastery of Surgery*. Boston: Little, Brown & Co.; 1992; 1115-1124.
3. Bornmann PC, Terblanche J, Kahn D, Jonker MA, Kirsch RE. Limitations of multiple injection sclerotherapy sessions for acute variceal bleeding. S Afr Med J 1986;70:34-36.
4. Burroughs AK, Hamilton G, Phillips A, Mezzanotte G, McIntyre N, Hobbs K. A comparison of sclerotherapy with stapler transection of the esophagus for the emergency control of bleeding from esophageal varices. N Engl J Med 1989;321:857-862.
5. Häring R. Notfallmäßige portosystemische Anastomosen bei der massiven Oesophagusvarizenblung. In: Siewart JR, Harder F, Allgöwer M, et al, eds. *Chirurgische Gastroenterolgie*. Berlin: Springer Verlag; 1990;1550-1557.
6. Wolff H. Elektive shuntsinklusive Warren-Shunt. In: Siewart JR, Harder F, Allgöwer M, et al, eds. *Chirurgische Gastroenterolgie*. Berlin: SpringerVerlag; 1990;1564-1573.
7. Ottinger LW. The Linton spleno-renal shunt in the management of the bleeding complications of portal hypertension. Ann Surg 1982;196:664-668.
8. Jarvinen H, Kallio H, Lempinen M. Interposition mesocaval shunt for bleeding esophageal varices in moderate and poor risk cirrhotics. Ann Chir Gynaecol 1981;70:45-49.
9. Warren WD, Henderson JM, Millikan WJ, et al. Distal splenorenal shunt versus endoscopic sclerotherapy for long-term management of variceal bleeding. Preliminary report of a prospective, randomized trial. Ann Surg 1986;203:454-462.
10. Rikkers LF. Prevention of recurrent bleeding: Selective shunt operations. In: Okuda K and Benhamou JP, eds. *Portal Hypertension. Clinical and Physiological Aspects*. Berlin: Springer Verlag; 1991;509-518.
11. Mosimann R, Marquis C, Mosimann F, Gertsch P. Long-term follow-up after a distal splenorenal shunt procedure. A clinical and hemodynamic study. Am J Surg 1983;145:253-255.
12. McCormick PA, Kaye GL, Greenslade L, et al. Esophageal staple transection as a salvage procedure after failure of acute injection sclerotherapy. Hepatology 1992;15:403-406.

TIPS: Concepts and Results

Goetz M. Richter[1], Gerd Nöldge[1], Thomas Roeren[1],
Guenter W. Kauffmann[1], Julio C. Palmaz[2]

[1]*Department of Diagnostic Radiology, University Hospital Heidelberg, Germany*
[2]*Department of Radiology, University of Texas Health Science Center, San Antonio, TX USA*

INTRODUCTION

In 1987 we submitted a pilot study application for the first clinical use of the transjugular intrahepatic portosystemic shunt (TIPS) procedure to the Institutional Revision Board of the University Hospital of Freiburg. The first successful procedure was accomplished in January, 1988 (1). Since that time, we have developed and improved the TIPS technique from the experience gathered in more than 200 patients (2-4). Initially, the study protocol restricted the use of the procedure to patients in whom conservative management with repeat sclerotherapy and vasoactive drugs failed to control bleeding and who were at a prohibitive risk for surgical shunts. Subsequent accumulation of technical and clinical experience encouraged a wider and more deliberate use of TIPS to include younger patients and patients with milder stages of liver disease.

STENTS FOR TIPS

There are currently several stents on the market which might offer promise for use in TIPS. Vascular stents are implanted as permanent devices and therefore, choice of material and design properties must be directed towards a maximum of intracorporeal endurability. In this regard, factors such as metal corrosion, structural weak points, or histologic inertness are of utmost importance. Stainless steel 316L has shown an excellent biocompatibility without any known corrosion problems. By contrast, tantalum alloys — the material used for the Strecker stent — are prone to relatively rapid intravascular corrosion. In addition to possible corrosion, specific design problems — or weak points — may add to failure in long-term durability. Therefore, in the design of a permanent vessel implant, crossing points with metal riding over metal (fretting corrosion) should be decreased to a minimum.

For the transjugular intrahepatic portosystemic stent shunt, two different stent types are widely used: the balloon-expandable Palmaz™ iliac stent (Johnson & Johnson Interventional Systems Co., Warren NJ) and the self-expandable Wallstent™ (Schneider, Zurich, Switzerland). The Palmaz stent consists of a single-segment, tubular stainless steel mesh, surgical grade 316L, with a wall thickness of 150 μm and an unexpanded length of 30 mm. Around its circumference, each stent has four staggered, offset slots that are 4.5-mm long. Its diameter in the non-expanded state measures 3.1 mm. Radial compression of the stent over a balloon catheter decreases this diameter by closure of the slots and, thus, firmly attaches the crimped stent to the catheter (7 Fr shaft). The Palmaz stent is a typical malleable stent that, when expanded, employs plastic forces to withstand hoop stress. Since it has no expansile force by itself, expansion of the coaxial balloon used for stent delivery will impose a force beyond the elastic limit of the metal mesh and thus, radially open the slots to quadrangles. It is because of this mode of action that this stent type has a wide range of possible luminal diameter which is solely dependent on the balloon size used for delivery. The Palmaz type is the only stent that allows such a variability. The size of the balloon applied for stent deployment determines the final expansion ratio.

By contrast, the Wallstent is a self-expandable vascular endoprosthesis which closely resembles a "Chinese finger". The basic metallic material from which the stent is manufactured is proprietary. A special delivery system is provided because of the spring load of the design. It consists of a 7 Fr catheter at the distal end by which the stent is both held in place and flattened down by a plastic membrane that covers the whole set. A sidearm is connected to the narrow interspace between the shaft and membrane. Immediately after the contrast medium is injected through this sidearm at a maximum limited pressure of 4 atm, friction between the membrane and the catheter shaft is minimized to allow pulling or rolling back of the membrane. This sets the stent free from distal to proximal as it pops up from its spring load. The Wallstent is very flexible and will open even when heavily bended or curved.

In addition to the above mentioned, two other stent types have been advocated for TIPS: the Gianturco™ stent (Cook, Bloomington IN) in the modified version by Rösch (5) and the Strecker™ stent (Boston Scientific Corp., Denmark). The Gianturco stent can be categorized as self-expanding and is made from spring-loaded, stainless steel wire which is bent into a zigzag pattern and soldered at the ends to form a closed circle. The thickness of the wire, its inherent spring load, the number of turns, and the angulation of the turns determine the final diameter and the resistance to hoop stress. Usually, a single stent cylinder is 2.5-cm long; for long segment stenting double or triple cylinders are available. For deployment, the stent can be pushed through a delivery cartridge in a compressed state. A specific feature of this stent is its availability in large diameters which is particularly useful in venous stenting. The Strecker stent is knitted from tantalum wire. As compared to the other stent types, it provides high flexibility but relatively low resist-ance to radial compression because of its loosely knitted loops.

TECHNIQUE

There were several complications during our early experience with TIPS. Many of these early problems have been published in detail (1-4). The following is a discussion of our current methodology which has reduced the procedural time from 7 hours to a little more than 2 hours in the majority of our cases.

Patient Preparation

A variety of appropriate clinical and laboratory tests should be performed before the TIPS procedure to allow for application of the Child and Turcotte classification of liver cirrhosis (6) in the modified version according to Conn (7). Subclinical hepatic encephalopathy can be diagnosed applying the Number Connection Test according to Conn (7) in an age-correlated version by Schomerus (8). Imaging procedures are performed to rule out malignant disease, infection, portal vein occlusion, and major anatomic abnormalities which might prevent successful performance of the procedure. Hence, abdominal ultrasound including Doppler sonography of the portal vein, chest radiography, and abdominal angiography are required. If hepatocellular carcinoma or portal vein occlusion is suspected, additional abdominal CT studies should be performed.

It is important to try to improve the clinical state of each individual patient before the TIPS procedure. This includes correction of hematocrit, protein, and coagulation deficits, bowel cleaning and sterilization, drainage of ascitic fluid, correction of electrolyte imbalance, and prophylactic broad-spectrum antibiotic therapy. Immediately before the procedure, 3 to 6 blood units should be cross-matched.

Anatomic Situation

We consider the creation of a wide, central, and more or less straight intrahepatic shunt tract as crucial for early and long-term success. In view of this consideration, the puncture tract should bridge the proximal part of either the right or the middle hepatic vein with the upper wall of either one of the main portal vein branches. Therefore, exact knowledge of the anatomic relationship between the portal bifurcation and the hepatic vein radicles is mandatory. In most patients the portal bifurcation is located anterior to the main stems of the hepatic veins, but there are several anatomic variants. Of particular interest is the discrimination of the origin and termination of the liver capsule in the course of the portal vein. An inadvertent puncture of the extracapsular part of the portal vein carries a high risk of life-threatening, intraabdominal bleeding. Both CT and ultrasound are helpful in identifying and defining the anatomic situation in each patient.

Transjugular Access

For sterility reasons the procedure is performed in the angiography suite on completely draped patients after careful skin preparation. Following sonographic documentation of the course of the right internal jugular vein and skin anaesthesia, a beveled 18-gauge cannula with a 5-mL syringe connected to the hub and filled with normal saline is introduced 4 to 5 cm cranial to the upper aspect of the clavicle at a very shallow angle to provide easy access for the large bore instruments to follow. When blood is drawn easily, a 0.035-inch J guidewire is inserted and manipulated down to the inferior vena cava under fluoroscopic control to allow insertion of a long 9 Fr sheath (Terumo, Tokyo, Japan). If the wire does not advance to the inferior vena cava, a selective catheter is used.

3-D Orientation

Most of the difficulties associated with punctures aimed centrally and medially towards the portal bifurcation have been eliminated by guiding the puncture simultaneously through fluoroscopy and ultrasound. It has to be understood that compared to a normal liver, the sonographic appearance of a cirrhotic liver is significantly changed and vascular structures are much less visible. Hence, only state-of-the-art ultrasound technology demonstrates the relevant structures, particularly when equipped with color Doppler sonography.

Sonographic guidance from an intercostal lateral view visualizes both the bifurcation of the portal vein and hepatic veins. By directing the beam anteriorly or posteriorly, the length and angulation of the shortest shunt tract between both venous systems may be easily determined. In connection with CT studies this also helps to determine the orientation of the portal bifurcation in relation to the hepatic veins.

Puncture and Shunt Tract Creation

After establishment of transjugular access, the hepatic veins are catheterized. A 5 Fr multipurpose catheter (Terumo) is generally used to find the right hepatic vein. Angiographic documentation with the catheter tip positioned distally in the vein demonstrates the morphologic situation. Particular attention is given to the size of the vein at its inflow into the inferior vena cava and its diameter should be at least 10 mm. In some instances there is retrograde sinusoidal flow which quickly identifies the portal bifurcation. A superstiff wire is then inserted which helps to visualize the vein by ultrasound. An 8 Fr guiding catheter from the TIPS set which we designed (Angiomed, Karlsruhe, Germany) is then introduced over the wire. A puncture device, specially designed for the TIPS procedure, is provided which features a blunt 50-cm long cannula that has a 15 G shaft tapered to 17.6 G at the tip. The cannula is pre-bent to 30° and is stiff for sufficient torque control. To function as a needle, an inner mandril made from nitinol is inserted into the cannula; this is extremely sharp and highly flexible and has a smooth transition from its tip to the cannula. The cannula can be inserted into the liver over a stiff wire or by using a blunt obturator which is also part of the set and made from nitinol. In most cases the curve of the needle is changed to adopt the angle at which the hepatic vein enters the inferior vena cava. If this happens to be near 90° angulation, heavy manual bending is required.

With the aid of ultrasound and fluoroscopy the optimal puncture site is chosen. Ultrasound usually helps to identify a position in the hepatic vein from which a short and straight course to the portal bifurcation is achieved. The cannula is then securely held in place and the sharp mandril inserted and locked to the hub of the cannula. The needle is rotated according to the predetermined puncture direction. Significant resistance is felt as soon as the needle reaches the portal vein wall and must be overcome with some pushing force. Correct portal access is confirmed as soon as the sharp mandril is removed and blood returns upon aspiration; contrast medium injection should confirm the situation. During this highly critical step, the needle must be held perfectly in place. With the needle tip pointing medially, a special stiff wire (0.035 inch) is passed, which generally travels down to the superior mesenteric vein because of its olive-shaped tip (also part of the puncture set). The guiding catheter is pushed over both the wire and cannula into the portal vein; this usually requires considerable force. In some cases the wire lodges in the peripheral portal branches instead of going centrally. A selective catheter must then be used to direct the wire centrally. In these cases a Terumo wire is more useful than our olive-shaped wire.

Once stable portal access is achieved, the shunt tract is pre-dilated to 8 mm utilizing low profile, 5 Fr angioplasty catheters. Typically, upon initial inflation a balloon waist forms at the entry site of the puncture tract into the portal wall. In most cases several minutes of inflation are needed for complete balloon expansion and effacement of the waist.

Stenting and the Hemodynamic Concept

It is generally accepted that an absolute portal pressure of higher than 20 mm Hg or a portosystemic gradient of greater than 15 mm Hg increases the risk of variceal bleeding. This is true both for spontaneously occurring bleeding episodes and for recurrence of bleeding after surgical shunts. Conversely, a low portosystemic gradient accompanied by high volume shunt flow may significantly increase the risk of hepatic encephalopathy. We prefer to lower the portosystemic gradient to approximately 12 mm Hg. Careful measurement of the portal pressure conditions is a crucial point in the procedure. We typically monitor the portosystemic gradient before pre-dilation of the above described shunt tract. The tract is then completely scaffolded from its entry site at the portal system into the liver vein using a technique identical to arterial stenting. Stenting is performed through a special 35-cm long sheath which is also part of the TIPS set. We use as many Palmaz stents as necessary with an overlap of several millimeters and an initial diameter of 8 mm. The flow conditions in the hepatic vein are very important and the "outflow" must be wide enough to accept the shunt flow. It may become appropriate, therefore, to stent the entire hepatic vein if it is too small. Upon completion of the stent shunt with an initial diameter of 8 mm, the portosystemic gradient is again monitored. Unless substantial portal decompression within a range of 10 to 13 mm Hg is measured, stepwise increase of the shunt diameter is performed by applying balloon dilation in 1-mm increments until the desired pressure level is reached. The stented segment within the liver is flared to a trumpet shape by dilating it with a 12-mm balloon which is performed to allow easier follow-up catheterization.

Variceal Embolization

The need for variceal embolization as an adjunct to a successful TIPS procedure in an acutely bleeding patient is a major concern and a somewhat unclear issue. In our opinion, simultaneous embolotherapy (by whatever means) in addition to creation of a well-functioning shunt, may potentially help to speed patient recovery. Acutely bleeding patients in whom medical treatment fails to control variceal hemorrhage usually present in a poor or critical clinical state because of substantial intestinal blood loss, coagulopathy (possibly worsened by mass transfusion), and hepatic encephalopathy. Failed intravenous therapy with vasopressin and prolonged inflation times of the gastroesophageal balloon add to the life-threatening situation.

Patient Monitoring During TIPS

Significant pain usually accompanies dilation of the shunt tract and stent deployment which should be alleviated by appropriate intravenous pain medication under oxygen saturation monitoring. Inadvertent catheter or wire passage into the right ventricle frequently happens at a variety of stages during the procedure and could activate severe arrhythmia. Constant ECG monitoring is therefore required, with antiarrhythmic medication ready at hand.

Specific Medication for TIPS and Post-Procedural Care

In elective procedures 3 to 6 units of whole blood are prepared depending on the patient's coagulation status, hemoglobin level, and total blood count. In cases of significant coagulation abnormalities (prolongation of the partial thromboplastin time [PTT] by more than 30% and/or decrease of the prothrombin time [PT] level to below 50% of normal), 4 to 8 units of fresh frozen blood are ordered to allow instantaneous infusion to treat any bleeding complication if necessary (also see below). Broad-spectrum antibiotic therapy is started on the day of the procedure and continued for an additional 2 days. Immediately prior to stent deployment, heparin is administered according to the coagulation status of the patient. Patients with PT levels of > 60% of control receive 5000 units while patients with PT < 60% and > 45% receive 2500 units. Therapeutic heparinization is maintained for an additional 2 days in patients with generally normal coagulation and antiplatelet medication is established for 3 months.

In emergency shunting the full range of conservative methods to control variceal hemorrhage should have been established and functioning (occlusion tubes, beta blockers, and vasoconstrictor infusions). General anaesthesia is required for patients in danger of aspiration or for those with severe encephalopathy who failed to cooperate during the procedure. In acutely bleeding patients, broad-spectrum antibiotic therapy should be initiated at least 1 day before the procedure along with medication and measurements for mechanical and biologic clearing of the bowel from blood and bacteria.

After successful completion of the TIPS procedure, patients are kept in the intensive care unit until a stable clinical situation is guaranteed and there are no signs of gastrointestinal hemorrhage, pulmonary infection, and renal and hepatic malfunction. The length of hospital stay depends on the general clinical status of the patient.

In the early post-procedural phase endoscopic reevaluation of variceal filling is confirmed to obtain baseline information as to visible changes in comparison with the situation before TIPS. If variceal reduction is not observed and there are no signs of hepatic encephalopathy, the patient may be rescheduled for shunt redilation. This is easily performed by simple re-expansion of the stent shunt with bigger balloons.

Normal nutrition is allowed for patients with near normal liver function. In patients with abnormal liver function, a low protein diet is instituted.

Direct portography is performed 3, 6, and 12 months after TIPS as part of our routine follow-up examination. The healing pattern of the stent shunt is examined and patients are observed for the possible onset of intimal hyperplasia (see below).

RESULTS

Changes in Study Population and Success Rates

More than 6 years have elapsed since our first TIPS procedure (1). Initially, only very high risk patients were selected. With promising results emerging from our first year of clinical application (2,3), TIPS application was expanded to include patients with failed surgical shunts, those refractory to medical treatment for severe ascites, and patients who were awaiting liver transplantation. With broadening of the inclusion criteria, difficulties arose in the interpretation of clinical benefit and long-term success of the procedure. As recently reported (4), the technical success rate in our first 24 patients was 75%. Failures resulted from an inability to puncture the portal vein because of equipment problems as detailed above. Since then, only one additional failure has occurred. Our total success rate is 92% with a technical success rate in 1993 of 97%.

30-Day Mortality and Complications

The 30-day mortality rate in the first 13 (out of 18) successful cases was 15% (2-4). This has completely changed with the advent of better materials and puncture techniques (see above). Among almost 200 procedures completed by simultaneous fluoroscopic and sonographic guidance, only four deaths occurred which were directly related to the procedure and resulted from inadvertent puncture of the extracapsular portal vein and onset of immediate exsanguination. The overall early mortality rate was 6.7%. Other deaths resulted from disease-related problems such as sepsis or hepatic failure. Minor complications included transient elevation of bilirubin and transaminases without unfavorable sequelae. Mild signs of hemolysis occurred in two patients which could not be sufficiently explained. In six patients, balloon rupture upon stent placement required sophisticated stent correction methods; all were successful.

30-Day Clinical Success

The total early clinical success rate was 93.3% while rebleeding was encountered in 6.7% during the 30-day period. Five patients rebled from pre-existing severe ulcerative and erosive esophageal and gastric mucosal disease, probably caused by extensive sclerotherapy trials accompanied by prolonged inflation times of occlusion balloons. Our very first patient in the series had widespread mucosal bleeding 2 days after TIPS which was most likely due to disseminated intravascular coagulopathy from accelerated absorption of ascites with imbalance of fibrinolysis. This was controlled by blood transfusions and fresh frozen plasma (1). In two other patients, bleeding events continued for approximately 2 weeks.

30-Day Encephalopathy

In addition to mortality and shunt occlusion, hepatic encephalopathy is one of the main problems associated with shunt surgery (9-16) and a crucial issue in TIPS. In nonselective shunts the post-operative rate of hepatic encephalopathy may rise to 50% (15-17). Even in selective shunts an incidence of hepatic encephalopathy as high as 20% has been reported (15-17). In our series, 14% developed *de novo* hepatic encephalopathy during the first 30 days which was controlled by appropriate medical treatment. More importantly, worsening of symptoms did not occur in any of our stage C patients; they almost invariably presented with hepatic encephalopathy before TIPS. Conversely, those patients who had hepatic encephalopathy attributable to severe acute bleeding and significant intestinal protein uptake improved as soon as the shunt was functional. These findings are reflected by variations in ammonia levels. Most of the patients with normal values before TIPS did not exceed the critical threshold during follow-up. In patients with increased values due to active bleeding, ammonia levels generally decreased after TIPS. At the present time, the number of patients appears to be still too small for final conclusions as to the definitive risk of hepatic encephalopathy in TIPS. The relatively low incidence of *de novo* hepatic encephalopathy should be considered as a positive trend favoring the concept of partial diversion of portal flow volume with small calibre interposition shunting TIPS.

Late Results

The actuarial 1-year survival rate is 70%, with a 3-year survival rate of 50%. Four patients have been referred for liver transplantation because of progressive decrease of liver function during a period of 5 months (4.1%).

De novo encephalopathy was seen in 4.7% of patients during late follow-up which was mostly attributable to failure to respond to protein uptake restriction. In all, adequate hydration and re-establishment of correct dietary schedules retained normal brain function.

Intimal hyperplasia during the first 6 months after the TIPS procedure is an important feature in patients with good liver function and normal or close-to-normal coagulation. In almost all patients with Child stage A liver disease, major intimal hyperplasia was seen both within the stented shunt segments and in the free area of the hepatic vein. It was never seen in the portal vein. When hemodynamically necessary, as determined by portosystemic pressure gradient monitoring, correction by either redilation or additional stenting of hepatic vein segments may be easily achieved. By contrast, such intimal hyperplasia is rare in patients with reduced liver function. This underscores the thrombogenic property of metallic stents, particularly in areas without functioning endothelium and well-functioning blood coagulation. The rate of reintervention for intimal hyperplasia is demonstrated in Table 1 according to Child's classification. These results also show that, after a certain time span, the shunt surface becomes inactive, ultimately leading to a safe intrahepatic neovascular channel.

Thrombogenicity and inadvertent intimal hyperplasia appear to be some of the unsolved problems of the TIPS procedure which warrant further research.

Table 1. Reintervention Rate After TIPS Procedure Because of Shunt Stenosis

Classification	3 Months	6 Months	12 Months
Child A	95%	41%	11%
Child B	62%	15%	4%
Child C	5%	1%	0%
Total	46%	17%	6%

INDICATIONS FOR TIPS

Six years have elapsed since our first successful TIPS application. This time span still appears too short to define "absolute" indications. Rather, we propose to consider indications for the procedure relative to well-established methods for the treatment of portal hypertension. Before a TIPS procedure is indicated, an experienced endoscopist should rule out further treatment options such as variceal eradication and/or medical treatment. The following indications seem appropriate for TIPS:

- Chronically recurring variceal bleeding despite sclerotherapy.
- Recurrent variceal bleeding and severe ulcerative or erosive disease from repeat sclerotherapy.
- Repeated bleeding episodes from major gastric varices inaccessible for sclerotherapy.
- Recurrent variceal bleeding from occluded surgical shunts.

When patients are admitted for TIPS because they pose an unacceptable risk for surgery, their presentation implies a negative case selection profile. For this particular subset of patients, no therapeutic choice other than TIPS exists. For patients in class A or B of the Child and Turcotte classification of liver disease (6) who are suitable for surgery, the classical therapeutic option has been the distal splenorenal shunt (DSRS, or Warren shunt). In such patients, TIPS seems to be competitive with surgery (12,16,18).

It is our belief that more time and experience with a much wider clinical background will be necessary to enable stage-related and risk-stratified analysis of patency rates, risk of encephalopathy, and both morbidity and mortality of the TIPS method in comparison with shunt surgery. To date, however, it seems safe to state that TIPS can be recommended for patients already enrolled in a liver transplantation program who are threatened by a high bleeding risk. In these patients, the performance of a TIPS procedure leaves the main vascular structures untouched contrary to shunt surgery. Previous shunt surgery is known to increase surgical difficulties and morbidity upon liver transplantation.

It is still unclear whether TIPS should be offered to patients with untractable ascites. Our long-term results in this particular subset of patients are still too limited to allow more than preliminary conclusions. It appears from our experience that TIPS is very beneficial for patients in whom ascites have been rapidly developing and are associated with a high portosystemic pressure gradient. By contrast, in patients with a long history of liver cirrhosis, borderline liver failure, and small organ size without a very pronounced pressure component, TIPS may lead to rapid liver failure from deprivation of portal blood nutrition. Therefore, it seems very critical to measure the venous occlusion pressure beforehand in patients referred for TIPS for treating intractable ascites. This may help to separate patients that will not benefit from the procedure and should be left untreated or transferred to a liver transplantation program.

CONTRAINDICATIONS

The contraindications for TIPS are not necessarily the same as those of shunt surgery because the radiological intervention is much less invasive. Four absolute contraindications exist, however, and include:

• Right heart failure or other cardiopulmonary factors contributing to substantial elevation of right ventricular pressure (chronic or acute left heart failure, cor pulmonale, etc.).

• Sepsis. Special attention must be paid to pulmonary infection as this may easily develop from aspiration pneumonia during bleeding episodes and sclerotherapy. Infected ascitic fluid can also be a pertinent feature in long-standing liver cirrhosis.

• Significant acute liver failure not attributable to active bleeding.

• Presence of hepatocellular carcinoma (HCC) engorging or infiltrating the vascular structures or the parenchyma of the liver neighboring the proposed shunt tract.

A relative contraindication is portal vein occlusion. With wider clinical application of the TIPS concept, more experience with this problem has emerged. In a recent update the San Francisco group reported a 70% initial success rate in such patients (E. Ring, personal communication). A final contraindication is peripheral small HCC in patients unfit for surgical resection.

REFERENCES

1. Richter GM, Palmaz JC, Nöldge G, et al. Der transjuguläre intrahepatische portosystemische stent-shunt (TIPSS). Radiologe 1989;29:406-411.

2. Richter GM, Nöldge G, Palmaz JC, et al. Transjugular intrahepatic portacaval stent shunt: preliminary clinical results. Radiology 1990;174:1027-1030.

3. Richter GM, Nöldge G, Palmaz JC, Rössle M. The transjugular intrahepatic portosystemic stent-shunt (TIPSS): results of a pilot study. Cardiovasc Intervent Radiol 1990;13:200-207.

4. Richter GM, Nöldge G, Palmaz JC, Rössle M. Evolution and clinical introduction of TIPSS, the transjugular intrahepatic portosystemic stent-shunt. Sem Intervent Radiol 1991;8:331-340.

5. Rösch J, Uchida BT, Putnam JS, et al. Experimental intrahepatic portacaval anastomosis: use of expandable Gianturco stents. Radiology 1987;162:481-485.

6. Child CG, Turcott JG. Surgery and portal hypertension. In: Child, CG ed. *The Liver and Portal Hypertension*. Philadelphia: WB Saunders; 1964.

7. Conn HO. Trailmaking and number-connection test in the assessment of mental state in portal systemic encephalopathy. Am J Dig Dis 1977;22:541-550.

8. Schomerus H, Hamster W, Reinhard U, Mayer K, Dölle W. Latent portosystemic encephalopathy. Dig Dis Sci 1981;26:622-630.

9. Galambos JT. Portal hypertension. Sem Liver Dis 1985;5:277-290.

10. Johansen K. Partial portal decompression for variceal hemorrhage. Am J Surg 1989;157:479-482.

11. Lafortune M, Patriquin H, Pomier G, et al. Hemodynamic changes in portal circulation after portosystemic shunts: use of duplex sonography in 43 patients. AJR 1987;149:701-706.

12. Millikan WJ, Warren WD, Henderson JM, et al. The Emory prospective randomized trial: selective versus non-selective shunt to control variceal bleeding. Ann Surg 1985;201:712-722.

13. Ohnishi K, Saito M, Sato S, et. al. Direction of splenic venous flow assessed by pulsed Doppler flowmetry in patients with large splenorenal shunts. Relation to spontaneous hepatic encephalopathy. Gastroenterol 1985;89:180-189.

14. Pagliaro L, Burroughs AK, Sorensen TIA, et al. Therapeutic controversies and randomized controlled trials (RCTs): prevention of bleeding and rebleeding in cirrhosis. Gastroenterol Intern 1989;2:71-84.

15. Spina GP, Galeotti F, Opocher E, et al. Selective distal splenorenal shunt versus side-to-side portacaval. Clinical results of a prospective controlled study. Am J Surg 1988;155:564-571.

16. Warren WD, Millikan WJ Jr, Henderson JM, et al. Ten years portal hypertensive surgery at Emory: results and new perspectives. Ann Surg 1982;195:530-542.

17. Palmaz JC, Garcia F, Sibbit SR, et al. Expandable intrahepatic portacaval shunt stents in dogs with chronic portal hypertension. AJR 1986;147:1251-1254.

18. DeLacy AM, Nevasa M, Garcia-Pagan JC, et al. Reversal of portal flow after distal splenorenal shunt (DSRS). Relationship to hepatic encephalopathy and impaired liver function. J Hepatology 1989;9(Suppl):S142.

Transjugular Intrahepatic Portosystemic Shunt with Strecker Stent

Antonio Echenagusia[1], Fernando Camuñez[1], Gonzalo Simó[1], Javier Peiró[2]

[1]Department of Radiology, General Hospital Universitario Gregorio Marañón, Madrid, Spain
[2]Department of Radiology, Hospital de Basurto, Bilbao, Spain

INTRODUCTION

The transjugular intrahepatic porto-systemic shunt (TIPS) procedure is a new, non-operative method of portal decompression. In animal studies, balloon-expandable and self-expandable metallic stents have demonstrated their ability to hold open the parenchymal tract between the portal and hepatic venous systems (1-4). The first clinical TIPS procedure using balloon-expandable metallic stents was reported by Richter et al (5); subsequently, several reports have stressed the clinical feasibility of TIPS using various types of stents (6-10). We report the results obtained with TIPS in 45 patients using Strecker stents.

MATERIALS AND METHODS

Prior to performing the TIPS procedure, arterial portography was performed to determine the patency and anatomy of the portal vein. Whenever possible, the diagnostic study was performed a few days before the procedure. In the first two patients the procedure was carried out using a combined transjugular and transhepatic approach. The transjugular approach was used alone in the subsequent patients. After selection of an appropriate hepatic vein, a 10 Fr, 41-cm long introducer sheath (Cook, Europe) was advanced into the vein. The intrahepatic puncture was performed using a coaxial catheter-needle system developed by Rösch (transjugular intrahepatic portosystemic shunt set, Cook). The components of this system and its mode of use have been reported elsewhere (11).

Once the portal vein was entered, portography and pressure measurements were carried out. Depending on the size of the stent to be inserted, the parenchymal tract was then dilated using a 7 Fr, 8- or 10-mm diameter high pressure balloon catheter. After dilation a portography was performed to document the hepatic tract, following which one or more stents were deployed. Strecker™ stents (Boston Scientific Corp., Denmark) were used in all cases. Stent diameter was 11 mm in 35 patients and 9 mm in 7 patients. After deployment of the stent, portography and pressure measurements were again performed (Figure 1). If the portography showed good flow and the portosystemic gradient fell to below 12 mm Hg, no subsequent operations were performed. If the portosystemic gradient remained high, the stent was dilated with a high pressure balloon 1-mm larger than the diameter of the prosthesis to achieve complete expansion of the stent. Follow-up examinations included clinical evaluation and Doppler ultrasound examination at 1, 3, 6, 9, 12, and 18 months. Portal venography was performed in any patient who developed recurrent bleeding. In asymptomatic patients elective portal venography and pressure measurements were performed after 2 to 5 and 7 to 12 months.

RESULTS

Patients

Between September, 1991 and February, 1993, 45 patients with variceal hemorrhage underwent treatment with the TIPS procedure. The patient population consisted of 29

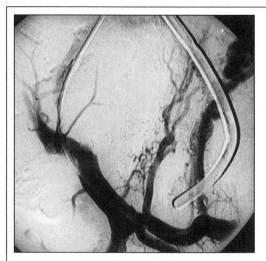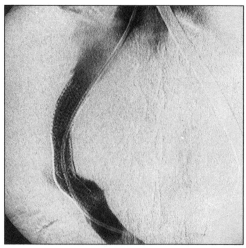

Figure 1. Images of a 52-year-old woman with acute variceal hemorrhage who underwent TIPS placement. Initial portal venogram *(left)* shows large esophageal varices. Portal venogram obtained after shunt creation *(right)* shows no filling of varices and good flow through the shunt.

men and 16 women ranging in age from 25 to 76 years (mean, 57 years). All patients presented with liver cirrhosis (alcoholic [N=28], post-necrotic [N=15], primary biliary [N=1], cryptogenic [N=1]) and portal hypertension with endoscopically confirmed gastric and/or esophageal varices. According to the Child-Pugh classification of hepatocellular disease, 6 patients had class A disease, 30 patients had class B disease, and 9 patients had class C disease. Prior to the procedure, ascites was detected in 23 patients and clinically apparent encephalopathy was recorded in 14 patients.

All patients underwent TIPS to treat acute or recurrent variceal hemorrhage that did not respond to sclerotherapy. In 12 patients the procedure was performed on an emergency basis because of continued bleeding, despite endoscopic and pharmacologic treatment. The procedure was performed electively in 33 patients after a period of at least 24 hours without hemorrhage. The average number of episodes of prior variceal bleeding was three.

Immediate Results

TIPS placement was technically successful in 42 (93.3%) of the 45 patients. Shunts were formed from the right or middle hepatic vein to the right portal vein in 31 patients, to the left portal vein in 7 patients, and to the portal bifurcation in 4 patients. The portosystemic pressure gradient was reduced from an average of 20.4 ± 5.4 mm Hg before creation of the shunt to 9.2 ± 4.1 mm Hg immediately afterwards. Following TIPS, bleeding was controlled in all 12 patients with acute variceal hemorrhage. The 60-day mortality rate was 4.7% (N=2). Color Doppler examinations performed during the first week after the procedure revealed a patent shunt in 41 of 42 patients.

Complications occurred in five patients. One patient developed right jugular vein thrombosis after the procedure. Post-procedural bacteremia was noted in another patient which was successfully treated with antibiotics. Acute thrombosis of the shunt occurred in two patients; the shunt was successfully reopened in one patient. In one case the stent was dislodged during withdrawal of the balloon catheter. The stent was removed through a 12 Fr sheath using retrieval forceps, and a new stent was successfully placed in the liver tract.

Follow-Up Results

Thirty-nine patients with patent shunts at discharge have been followed for periods ranging from 3 to 18 months (mean, 8.9 months). Six patients (15.3%) experienced variceal rebleeding due to shunt stenosis or occlusion. These patients were treated percutaneously by balloon angioplasty and/or stent placement with good angiographic and clinical immediate results. During the follow-up after shunt revision, four patients experienced a second episode of variceal rebleeding, and two patients died of these causes (see below). A further two patients remain asymptomatic at 3 and 8 months, respectively.

Three patients died during the follow-up period. Two died of variceal bleeding 4 and 8 months after TIPS placement while the third patient died of cerebral hemorrhage 14 months after TIPS. New or worsened encephalopathy developed in six patients after TIPS. In five of these patients the encephalopathy was well controlled with conventional medical therapy. Twenty-one patients presented with clinically evident ascites prior to TIPS; 16 of these patients experienced a significant improvement after TIPS placement.

During follow-up, the shunt was controlled by direct portal venography in 33 asymptomatic patients. Fourteen patients (42.4%) presented hemodynamically significant stenoses requiring further intervention. Stenoses were located within the stent in two patients and in the hepatic vein in 12 patients (Figure 2). All 14 patients were successfully treated by balloon dilation (N=4) or by repeat stent placement (N=10). After shunt revision all patients remained asymptomatic at a mean follow-up time of 4.1 months.

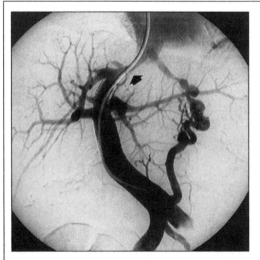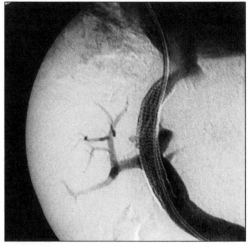

Figure 2. Follow-up portogram *(left)* taken in an asymptomatic patient 4 months after TIPS placement showing marked narrowing of the hepatic vein (arrow). Note filling of the large coronary vein. The portosystemic gradient was 17 mm Hg. Good flow was achieved after balloon dilatation and deployment of a new stent *(right)*, with the portosystemic gradient falling to 9 mm Hg.

DISCUSSION

The TIPS procedure is a new, non-operative method of treating variceal hemorrhage. Previously, both Palmaz stents and Wallstents have been used in the clinical creation of shunts (6,7,9). In our opinion, the Strecker stent is a satisfactory alternative for the TIPS procedure because it offers good visibility during fluoroscopy, has a high degree of longitudinal flexibility, and shortening of the stent during placement is negligible. These qualities enable the stent to be precisely deployed in hepatic tracts of any shape, thus simplifying the procedure.

In our series, the mean percentage reduction in the portosystemic gradient attained after the TIPS procedure was 55%. This decrease was similar to that reported by Adam et al (12) for 10-mm portacaval H-grafts and indicates that TIPS is an effective method of achieving portal decompression. Thus, in our experience the TIPS procedure has proven to be a highly efficacious treatment for acute variceal hemorrhage.

An essential aspect of any therapy for variceal hemorrhage is its ability to prevent subsequent rebleeding episodes. The incidence of recurrent bleeding in our series was 15.3%, but our follow-up has still been too short for comparison of our results with the results of other treatments.

The incidence of new or more severe encephalopathy following TIPS was 15.3% in our series which is within the range of 10 to 20% reported by others (9,10,13). It should be underscored that in most cases the encephalopathy was mild and easily managed; only 2.5% of our patients developed severe encephalopathy. Control of ascites improved after TIPS in 76% of the patients who presented with ascites in our series. These results suggest that the TIPS procedure may be beneficial in controlling ascites. None of our patients, however, underwent TIPS placement for refractory ascites; hence, final conclusions cannot be drawn from our data. In our experience, only direct portography furnished sufficient information for assessing shunt patency in asymptomatic patients. Hemodynamically significant stenoses, mainly in the hepatic vein, were found in 42% of our asymptomatic patients. This finding indicates that intimal hyperplasia is a commonly occurring complication subsequent to TIPS placement and a cause of shunt dysfunction in a substantial proportion of patients. It is our opinion that direct portography should be employed to monitor shunts and verify shunt patency in asymptomatic patients.

CONCLUSIONS

In conclusion, the TIPS procedure is an effective method of achieving portal decompression and is particularly effective in the treatment of acute variceal hemorrhage. TIPS placement is also useful in the short-term prevention of variceal rebleeding. The TIPS procedure can be performed in most patients with low morbidity and mortality. Intimal hyperplasia after TIPS placement is a commonly encountered complication requiring reintervention in a substantial number of patients.

REFERENCES

1. Palmaz JC, Sibbit RR, Reuter SR, Garcia F, Tio FO. Expandable intrahepatic portacaval shunt stents: early experience in the dog. AJR 1985;145:821-825.
2. Palmaz JC, Garcia F, Sibbit RR, et al. Expandable intrahepatic portacaval shunt stents in dogs with chronic portal hypertension. AJR 1986;147:1251-1254.
3. Rösch J, Uchida BT, Putnam JS, Buschman RW, Law RD, Hershey AL. Experimental intrahepatic portacaval anastomosis: use of expandable Gianturco stents. Radiology 1987;162:481-485.
4. Cwikiel W, Stridbeck H. Experimental transjugular portacaval shunt: use of a fine-needle puncture device for the implantation of Strecker stents. Acta Radiol 1992;33:356-359.

5. Richter GM, Nöldge G, Palmaz JC, et al. Transjugular intrahepatic portacaval stent shunt: preliminary clinical results. Radiology 1990;174:1027-1030.

6. Richter GM, Nöldge G, Palmaz JC, Rössle M. The transjugular intrahepatic portosystemic stent-shunt (TIPS): results of a pilot study. Cardiovasc Intervent Radiol 1990;13:200-207.

7. Zemel G, Katzen BT, Becker GJ, Benenati JF, Sallee DS. Percutaneous transjugular portosystemic shunt. JAMA 1991;266:390-393.

8. Ring EJ, Lake JR, Roberts JP, et al. Using transjugular intrahepatic portosystemic shunts to control variceal bleeding before liver transplantation. Ann Intern Med 1992:116:304-309.

9. LaBerge JM, Ring EJ, Gordon RD, et al. Creation of transjugular intrahepatic portosystemic shunts with the Wallstent endoprosthesis: results in 100 patients. Radiology 1993;187:413-420.

10. Maynar M, Cabrera J, Pulido-Duque JM, et al. Transjugular intrahepatic portosystemic shunt: early experience with a flexible trocar/catheter system. AJR 1993;161:301-306.

11. Rösch J, Uchida BT, Barton RE, Keller FS. Coaxial catheter-needle system for transjugular portal vein entrance. JVIR 1993;4:145-147.

12. Adam R, Diamond T, Bismuth H. Partial portacaval shunt: renaissance of an old concept. Surgery 1992;111:610-615.

13. Conn HO. Transjugular intrahepatic portal-systemic shunts: the state of the art. Hepatology 1993;17:148-158.

TIPS with Self-Expandable Z-Stents

Josef Rösch, Robert E. Barton, Bryan D. Petersen,
Richard R. Saxon, Barry T. Uchida, Frederick S. Keller

*Dotter Interventional Institute, Oregon Health Sciences University and
Veterans Affairs Medical Center, Portland, OR USA*

Self-expandable Z-stents were used for creation of a transjugular intrahepatic portosystemic shunt (TIPS) in 28 patients with acute or recent gastroesophageal or stomal variceal bleeding. Ten-millimeter diameter stents placed in four patients resulted in suboptimal shunts. An effective portal decompression was later achieved in 24 patients with the use of 12-mm diameter stents. The Z-stent alone was sufficient for creation of a centrally-placed shunt in 19 of these patients. In the other five patients with shunts established more peripherally, a Wallstent had to be added to completely open the Z-stent which was narrowed at the portal vein entrance. Clinically, TIPS controlled variceal bleeding in all seven patients with acute hemorrhage and prevented recurrence of bleeding in 22 patients. Bleeding recurrence occurred in six patients, mainly in those with suboptimal shunts. Routine follow-up venographic studies at 6-month and 1-year intervals revealed shunt narrowing in a high percentage of patients, particularly in the hepatic vein, with good response to balloon dilation or new stent placement. All shunts were kept wide open and well functional with these additional interventions. The 12-mm diameter Z-stents are suitable devices for creation of centrally-placed TIPS.

INTRODUCTION

Transjugular intrahepatic portosystemic shunts (TIPS) have been performed mostly with self-expandable Wallstents (1-4) or balloon-expandable Palmaz stents (5-8). The first experience with TIPS created with Strecker balloon-expandable stents has been recently reported (9-10). In our series of 160 TIPS patients at the Dotter Interventional Institute, self-expandable Z-stents were used in 28 patients, mainly in our early experience. The other patients received Wallstents.

SELF-EXPANDABLE Z-STENTS

In 25 patients the biliary type Gianturco-Rösch™ self-expandable Z-stents were used (GRZ stents). The earlier patients received GRZ stents which were made in our research laboratory; the latter patients received stents obtained from Cook Surgical (Bloomington IN). The stents were 6- to 7.5-cm long and consisted of four to five 1.5-cm long stent bodies connected together with a monofilament suture. Early in our series, 10-mm diameter stents were used in four patients, in the latter 21 patients 12-mm diameter stents were used (Figure 1A). In the last three patients we created shunts with a new Z-stent modification — spiral Z-stents. These were also made in our research laboratory, had a 12-mm diameter, and were 6- to 8-cm long (Figure 1B) (11).

Both the biliary GRZ stents and the spiral Z-stents expanded spontaneously to a diameter about 2 mm smaller than their original size after introduction. They could be fully expanded to their original diameter, however, using an appropriate size balloon catheter. The Z-stents are very opaque, can be easily positioned, and their expansion can be followed under fluoroscopy, even in patients with ascites.

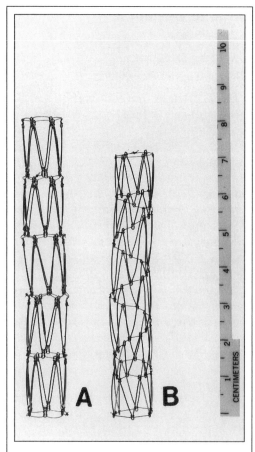

Figure 1. Self-expandable Z-stents used for creating TIPS.

A. Gianturco-Rösch biliary Z-stent
B. Spiral Z-stent

TECHNIQUE

A coaxial catheter needle set (RUPS-100, Cook) was used for transjugular liver puncture, portal vein entrance, and stent placement (12). The combination of the 10 Fr sheath, 10 Fr Teflon catheter, and metal cannula gives the set rigidity with good torque control and enabled us to select a suitable site for liver puncture. The puncture was performed with a 0.038-inch diameter needle inside a well-tapered 5 Fr Teflon catheter. From the proximal portion of the right hepatic vein the set was turned anteriorly and

the needle aimed distally to puncture the proximal portion of the right main portal vein. After gaining entrance into a portal branch and establishing good position of the 5 Fr catheter in the portal system, an Amplatz superstiff™ guidewire (Boston Scientific Corp., Watertown MA) was inserted. The 10 Fr Teflon catheter was then advanced with a leading 5 Fr catheter into the portal vein to dilate the liver puncture tract. A 5 Fr pigtail catheter was then inserted into the portal system for pressure measurement and portal venogram. Systemic pressure was simultaneously measured with the portal pressure of a 10 Fr sheath withdrawn into the inferior vena cava. Dilation of the liver puncture tract and portal and hepatic vein walls followed with a 10-mm diameter and 6-cm long balloon catheter (Cook). After dilation, the 10 Fr sheath was advanced together with a partially deflated balloon into the portal vein for stent deployment.

The stent was placed in the parenchymal liver tract with its ends protruding about 2 to 3 cm into both the portal and hepatic vein and its lumen oriented along the lumen of the veins. In six patients where the stent did not cover the entire liver tract or did not extend sufficiently into the hepatic or portal vein, another 4- to 6-cm long Z-stent was placed, partially overlapping the first stent. With insufficient stent expansion, usually at the portal vein entrance, a 10- or 12-mm dilation balloon was used for further expansion. In five patients where the Z-stent showed persistent narrowing and/or a kink even after balloon dilation or did not curve well into the portal or hepatic vein and was oriented against their wall, a 6.8-cm long, 10-mm diameter Wallstent™ (Schneider, Minneapolis MN) was added to further expand, extend, or better orient the inserted Z-stent. After stent placement, pressure measurements were taken and follow-up portograms obtained. Because we wanted to assess the efficacy of TIPS on control of variceal bleeding without additional interventions, we did not embolize gastroesophageal varices after TIPS, even when the patient was recently or actively bleeding during the study or when they were partially filled on follow-up portograms.

PATIENTS

Of the 28 patients, 18 were men; ages ranged from 29 to 80 years with a median of 56.2 years. Four were Child-Pugh class A, 11 were class B, and 13 were class C. At the baseline examination, encephalopathy was present in 16 patients and clinically apparent ascites was present in 21. TIPS was indicated for recurrent bleeding from gastroesophageal varices in 26 patients; 2 had the procedure performed for recurrent bleeding from varices around an ileostomy. Seven patients were acutely bleeding during the procedure; the others had several recent bleeding episodes after previous sclerotherapy.

RESULTS

The TIPS procedure was successfully established in all 28 patients and no complications related to the procedure were encountered. Three to four hours were necessary for the procedure in the early patients; after gaining experience and refining the technique, most of the procedures were completed in 60 to 90 minutes. In 22 patients, the portal system was entered and the shunt established in the right main portal branch, 1 to 4 cm from the portal vein bifurcation. The left main portal branch was the site of the shunt in four patients and the portal bifurcation in two patients.

With use of 10-mm diameter GRZ stents in four patients, a suboptimal shunt was created with a decrease in portal pressure ranging from 5 to 13 mm Hg (mean, 8 mm Hg). Follow-up venograms in these patients showed persistent moderate variceal filling. The portosystemic gradient was not evaluated in these early patients. The 24 patients who received 12-mm diameter stents had more effective shunts with portal pressure decreas-

ing from 10 to 25 mm Hg (mean, 15 mm Hg). An average portosystemic gradient after TIPS in these patients was 11 mm Hg (range, 6 to 14 mm Hg). Varices in these patients were not filled or showed only very slow, proximal visualization with stagnant flow on follow-up portograms.

The TIPS procedure was clinically successful and led to immediate arrest of bleeding in all seven actively bleeding patients with no recurrence of bleeding in 22 patients. In 13 patients, bleeding has not recurred up to the present time (15 to 42 months), in four patients until their liver transplant (1 to 15 months), and in five patients until their death (10 days to 20 months after TIPS). Bleeding recurred from 1 day to 4 months after TIPS in six patients. In two patients who had TIPS created with 12-mm diameter GRZ stents, bleeding recurred either due to inadequate stent length (1 day after TIPS) or secondary to persistence of large varices (5 days after TIPS). The addition of another stent and variceal embolization prevented recurrent rebleeding in these patients until the present, 18 and 27 months, respectively. The other four patients with recurrent bleeding had an inadequate TIPS with 10-mm diameter GRZ stents. One of these patients died 10 days after TIPS from liver failure and bleeding; his shunt was found thrombosed at autopsy. Another patient died 2 months after TIPS due to severe bleeding from a recurrent esophageal ulcer after sclerotherapy performed prior to TIPS. This patient did not have an autopsy. The other two patients with shunts created using a 10-mm diameter stent had recurrent bleeding 2 and 3 months, respectively, after TIPS; follow-up venograms revealed irregular stenoses of the parenchymal tract. They were successfully treated with balloon dilation and new stent placement; bleeding recurred several months later. These patients were subsequently treated with a liver transplant and surgical shunt, respectively.

The 30-day mortality rate was 14% (four patients). One patient died of ARDS, two of liver failure (in one combined with severe rebleeding), and the fourth patient of causes unrelated to TIPS. This latter patient had a pulmonectomy for bronchial carcinoma 2 weeks after successful TIPS and died of surgical complications. Three other patients died 2 to 21 months after TIPS. One aforementioned patient died of esophageal ulcer hemorrhage, another of myocardial infarction 8 months after TIPS, and the third due to liver failure 21 months after TIPS. Total mortality in our 28 patients was 25% with a follow-up period of up to 42 months.

Pre-existing encephalopathy and ascites responded well to TIPS and disappeared or significantly improved after the procedure. Of the 21 patients followed 3 and 6 months after TIPS, only five (24%) had mild to moderate encephalopathy which is well below the 57% occurrence rate prior to the procedure; all responded well to lactulose treatment. Mild ascites, detectable on physical examination, was present in only two patients (10%), again well below the 75% occurrence rate prior to TIPS. Child-Pugh classification also significantly improved after TIPS and the majority of the patients (13 of 21) were classified as Child-Pugh class A after TIPS with the others classified as Child-Pugh class B. Hepatic synthetic function improved after TIPS, particularly with regard to albumin which rose from 2.9 to 3.2 g/dL at 3- and 6-month follow-up evaluations. Slight but not statistically significant decreases in prothrombin time (14.8 to 14.1 sec) and total bilirubin (2.4 to 2.3 mg/dL) were noted.

Stent patency was evaluated in five patients with liver transplants by gross and histologic examination of the explanted liver and in 16 patients by routine follow-up venography. In three patients who received transplants from 1 to 6 months after TIPS, the shunts were well patent and stents diffusely covered with a thin pseudointima (Figure 2). Shunts in two patients transplanted 13 and 15 months after TIPS, respectively, were also patent but narrowed by an exuberant pseudointima. In the patient with the shunt created with a 10-mm diameter GRZ stent,

luminal narrowing exceeded 50%; in the other patient who had a 12-mm stent, narrowing was about 30% of the lumen.

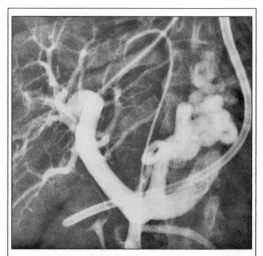

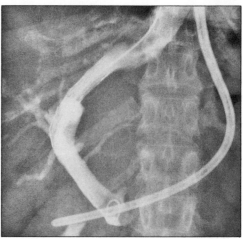

Figure 2. A 63-year-old woman with idiopathic cirrhosis and recurrent massive bleeding from large gastric varices. Her bleeding ceased immediately after the TIPS procedure and did not recur for 6 months at which time she received a liver transplant. Her shunt was widely patent at inspection and covered with fine pseudointima. Portal venogram after puncture of the left portal vein *(top)* reveals extensive gastric varices and retrograde filling of mesenteric veins. Portal pressure was 43 mm Hg. Portal venogram after TIPS *(bottom)* reveals almost complete shunting of the portal flow into the inferior vena cava. Portal pressure was 29 mm Hg; the patient had considerable splenomegaly.

Routine follow-up venographic studies in the 16 asymptomatic patients were scheduled every 6 months in the first 2 years after TIPS and yearly afterwards, but not all patients complied with this schedule. Fourteen patients had a follow-up examination at 6 months, nine patients at 12 months, six at 18 months, four at 24 months, and one at 36 months. Results of these examinations are summarized in Table 1. At the 6- to 18-month follow-up examinations, only 11 to 21% of shunts were considered to be well open with a lumen larger than 50% of stent diameter and a portosystemic gradient under 14 mm Hg. In 78 to 89% of our patients, shunts were narrowed to more than 50% of stent diameter and their portosystemic gradient was above 14 mm Hg. At 6 months, narrowings were localized more frequently in the hepatic vein portion of the shunt or hepatic vein above the stent than in the parenchymal tract. No portal vein narrowing was encountered. Most of the stenoses (64%) responded well to simple balloon dilation; the other stenoses needed additional stent placement for their correction. At follow-up examinations performed at 12 months and later, there was a trend towards increasing incidence of hepatic vein stenosis

and decreasing incidence of parenchymal tract narrowing with good response of stenoses to balloon dilation; the need for additional stents decreased (Figures 3 and 4).

Histologic studies of the stenotic shunt areas and narrowed hepatic veins revealed excessive pseudointimal and intimal proliferation with predominant collagen tissue formation. No ingrowth of liver tissue was observed inside the stent.

DISCUSSION

The biliary GRZ self-expandable stents have both advantages and disadvantages compared with the other expandable stents used for TIPS. Their placement is predictable because they do not shorten after delivery and, because of their opacity, are easy to follow fluoroscopically. Another advantage is their incomplete spontaneous expansion at delivery. After being pushed through the introducing sheath, their diameter is about 2-mm smaller than the original size. When needed, however, they can be fully expanded to their original diameter using an appropriate size dilation balloon. This can be done immediately after stent placement when portal

Table 1. Routine Follow-Up Portographic Studies in 16 Asymptomatic Patients

Follow-up	No. of Patients	Well-Functioning Shunt[a]	Compromised Shunt[b]	Location of Shunt Stenosis			Treatment	
				Tract	Tract + Hepatic Vein	Hepatic Vein	PTA	New Stent
6 months	14	21%	79%	18%	36%	45%	64%	36%
12 months	9	11%	89%	12%	25%	63%	75%	25%
18 Months	6	17%	83%	-	20%	80%	100%	-
24 months	4	75%	25%	-	-	100%	100%	-
36 months	1	1	-	-	-	-	-	-

[a] Well-functioning shunt: shunt lumen wider than 50% of the stent diameter and portosystemic gradient below 14 mm Hg.

[b] Compromised shunt: shunt lumen narrower than 50% of stent diameter and portosystemic gradient higher than 14 mm Hg.

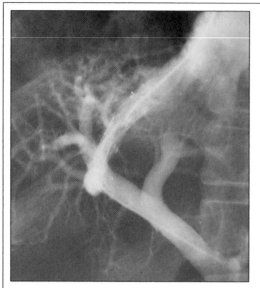 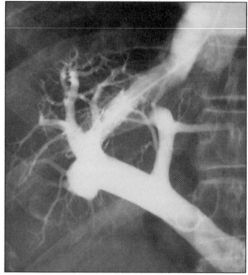

Figure 3. A 47-year-old man with Child-Pugh class C cirrhosis and massive bleeding from gastroesophageal varices. Bleeding immediately ceased after the TIPS procedure and has not recurred for 30 months. His routine follow-up ultrasound studies at 6-month intervals have shown a well-patent shunt. Portogram immediately after TIPS procedure *(left)* reveals excellent shunting with persistent filling of hepatic radicles. Portosystemic gradient was 13 mm Hg. Follow-up portogram 6 months after TIPS *(right)* shows continuous excellent shunting with persistent filling of hepatic radicles. There is only a minor amount of pseudointimal tissue in the shunt. Portosystemic gradient was 13 mm Hg.

decompression is not sufficient or later when follow-up studies reveal decreased shunt diameter due to pseudointimal proliferation. GRZ stents also cost less than other stents.

The need for introduction of the 10 Fr sheath into the portal vein for stent placement, low flexibility, and uneven expansile force along the stent length are disadvantages of the GRZ stents for TIPS creation. The GRZ stents, consisting of four to five bodies connected with sutures, flex only slightly while maintaining their lumen. Connections between individual stent bodies have decreased expansile force and when placed at the level of the portal vein (the point of maximum resistance in the tract), the stent may remain slightly narrowed and possibly kinked. Placement of another GRZ stent or a Wallstent inside the first stent usually solves this problem. The spiral Z-stent which has a more even expansile force along its length should not have such a problem, and its use in three of our cases is promising.

Figure 4. A 72-year-old man with cirrhosis and massive bleeding from gastric varices. He was previously treated by sclerotherapy of esophageal varices and distal splenorenal shunt which occluded. Bleeding immediately ceased after the procedure and has not recurred for 42 months; the patient has been doing well. Follow-up venographic studies revealed intimal hyperplasia in the shunted hepatic vein responding well to balloon dilations. A 12-month follow-up portogram *(top left)* reveals severe narrowing of the stented hepatic vein and filling of hepatic radicles and varices. Portosystemic gradient was 24 mm Hg. A 12-month portogram after balloon angioplasty *(top right)* of the stenotic area shows well-open shunt. Portosystemic gradient decreased to 5 mm Hg. A 24-month follow-up venogram *(middle left)* reveals moderate recurrence of the hepatic vein stenosis. Portosystemic gradient was 8 mm Hg. A 24-month venogram after balloon angioplasty *(middle right)* shows good response of stenosis to dilation. Gradient decreased to 6 mm Hg. A 40-month follow-up venogram *(bottom center)* shows stabilization of the stenosis with a low portosystemic gradient of 4 mm Hg. (See page 159.)

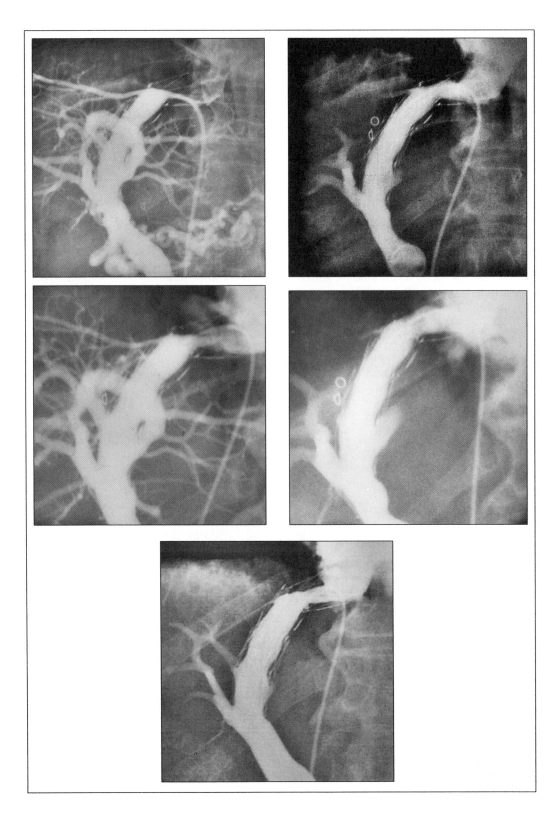

The GRZ stents are well suited for centrally-placed shunts connecting proximal portions of the hepatic vein with the proximal portion of the right or left portal vein branch. They are optimal for vertically-oriented portal veins where the centrally-established shunt forms its continuation. The GRZ stents, however, are not suitable for more peripherally located shunts. The 10-mm diameter stents used in our four early patients did not allow sufficient decompression and exhibited problems in long-term patency. We therefore abandoned their use and instead have used 12-mm diameter GRZ stents. We have achieved excellent shunts with these stents in 19 of 24 patients (79%). In the remaining five patients a Wallstent was added for creation of a well-functioning TIPS. The GRZ stents alone did not result in adequate shunting in these five patients because of peripheral stent position resulting in focal stent narrowing or kinking.

Clinical results in our series are similar to those reported with the use of other stents for TIPS creation. TIPS controlled acute bleeding in all seven of our actively bleeding patients; bleeding did not recur in 79% of our 28 patients even when the varices were not embolized after the TIPS procedure. The 30-day mortality rate was 14% and total mortality with up to 42 months of follow-up was 25%. Both of these rates are quite low for the advanced types of liver disease present in the majority of our patients. Pre-existing encephalopathy in 51% of our patients decreased to 24% and could be well-managed medically. Similarly, the occurrence of ascites decreased from 75% to 10% and hepatic synthetic function improved after TIPS.

Long-term shunt patency, however, was compromised in a high percentage of our patients, particularly in the first year after TIPS. This was secondary to exuberant pseudointimal tissue formation in the parenchymal tract and intimal hyperplasia in the draining hepatic vein. Stenoses with the Z-stents were found more often in the hepatic vein than in the shunt's parenchymal tract, similar to the Palmaz stent (1,5,7) but contrary to the Wallstent (2,4). The general incidence of shunt stenoses with the Z-stents was somewhat higher than that reported with other stents (1,2,4,7). This was also true in our series comparing Z-stents and Wallstents in the 6- and 12-month venographic follow-up. All stenoses, however, responded well to balloon dilation alone (64%) or to the addition of a new stent (36%). Single intervention at 6 months was sufficient to keep the shunt open at later follow-ups in 21% of patients. The other 79% of patients required another form of intervention, mainly balloon angioplasty at 12 and/or 18 months. Repeated balloon dilations appeared to stabilize growth of pseudointimal tissue in the tract and intimal hyperplasia in the hepatic vein and appeared to decrease recurrence of stenoses.

One may question why we have recently used mainly Wallstents for TIPS even when the Z-stents are more radiopaque, easier to place in a precisely desired location, and are less expensive. The majority of our recent TIPS patients have been transplant candidates and a more peripherally-established shunt is preferable in these patients to avoid stent extension deep into the portal vein and into the inferior vena cava. More peripherally-established shunts may also avoid injury of a major hepatic artery or bile duct. Based on these reasons we have recently preferred using Wallstents which are more flexible, faster to place, and have a wider range of applications compared to the GRZ stents.

CONCLUSIONS

The 12-mm diameter GRZ self-expandable stents are suitable devices for creation of centrally-located TIPS connecting proximal portions of the hepatic vein and proximal portions of the right or left portal vein branch. The established shunts have a tendency for gradual narrowing, particularly in the hepatic vein, and their maintenance with repeated balloon dilations or additional stent placement is necessary for continued wide patency and good function.

REFERENCES

1. Katzen B, Becker GJ, Benenati JF, Zemel G. TIPS: The Miami Vascular Institute experience. Presented at Annual Meeting of Western Angiographic and Interventional Society, Portland, Oregon, October 2, 1993.

2. LaBerge JM, Ring EJ, Gordon RL, et al. Creation of transjugular intrahepatic portosystemic shunts with the Wallstent endoprosthesis: results in 100 patients. Radiology 1993;187:413-420.

3. Maynar M, Cabrera J, Pulido-Duque JM. Transjugular intrahepatic portosystemic shunt: early experience with a flexible trocar/catheter system. AJR 1993;161:301-306.

4. Rousseau H, Binel JP, Bilbao JI, Joffre F. TIPS with Wallstent endoprostheses, histological study. Presented at Annual Meeting of Western Angiographic and Interventional Society, Portland, Oregon, October 2, 1993.

5. Nöldge G, Rössle M, Richter GM, Perarnau JM, Palmaz JC. Die modellierung des Transjugulären Intrahepatischen Portosystemischen Shunts (TIPSS) mittels metalprothese: andorderungen an den stent. Radiologe 1991;31:102-107.

6. Richter GM, Nöldge G, Palmaz JC, et al. Transjugular intrahepatic portacaval stent shunt: preliminary clinical results. Radiology 1990;174:1027-1030.

7. Richter G. TIPS: The Heidelberg University experience. Presented at Annual Meeting of Western Angiographic and Interventional Society, Portland, Oregon, October 2, 1993.

8. Zemel G, Katzen BT, Becker GJ, Benenati JF, Sallee S. Percutaneous transjugular portosystemic shunt. JAMA 1991;266:390-393.

9. Maynar M, Cabrera J, Gorriz E, Reyes R, Pulido-Duque JM, Rublo P. Preliminary experience with Strecker stents in TIPS procedures. Presented at Annual Meeting of Western Angiographic and Interventional Society, Portland, Oregon, October 2, 1993.

10. Rossi P. TIPS: indications and results. Presented at Annual Meeting of Western Angiographic and Interventional Society, Portland, Oregon, October 2, 1993.

11. Maeda M, Timmermans HA, Uchida BT, Uchida H, Keller FS, Rösch J. In vitro comparison of the spiral Z-stent and the Gianturco Z-stent. JVIR 1992;3:565-569.

12. Rösch J, Uchida BT, Barton RE, Keller FS. Coaxial catheter-needle system for transjugular portal vein entrance. JVIR 1993;4:145-147.

Nitinol Strecker Stents in TIPS

Plinio Rossi, Francesca Maccioni, Laura Broglia, Paolo Ricci

Department of Radiology, III Cattedra, University "La Sapienza", Rome, Italy

To evaluate the validity of the new nitinol Strecker stents in transjugular intrahepatic portosystemic shunts (TIPS), we performed the TIPS procedure in 24 patients using 34 new metallic stents made of a nickel-titanium alloy wire. In 13 patients we used a single nitinol Strecker stent, while in 6 patients we used more than one. In the remaining five patients a nitinol stent was combined with other types of metallic stents. Stent placement was successful in all 24 patients. The average portosystemic gradient decreased from 16.5 to 11 mm Hg after the procedure. A further decrease to 10 mm Hg was observed in those patients in whom a 5-day angiographic control was performed. No major complications or procedure-related mortality were encountered during this clinical trial. Early reintervention after 5 days with balloon dilation was necessary in four patients: in three because of small thrombi within the stent and in one for complete obstruction. In late angiographic control, stenosis was present in three patients. Recurrent bleeding occurred in one patient and temporary crises of mild encephalopathy were present in 24% of cases. Four patients received a liver transplant and one patient died. In conclusion, TIPS procedures are easily performed using nitinol stents because of the excellent decrease in portosystemic gradient. The incidences of stent-related complications, encephalopathy, rebleeding, and stenosis were not different from those observed with other types of uncovered metallic stents.

INTRODUCTION

In performing a transjugular intrahepatic portosystemic shunt (TIPS) procedure, stent selection is one of the most important factors. The adequate length, correct diameter, flexibility, ease of placement, and the possibility for redilation of the stent are essential aspects for achieving success.

Among the metallic endoprostheses currently available for the treatment of vascular, esophageal, gastrointestinal, and biliary stenosis or obstruction, the nitinol Strecker stent is a new type of self-expandable stent. These stents were initially provided to us on an investigational basis for biliary application (1).

In the last 2 years we performed 75 TIPS procedures using different types of metallic stents. Herein we report our clinical experience in 24 patients in whom a TIPS procedure was performed with nitinol Strecker stents alone or in combination with other types of metallic stents.

MATERIALS AND METHODS

In the last 13 months we have placed a total of 34 nitinol Strecker™ stents (Boston Scientific Corp., Denmark) (length: 6 cm; diameter: 10 mm) in 24 patients. A single stent was placed in 13 patients, while in 11 more than one stent was placed, in 5 of whom the nitinol stent was combined with another type of metallic stent.

The need for multiple stent placement in the same patients was determined either by the length of the intrahepatic tract or by the necessity to extend the stented portion into the hepatic vein or distally into the portal vein.

As previously described (1), this new type of self-expandable stent is made of a 0.13-mm thick nickel-titanium alloy wire (Elastalloy™, Boston Scientific Corp., Denmark) (Figure 1). The delivery system is comprised of an introducer shaft with three radiopaque markers and a cover sheath which upon retraction releases the stent. The distance between the distal and the middle marker represents the actual length of the stent after release. Also provided with the stent is an anchoring system (Figure 2) which in theory should prevent shortening of the distal end of the stent after deployment.

Our technique for performing the TIPS procedure can be summarized as follows:

- Catheterization of the hepatic vein using a transjugular approach.
- Portal vein puncture and atrio-portal pressure gradient measurement.
- Intrahepatic tract dilation.
- Stent placement and measurement of the post-procedure atrio-portal pressure gradient.
- Additional stent positioning if necessary.

The most important of these is the localization and puncture of the main portal vein because the anatomy and consistency of the liver parenchyma varies from patient to patient. In patients with a large liver and previously documented anatomy of the portal system, we proceed with blind puncture. In a small fibrotic liver where ascites is present, we localize the portal system by introducing a 0.018-inch guidewire with a platinum tip using a left portal branch approach. In cases with portal vein thrombosis the procedure is often performed under ultrasound guidance (3).

In the few days following the TIPS procedure, patients are studied by endoscopy to evaluate the status of esophageal varices by Eco-color Doppler which measures portal and stent blood flow. These studies are repeated every 2 to 3 months after TIPS.

In addition, serial angiographic controls are usually performed after 5 to 7 days and, when possible, every 3 to 6 months thereafter, both in symptomatic patients and in those without clinical evidence of recurrent disease.

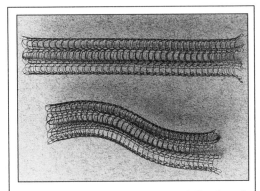

Figure 1. The nitinol Strecker stent fully released. Note the looped ends and the flexibility.

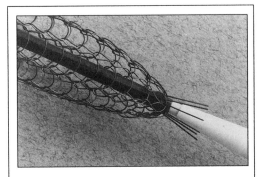

Figure 2. The nitinol Strecker stent kept in position by the anchoring system.

RESULTS

Technical Results

We successfully completed all 75 cases performed at the University of Rome "La Sapienza". In the early cases we encountered many difficulties and the procedure lasted 2 to 3 hours. With increased experience, however, the procedure time has decreased to 30 to 40 minutes in easy cases, i.e., in patients with large livers. In patients with small fibrotic livers, the puncture is more difficult and the procedure time is longer.

On the basis of our experience using various types of metallic stents such as the Wallstent, nitinol Strecker, Palmaz, and Angiomed nitinol stents, we have established a scoring system, grading the quality of each type of stent. Scores for the nitinol Strecker stent are shown in Table 1.

Table 1. Nitinol Strecker Stent Scores

Diameter	+ + + +
Length	+ +
Flexibility	+ + + +
Shortening	+ + +
Radial Force	+ + +
Radiopacity	+
Stent Profile	+ + +
Removal Ability	+ + + +
Reentry	+ + + +
Dislodgment	Possible

Clinical Results

In all patients treated with nitinol Strecker stents the average portosystemic gradient decreased from 16.5 to 11 mm Hg soon after the procedure (Figures 3 and 4). The esophageal and gastric varices disappeared in all but one patient in whom the stent was completely obstructed because of shortening into the distal end of the intrahepatic tract. In this case the varices were successfully embolized 8 days after the procedure and an additional stent was placed.

Only one patient died 3 days after the TIPS procedure. Four patients received liver transplants and therefore did not undergo further control measures. Among the remaining 19 patients, 5-day angiographic controls were performed in 12 patients, and 6- to 12-month controls were performed in five.

In the 12 patients who were angio-graphically-controlled after 5 days, reintervention with balloon dilatation was performed in four patients (21%) because of small thrombi within the stent (N=3) and complete obstruction (N=1).

Intimal hyperplasia was the most common finding upon late angiographic controls (3 to 12 months). Two patients presented with three stent stenoses. In one, dilatation was necessary after 9 and 12 months, while in the other a single dilatation was performed after 10 months.

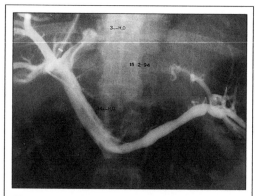

Figure 3. A 46-year-old man with post-hepatic cirrhosis (Child-Pugh class A) awaiting liver transplantation. Puncture of the portal vein through a transjugular approach with opacification of the portal system. Atrial pressure was 3 cm H_2O (2.2 mm Hg) and portal pressure measured 34 cm H_2O (24 mm Hg).

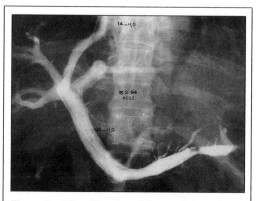

Figure 4. After dilatation of the parenchymal tract with a 10-mm balloon catheter, a nitinol Strecker stent was placed between the hepatic vein and the right portal branch. After the procedure the atrial pressure increased to 14 cm H_2O (10.3 mm Hg) while the portal pressure decreased to 26 cm H_2O (19 mm Hg) and the portosystemic gradient = 9 mm Hg.

A long follow-up for all patients is not possible because insufficient time has elapsed since the TIPS procedure. Temporary crises of mild, *de novo* encephalopathy were observed in 24% of cases and were easily controlled with lactulose. One patient experienced rebleeding despite a low portosystemic gradient.

DISCUSSION

Stents are important tools for interventional radiology because they have multiple applications in vessels, the biliary tree, and the gastrointestinal tract (1,4-8). Despite industry's efforts to improve stent quality, an ideal stent is still not available. The major disadvantage with uncovered stents is that inflammatory, reactive, or neoplastic tissue grows into the stent producing a progressive obstruction (9). Covered stents, on the other hand, present many difficulties, such as biocompatibility, migration, and increased size of the delivery system.

We obtained good results after using nitinol Strecker stents in malignant obstructions of the biliary system and have reported a patency rate longer than that reported with another similar stent (1).

Our overall clinical results with the TIPS procedure are very good and are similar to those reported by others (4-8,11). After comparing the results of nitinol stents to the other stents we used in our 75 cases, there was no increase in shunt or hepatic vein complications. During follow-up, the incidence of rebleeding and of encephalopathy was similar to that observed with other stents (10). For a correct evaluation, a longer follow-up period would be more helpful.

On the basis of our experience in using these stents, we make the following suggestions and comments.

The low radiopacity of the device makes it mandatory to rely on the three radiopaque markers of the delivery system. Even with the best high resolution fluoroscopic equipment, nitinol Strecker stents are rarely seen in patients of average or large size (Figure 5). Therefore, a greater radiopacity would improve the exactness of stent deployment.

The size of the stent (10 mm) seems adequate, although an 8-mm balloon is sometimes used for initial dilation.

The length of the stent is an important aspect to consider because it should be selected according to the patient's anatomy.

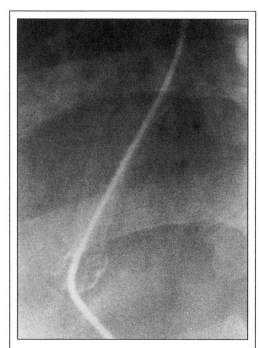

Figure 5. Radiogram of the nitinol Strecker stent. Note the low radiopacity, the complete expansion of the stent and the indentation at the level of the crossing of the portal vein.

For example, the 6-cm length of the nitinol stent, although sufficient for short intrahepatic tracts (2 to 3 cm), does not seem adequate for long tracts in which you have to cover from the portal vein almost up to the junction between the hepatic vein and the inferior vena cava. For this reason several stents were used in 11 of our patients. In 5 of the 11 patients we used different types of stents because nitinol stents were no longer available or because of the need for a shorter stent. The procedure thus becomes more expensive. Moreover, by having two stents, one inside the other, the inner lumen is considerably decreased and not dilatable.

Considering the predictable shortening of the stent on the distal end, about 0.5 to 1 cm, we place the introducer with the distal radiopaque marker 1 to 1.5 cm inside the portal vein so that, regardless of the shortening, enough stent remains within the lumen of the portal vein. If needed, additional stents can be deployed.

Upon release, the stent sometimes does not expand completely even though the tract has been dilated to 10 mm. Full expansion is achieved only after 24 to 48 hours, except at the level of the portal vein crossing where a characteristic narrowing is often present (Figure 5). This is observed at the 5-day angiographic control and can be resolved by balloon dilatation.

The stent presents a good radial force which lets the stent adhere tightly to the intrahepatic tract immediately after deployment. If additional balloon dilations are required, however, we suggest that they not be performed on the same day as the TIPS procedure because working inside the stent can cause dislodgment. This happened to us on two separate occasions and prompted immediate removal. We therefore prefer to dilate the stent at the 5-day angiographic control.

Stent removal can be performed with grasping forceps or with a loop technique during the procedure if the deployment is not correct. The presence of looped ends is another important stent characteristic (Figure 1) and allows for easy reentry if the deployment is incorrect.

CONCLUSIONS

In conclusion, the nitinol Strecker stent has made the TIPS stent procedure very easy and offers a self-expandable tool characterized by an easy deployment system and good flexibility, along with the possibility for removal and reentry without complications.

We have not observed any difference in the overall clinical results or complication rates for obstruction, partial thrombosis, rebleeding, and encephalopathy using these stents. Therefore, we feel confident that the nitinol stents are excellent for both biliary and TIPS procedures.

REFERENCES

1. Bezzi M, Orsi F, Salvatori F, Maccioni F, Rossi P. Self-expandable nitinol stent for the management of biliary obstruction: long-term clinical results. JVIR 1994;5:287-293.
2. Rossi P, Ricci P, Natali G, et al. TIPS: aspetti tecnici. La Radiologica Medica 1994; in press.
3. Bilbao JI, Longo JM, Rousseau H, et al. Transjugular intrahepatic portacaval shunt after thrombus disruption in partially thrombosed portal veins. Cardiovasc Intervent Radiol 1994;17:106-109.
4. Zemel G, Katzen BT, Becker JG, Benenati JF, Salee D. Percutaneous transjugular portosystemic shunt. JAMA 1991;266:390-393.
5. Maynar M, Cabrera J, Gorriz E, et al. Transjugular intrahepatic portacaval shunt. JVIR 1993;4:63.
6. Rousseau H, Puel J, Joffre F, et al. Experimental portohepatic shunt with the Wallstent endoprosthesis. JVIR 1991;2:12.
7. Ring EJ, Lake JR, Roberts JP, et al. Using transjugular intrahepatic portosystemic shunts to control variceal bleeding before liver transplantation. Ann Intern Med 1992;116:304-309.
8. Zemel G, Becker GJ, Bancrott JW, Benenati H, Katzen BT. Technical advances in transjugular intrahepatic portosystemic shunts. Radiographics 1992;12:615-622.
9. Palmaz JC. Intravascular stents: tissue-stent interactions and design considerations. AJR 1993;160:613-618.
10. Rossi P, Maccioni F, Salvatori FM, et al. TIPS: indicazioni e risultati dopo 22 mesi di esperienza. La Radiologica Medica 1994; in press.
11. Rössle M, Haag K, Ochs A, et al. The TIPS procedure for variceal bleeding. N Engl J Med 1994;330:165-171.

Memory Alloy Endoprostheses and TIPS: Initial Results

D. Liermann[1], J. Berkefeld[1], M. Grosso[2], J. Kollath[1]

[1]Department of Radiology, J.W. Goethe University Hospital, Frankfurt am Main, Germany
[2]Department of Radiology, University Hospital Turin, Turin, Italy

INTRODUCTION

Portal hypertension usually develops as a consequence of cirrhotic metaplasia of the liver from various causes. The main origin, apart from toxic alcoholic processes, is a chronic, frequently aggressive form of viral hepatitis (1-3). A rarer cause can be direct obstructions or occlusions of the root of the portal vein in the hepatic area caused by tumor infiltration or impression, or iatrogenic thromboses and occlusions caused by laying a catheter in the umbilical vein in premature babies (1,4). Regardless of the genesis of the original disease, the consequences of the resulting portal hypertension become evident in the development of collateral circulation with an extended venous plexus in the area of the stomach fundus, esophagus, and porta of the liver. The consequences of collateral circulation impose on the abdominal wall in the form of caput medusae. The increasing rise in pressure on this venous plexus finally results in a tearing of the frequently paper-thin vessel wall of the convoluted veins in the esophagus or stomach, with consecutive variceal bleeding.

The therapeutic approach for acute treatment of such bleeding is usually the initial application of an endoluminal cuff, the so-called Sengstaken probe (1-7). This probe has only a limited service life because of the generation of pressure ulceration, so that scabbing the source of the bleeding using lasers has become established as the preferred method of treatment. Additional medication supports this purely symptomatic measure (5,8-11). In order to achieve effective pressure reduction in the portal system, the only possible treatment up to now was to perform surgery with the artificial application of a bypass, or elimination of the cause of portal hypertension by implantation of a new liver. The choice for artificial bypasses for reducing pressure on the liver has been limited to several surgical techniques for shunt systems such as direct anastomosis of the splenic vein with the vena cava or the splenic vein with the left renal vein (Warren shunt) (12-25). Such operations were frequently supplemented by skeletization of convoluted veins in the esophagus and stomach fundus in order to avoid recurrent bleeding (26). Depending on the particular stage of hepatic disease, such operations were either successful or accompanied by a high peri-operative mortality rate (20,21,24,25,27-33). Patients with Child stage C disease in particular often showed only short-term success with poor prognosis, in spite of the surgical approach.

In view of these unfavorable circumstances, the search for alternatives started at an early stage. Initial attempts to apply an intrahepatic portacaval shunt by means of balloon dilatation began in 1969 (1,34,35). Unfortunately, the clinical success of the technically complicated, but successfully implemented project, was only short-lived, as it was not possible to obtain sufficient flow in the anastomosis due to a lack of stability in the diameter of the artificially-created lumen. We carried out our own tests with successful canalization between the hepatic and portal veins without sufficient stability in the canal and with correspondingly unfavorable progress. The technique we used for transjugular intrahepatic puncture from the pre-stent age has, in fact, been shown to be the appropriate approach. Failure of this method was caused by the lack of support in the newly created canal, which recollapsed after a single percutaneous transluminal angioplasty (PTA) procedure. In contrast to Nöldge and Richter, we have only used the transjugular access and have oriented ourselves according to anatomic facts during puncture of the liver from the vein to the portal vein. When in doubt, we detect the course of the portal vein by ultrasonic scan, mark the same, and proceed with puncture under x-ray control. This technique reduced the procedure to under 4 hours, whereas Nöldge and Richter had to accept operating times of around 8 hours because of the additional percutaneous puncture of the portal vein system with the basket method (36). The complicated additional percutaneous puncture of the portal vein has been neglected in favor of purely ultrasonic scan-based transjugular puncturing (36). Modification of this method has reduced the time involved to 1.5 to 3 hours for an experienced surgeon.

The splinting mechanisms available in the "pre-stent" age after creating a canal between vein and portal vein included "stents" which had originally been designed for other uses. In one of our first cases, we treated a patient with a "double mushroom" stent known from splinting of the biliary tract, which required a maximum lumen of 4 mm with an implant set of more than 14 Fr (Figure 1). In retrospect, it is possible to understand that the resulting loss in pressure was not adequate. In another case, we implanted a double helix spiral as per Maas, which could be positioned with a considerably larger lumen diameter. Although the spiral structure was able to guarantee an open lumen in the vascular system, it was not suitable to function as a bridge in an artificially "parenchymatous" canal. On the second day following technically successful implantation, the control revealed disintegration of the spiral filaments. This led to occlusion in the stent which was detected in the digital subtraction angiography (DSA) control and which, as revealed by the autopsy later on, was not caused by thrombosis but by parenchyma bridges which had prolapsed into the lumen between the helix filaments.

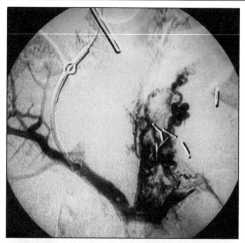

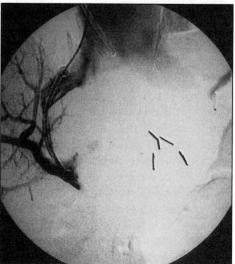

Figure 1. Our first attempt at applying a transjugular, intrahepatic portacaval shunt (TIPS) in the mid 1980s. *Top:* Following puncture by means of a needle introduced into the transjugular together with canalization and dilatation of a canal between the hepatic and portal veins, a "double mushroom" prosthesis with a diameter of 13 Fr was implanted, as normally used in percutaneous internal biliary tract splinting. *Bottom:* The prosthesis initially produced great relief but thrombosed due to the small diameter.

A representative case in a third group consisted of a patient with esophageal variceal bleeding who developed portal hypertension on the basis of post-infection liver cirrhosis with a pre-embolized liver tumor. The attempt to implant a portacaval shunt succeeded in this case, although it was ineffective from the start because the portal hypertension did not have an intrahepatic cause but was the result of an extrahepatic metastasis blocking the lumen of the portal vein. Stent implantation was ruled out in this case in view of the negligible difference in pressure between the intrahepatic portal system and the venous system.

Following a series of failures in patients with Child stage C disease who were classified as inoperable, surgeons' confidence in using percutaneous transjugular portosystemic shunts was limited, so that the development of metallic stents of various types did not result in a new version of the portacaval shunt. A further factor was the fact that the Strecker stent type at our disposition was thought to be relatively easily compressed on the basis of our experimental studies, so that compression by the usually firm cirrhotic liver tissue seemed highly probable. At that time, we did not have access to a reinforced version with a wire filament diameter of 0.15 mm or to the Palmaz endoprosthesis (35,37). Moreover, apart from the Freiburg group, no surgeons at that time had shown any interest in implanting stents as a therapy for portal hypertension.

It was not until endoprostheses were developed with sufficient rigidity, accompanied by simplification of the technique, that stent implantation was again discussed as an alternative to the surgical shunt. Following exemplary successes in implanting stents in other organ systems, interest also grew in various other medical centers. In Germany, this happened initially in Heidelberg, continuing the Freiburg technique with implantation of the Palmaz stent (36). In Frankfurt, the increase in liver transplants and the increasing number of patients waiting for donor livers gave rise to the need for a non-surgical method for creating an intrahepatic portacaval shunt as a temporary therapy for portal hypertension which at the same time preserved the extrahepatic structures still required for the

transplant (38,39). In light of the successes in Freiburg and Heidelberg (36), as well as in the US (40), the method was reintroduced in Frankfurt at the Radiology Center using improved material. The purpose of these first stent-based applications was to examine how far the stent implantation technique could make a contribution to achieving a sufficient clinical result. In doing so, special attention was given to a new, particularly rigid but also flexible memory metal stent prototype.

MATERIALS AND METHODS

Following puncture of the right internal jugular vein, partly under ultrasonic scan control and with Valsava's maneuver by the patient to improve puncturing the vein, a sheath, 10- to 12-Fr wide and 30-cm long, was introduced by wire. The equipment used here consisted mainly of sets produced by Angiomed (Karlsruhe, Germany) or Cook (Europe) which differed in the mechanism of the set puncture needle (41,42). Following heparin therapy, a catheter with a slightly bent tip was delivered through the sheath via a Terumo wire through the right vestibule into the lower vena cava. From this point, a corresponding large hepatic vein, usually in the right lobe of the liver, was probed and a special, particularly strong guidewire was inserted. An attempt was made to make a so-called "Wedgogram" by sliding a catheter right into the periphery (30). Contrast medium was injected under great pressure to achieve oversplashing and thus retrograde filling so that the intrahepatic portal system could be shown. The process was carried out using the road mapping technique with the actual x-ray being faded into the still of the portal system. This x-ray mode made it possible to achieve a more precise puncture from the hepatic vein towards the intrahepatic portal vein. This was not successful in every case, however, so that the puncture frequently had to be carried out using ultrasonic scan or, if available, color-coded Doppler. Depending on experience available, the puncture could be carried out under direct ultrasonic scan control or under x-ray control based on a metal marking previously applied under ultrasonic scan control, corresponding to the course of the portal vein. Without a doubt, profound anatomic knowledge played a vital role here.

A corresponding puncture set consisting of plastic catheters and a rigid steel needle was then inserted via the positioned wire (41-43), after the set had been bent by hand to match the course of the hepatic vein to the portal vein. The puncture was then carried out depending on the position of the blood vessels in relation to each other from the hepatic vein towards the portal vein. Following successful puncture in the intrahepatic course of both blood vessels, the precise position was checked by injecting contrast medium, and the guidewire was inserted further into the portal vein. A 5 Fr catheter was positioned to allow for pressure measurement in the portal system, checking to see whether there really was a pressure gradient which would justify stent implantation. The wire was then replaced by a stronger version (Amplatz superstiff™ 0.035-inch or 0.038-inch, Boston Scientific Corp., Watertown MA or a 0.035-inch nitinol guidewire, Angiomed), followed by insertion of a PTA catheter. The canal was then initially dilatated in the area of the parenchyma bridge.

Initially, balloon-dilatating Palmaz™ (Johnson & Johnson Interventional Co., Warren NJ) and Strecker™ (Boston Scientific Corp., Denmark) endoprostheses were used together with the self-expanding Wallstent™ (Medinvent, Lausanne, Switzerland). Subsequently, the first 10 nitinol (Memotherm®, Angiomed) endoprostheses were implanted. In these cases, after positioning of the implant system, a sheath was withdrawn allowing the stent to expand. The memory metal properties mean that the stent finally reaches its predetermined diameter. In such cases, the stent must be given at least 5 minutes to develop fully before safe removal of the system, even along the curved course of the vein without any interaction.

The canal was previously dilatated to 10 mm for all stent types. When treatment was performed under sedation, it was necessary for the patient to receive strong analgesic medication.

Revision of the stent diameter for the above types of prostheses was only possible for the Palmaz and nitinol endoprostheses. The Palmaz stent fixed on the balloon catheter was positioned in the anastomosis area and released by expanding an 8-mm balloon catheter. With the nitinol stent, a 12-mm stent was delivered which then only expanded to 10 mm because of the previous dilatation of the canal. After performing an angio-cardiogram of the shunt, the pressure was measured. On evidence of an excessive pressure gradient, the stent was dilatated further to a larger lumen by a larger balloon until the pressure gradient had fallen below 20 mm Hg. The pressure gradient was measured again by means of a catheter introduced through the stent into the portal vein. A final angiogram was taken on at least two levels. The implant set was then removed, and the results verified either by endovascular ultrasonic scan or by a color-coded Doppler. The prototypes of the nitinol memory metal stent we used were available in lengths ranging from 6 to 10 cm, with diameters between 10 and 12 mm. Experimental delivery of the system was tested on cadaver organs before being used on humans. The stents had to be rinsed with hot water to activate the memory effect and permit the stents to expand fully.

INDICATION

The indication to insert a portacaval shunt with stent implantation was initially limited to patients waiting for liver transplants and who had developed portal hypertension as a result of their liver disease, with bleeding and threatening recurrence or threatening bleeding. On a parallel basis, in addition to this purely temporary relief of the portal circulation while awaiting transplantation, one implantation was carried out as an alternative to surgical methods. A relative contraindication for implanting a portacaval shunt during this study was an alcoholic liver cirrhosis with poor compliance between the patient and doctor.

PATIENT DATA

This study considered patients implanted with a prototype nitinol memory metal stent. Altogether, we treated a total of seven men and three women in a 6-month period, aged between 38 and 73 years (mean, 59.3 years). In all cases, liver cirrhosis was the cause of portal hypertension. In two cases, the treatment was performed as therapy for ascites which had not responded to previous interventions. In four cases, the treatment was seen as a prophylactic measure to avoid recurrent bleeding prior to planned transplants, in two cases under acute bleeding which would not respond to treatment, and in two cases as a prophylactic measure under stable conditions in an interval free of recurrent bleeding. Two patients were in Child stage A disease, four were in Child stage B, and four were in Child stage C. Precise control of laboratory parameters and clinical examination of the treated patients was performed on a weekly, then monthly basis, and later at 6-month intervals. In addition, sonographic control was planned in the color Doppler at 3-month intervals together with angiographic control every 6 months. Apart from these fixed schedules, immediate examination was also carried out at the slightest suspicion of a shunt thrombosis or recurrent stenosis.

RESULTS

In all patients it was possible to apply a transjugular intrahepatic portosystemic shunt with implantation of the nitinol stent. In two patients there was no sufficient pressure gradient after application of the shunt, particularly in the cases with ascites not responding to treatment. In two cases the outflow via extremely wide varices was so large that the application of the shunt initially appeared to be without any notable effect on the pressure gradient. In one case, adequate flow in the shunt could not be detected, making reintervention necessary. In one of the nitinol stents, a thrombosis developed only a few hours after implantation and was successfully removed again.

Virtually all other stent types which we had previously implanted had to be revised at some point because of dislocation, compression from the outside, or migration (Figure 2). Here the Palmaz stent in particular revealed a greater than average tendency to shorten in length, resulting in a drifting apart of stents which had initially been inserted in overlapping mode. Use of these stents in curved blood vessels was practically impossible. As far as the Wallstent was concerned, problems developed more frequently than average in the deployment of the self-expanding stent from its implant system, so that in several cases, the stent was removed again with the implant system. This meant that the whole procedure practically had to be started all over again, as the partially deployed stent could only be removed together with the entire implant system, including the guidewire. The reinforced tantalum stent turned out to be insufficiently rigid in all cases, in spite of the wire filament being thickened from 0.1 to 0.15 mm; it was easily squashed or dislocated by manipulation of the catheter and guidewire material.

These severe complications were not observed following implantation of the Memotherm stent. It appears that the enormous expansion capacity of the stent was of great significance here. Naturally, all canals had to be dilatated in advance before the stent was applied. In addition, an expansion time of at least 5 minutes had to be taken into account to avoid any interaction with the implant set on removing the latter. Both implantation in markedly curved canals and subsequent deployment upon expansion were

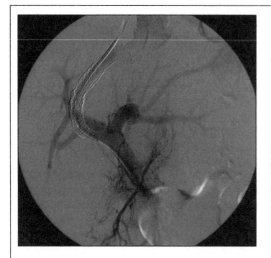

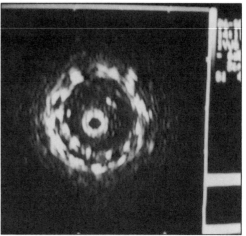

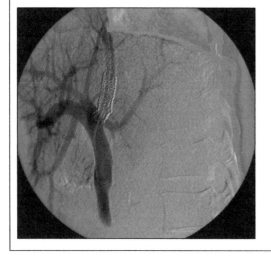

Figure 2. In the lengthy, complicated TIPS anastomosis, bizarre situations can develop after deployment of the stent until the lumen is finally open. The long, acutely bent canal means that the stent being implanted is released early and has to expand in untypical places. Two Strecker stents were implanted because of their flexibility, but showed clear compression phenomena from the outside. In the end, a self-expanding Wallstent was inserted coaxially through the other stents and expanded. It was responsible for the actual openness of the anastomosis. View of the open anastomosis (anteroposterior) *(top left)*. Lateral view of the open anastomosis *(bottom left)*. Cross section of the endovascular ultrasonic scan (the probe is the inner ring) showing from the inside outwards filaments of the Wallstent (inner ring) and the filaments of the two Strecker stents. Strecker stents (two outer rings) with free passage through the lumen in the anastomosis *(top right)*.

possible without any problems. Meanwhile, problems were encountered in attempts to revise the position of the stent during the deployment phase when the stent was partially expanded, as it can be squashed in various places here. Such processes can result, on the one hand, in too large meshes. Alternatively, forces pulling apart a section of the stent which is still expanding, while the expanded part is already fixed, can result in a relative narrowing of the lumen; the special elastic properties of the material indicate that it cannot be permanently expanded by a balloon (restoring forces). A version with narrower mesh gauge has been developed to overcome tissue prolapse through the mesh. Any shifting manipulation during deployment should be avoided at all costs. During the relatively short period available for post-treatment observation, no cases of intimal hyperplastic stenosis have occurred. Simultaneous embolization in the case of larger, severely draining varices also seems to play an important role in obtaining adequate flow on the shunt (Figure 3).

DISCUSSION

The initial results obtained from application of portacaval shunts with memory metal

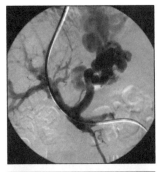

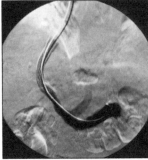

Figure 3. Sequence of implanting a nitinol Memotherm stent after canalization and probing a connection between the hepatic vein and the portal vein. Persistence of drainage via a large varices in spite of the stent *(top)*. Embolization of the varices by means of a spiral was required before very good flow was possible on the shunt *(bottom)*.

endoprosthesis support already indicate a clear tendency. Compared to other interventional measures, the TIPS procedure requires a higher than average learning curve (36,44) as demonstrated by the initially high rate of complications and the restricted success rate. Intensive monitoring of the patients is necessary, both during and after the treatment. The cost and time involved appear extremely high at first, and can only be justified from the point of view of the learning curve. This conclusion seems appropriate, particularly when our results are seen in the context of those obtained by other authors, who have now developed a sufficient routine to produce much more favorable statistics with correspondingly larger numbers of cases (36,40,43-46). The application of shunts has

the greatest success in patients awaiting transplantation. Prophylactic therapy in recurrence-free intervals show poorer results, with a tendency towards restenosis following intimal hyperplasia compared to operative shunts. Statistics for patients with Child stage C and for shunts applied under conditions of acute bleeding show good middle-term results (36,40). Depending on the indication involved, doubts remain as to whether application of a shunt is a suitable therapy for previously untreatable ascites, as the pressure gradient here is frequently too low to maintain good flow in the artificial shunt. Under these conditions, stasis and thrombosis of the shunt easily occur.

Our results agree with the experiences of other authors, suggesting a reserved indication for this procedure. In addition to the learning curve mentioned above, the role played by material insufficiencies should not be underestimated in failures observed in intrahepatic portosystemic shunts. It is worth mentioning the frequently difficult puncture phase because of the acute angle between the hepatic vein and the portal system, with resulting damage to the catheter material and guidewires.

The relatively high rate of failure in positioning various stent types is also a striking aspect, which is not seen with the same frequency when stents are implanted in other locations. Initially, it seemed that clear preference must be given to implantation of the apparently most rigid Palmaz stent in the treatment of portal hypertension, but the results with the nitinol Memotherm prototypes led to revision of this assumption. Compared to the other stent types, this stent can still be reliably positioned and deployed even under extremely difficult conditions. Its use increased the initial success rate to a decisive extent because of the clear reduction in the need for repeated intervention. Results obtained up to now indicate that this stent type provides a combination of the most positive characteristics of TIPS therapy.

In Europe, other stent types have also become established under study conditions.

For example, Maynar et al (46) reported on the successful implantation of Wallstents to apply a portacaval shunt. Rösch et al reported on the successful use of a modified Gianturco chain stent (40). Results have also been presented by a working group in Madrid about the favorable implantation of tantalum stents without complications (45). This was not the classical vascular tantalum stent, however, but a special stent made of considerably thicker tantalum wire. It would appear that contrary to initial assumptions, there are indeed arguments in favor of using different stent types when applying a portacaval shunt.

It seems worth mentioning that, in spite of the relatively complicated implantation technique and risky implantation, a malpositioned stent does not have the same fatal consequences as in other high risk areas. Apparently, no problems are posed by application of a second or third shunt in the event of failure of the first (36,40). This is already a reason not to attribute as much importance to the argument of stent removability for this indication as in the arterial system. The hypercoagulation argument is also not as important here, while the problem of sustained inflammation persists (36,40,46).

The lack of long-term experience means that here the results of already published experience with different stent types must be discussed. It appears that similar to the reactions of the vascular wall in the arterial system, hyperplastic wall reactions are possible at the transition point from the stent to the venous vascular section. These changes occur regardless of stent type (36,40,45,46) and can be eliminated by PTA as in the arterial system. A further problem in the context of stent implantation is the occurrence of encephalopathy caused by selection of an excessively high shunt volume. With the exception of the Palmaz stent and the nitinol stent featured in our study, the other stent types have a disadvantage in that revision is *de facto* no longer possible after selection of the stent diameter (and thus shunt volume) prior to implanta-

tion. In the Palmaz stent, this problem can be solved by gradual expansion, starting with a smaller diameter and progressing further until an acceptable pressure gradient is achieved (21,22,27,31,43,47). This also applies to the nitinol stent when a larger stent with subdilatation is selected. There are also no problems in implanting a tantalum stent, starting initially with a smaller diameter stent and then when the pressure gradient is no longer adequate, removing it and substituting a new stent with a larger diameter; however, implantation of several stents makes the procedure considerably more expensive and time-consuming. At the current time, we are of the opinion that the implantation of nitinol memory metal stents is the technique with the greatest efficiency and lowest possible rate of complications.

REFERENCES

1. Okuda K, Benhamou JP. *Portal Hypertension. Clinical and Physiological Aspects.* Berlin: Springer; 1991.
2. Palmaz JC, Garcia P, Sibbit SR, Chang P. Expandable intrahepatic portocaval shunt stent in dogs with chronic portal hypertension. AJR 1986;147:1251-1254.
3. Echenagusia A, Camunez F, Simo G, Peiro J, Banares R. Transjugular intrahepatic portosystemic shunts using Strecker stents. In: Liermann D, ed. *Stents.* New York: Marianne Liebert; 1993; in press.
4. Starzl TE, Demetris AJ. Liver transplantation: a 31-year perspective. Curr Probl Surg 1990;4:180.
5. Child CG. *The Liver and Portal Hypertension.* Philadelphia: WB Saunders; 1964.
6. Karavias T, Weber D, Hopfenmüller W, Häring R. Folgeerscheinungen und Langzeitergebnisse nach portosystemischen Anastomosen und Bedeutung der ambulanten Nachsorge. Langenbecks Arch Chir Suppl, Kongressbericht 1990:391-396.
7. Pagliaro L, Burroughs AK, Sorensen TIA. Therapeutic controversies and randomized controlled trials (RCT's): prevention of bleeding and rebleeding in cirrhosis. Gastroenterol Int 1989;2:71-84.

8. Peiper HJ, Siewert R. Chirurgische Erkrankungen der Speiseröhre In: Zenker R, Deutscher F, SchinkW, eds. *Chirurgie der Gegenwart*. München: Urban & Schwarzenberg; 1974.

9. Niebel W, Schax M, Brand MA, Eigler FW. The direct mesocaval shunt. In: Reiser M, Steudel A, Hirner A, Kania U, eds. *Lebertumoren und Portale Hypertension*. Berlin: Springer; 1993;3.4:417-421.

10. Murray JF, Mulder DG, Nebel L. The effect of retrograde portal venous flow following side-to-side portocaval anastomosis. J Clin Invest 1961;40:1413-1420.

11. Laberge JM, Ferrel LD, Ring EJ. Histopathologic study of transjugular intrahepatic portosystemic shunts. JVIR 1991;2:549-556.

12. Pandian N, Kreis A, O'Donnel T, Sacharoff A, Boleza E, Caro R. Intraluminal two-dimensional ultrasound angioscopic quantitation of arterial stenosis: comparison with external high frequency ultrasound imaging and anatomy. J Am Coll Cardiol 1989;13:2-5.

13. Kolvenbach H, Hirner A. Sklerosierungstherapie von Oesophgagusvarizen bei der Behandlung der Oesophagusvarizenblutung. *Lebertumoren und Portale Hypertension.* In: Reiser M, Steudel A, Hirner A, Kania U, eds. Berlin: Springer; 1993;345-351.

14. Conn HO, Resnick RH, Grace ND. Distal splenorenal shunt versus portal-systemic shunt: current status of a controlled trial. Hepatology 1981;1:151-160.

15. Kieninger G, Böhm T. Der distale splenorenale Shunt als Elektiveingriff bei portaler Hypertension. In: Reiser M, Steudel A, Hirner A, Kania U, eds. *Lebertumoren und portale Hypertension*. Berlin: Springer 1993;221-230.

16. Sarfeh IJ, Rypins EB, Conroy RM, Mason GR. Portocaval H-graft: relationships of shunt diameter, portal flow patterns and encephalopathy. Ann Surg 1983;197:422-426.

17. Warren WD, Zeppa R, Formon JJ. Selective transsplenic decompression of gastroesophageal varices by distal splenorenal shunt. Ann Surg 1967;166:437-455.

18. Redecker AG, Geller HM, Reynolds TB. Hepatic wedge pressure, blood flow, vascular resistance and oxygen consumption in cirrhosis before and after end-to-side portocaval shunt. J Clin Invest 1985;37:606-618.

19. Sarfeh IJ, Rypins EB, Raiszadeh M, et al. Serial measurement of portal hemodynamics after partial portal decompression. Surgery 1986;100:52-58.

20. Whipple AO. The problem of portal hypertension in relation to the hepatosplenopathies. Ann Surg 1945;122:449-467.

21. Berdal P. Die Verätzungsfolgen in der Speiseröhre und deren Behandlung. HNO 1973;21:264-267.

22. Maynar M, Cabrera J, Pulido-Duque JM, Reyes R, Gorriz E. Percutaneous transhepatic portocaval shunt. In: Liermann D, ed. *Stents*. New York: Marianne Liebert; 1993; in press.

23. Laberge JM, Ring EJ, Gordon RL. Percutaneous intrahepatic portosystemic shunt created via a femoral vein approach. Radiology 1991;181:679-681.

24. Gordon JD, Colapinto RF, Abecassis M. Transjugular intrahepatic portosystemic shunt: a nonoperative approach to lifethreatening variceal bleeding. Can J Surg 1987;30:45-49.

25. Rösch J, Uchida BT, Putnam JS. Experimental intrahepatic portocaval anastomosis: use of expandable Gianturco stents. Radiology 1987;162:481-485.

26. Pichlmayr R, Wilfiihr KU, Böker K, Gerstenkorn C. Liver transplantation in chronic liver failure. In: Reiser M, Steudel A, Hirner A, Kania U, eds. *Lebertumoren und Portale Hypertension*. Berlin: Springer; 1993;293-296.

27. Häring R, Hirner A, Karavias TH. Portale Hypertension: Stellenwert der portosystemischen Shunt-Operation und der Notfalleingriffe. Chirurg 1985;56:425-431.

28. Rössle M, Haag K, Nöldge G. Hämodynamische Konsequenzen der portalen Dekompression: Welches ist der optimale Shunt? Z Gastroenterol 1990; 28:630-634.

29. Warren WD, Millikan WJ, Henderson JM. Ten years portal hypertensive surgery at emory: results and new perspectives. Ann Surg 1982;1295:530-542.

30. Steegmüller KW, Schmidt D, Junginger T. Zur Therapie der Oesophagusvarzenblutung

in der BRD - Ergebnisse einer Umfrage. Arch Chir 1991;376:273-279.

31. Rösch J, Barton RE, Keller FS, Uchida BS, Petersen BD. TIPS with self-expandable Z-stents. In: Liermann D, ed. *Stents*. New York: Marianne Liebert; 1993; in press.

32. Hanafee W, Weier M. Transjugular percutaneous cholangiography. Radiology 1967;88:35-39.

33. Foster JH, Ellison LH, Donovan TH, Anderson A. Quantity and quality of survival after portosystemic shunts. Am J Surg 1971;12:490-501.

34. Sandritter W, Thomas C, eds. *Makropathologie*. Stuttgart: Schattauer; 1977.

35. Colapinto RF, Stronell RD, Birch SJ. Creation of of an intrahepatic portosystemic shunt with a Grüntzig balloon catheter. Can Med Assoc J 1982;126:267-271.

36. Burgener FA, Gutierrez OH. Nonsurgical production of intrahepatic portosystemic venous shunt in portal hypertension with the double lumen balloon catheter. Förtschr Roentgenstr 1979;130:686-688.

37. März E, Ungeheuer E, Berkhoff W. Therapie der Oesophagusvarizenblutung durch Venensperroperation. In: Paquet J, Denck H, Berchthold R, eds. *Portale Hypertension*. Basel: Karger 1982;164-170.

38. Otte JB, Gigot J, Reynaert M. Arterialisation der Pfortader in Kombination mit einemtherapeutischen porto-cavalen Shunt — Gibt es noch Platz für dieses Verfahren? Vorläufige Ergebnisse einer pospektiven, kontrollierten, randomisierten Studie. Chir Gastroenterol 1987;3:75-89.

39. Pichlmayr R. Technical developments in liver trasplantation. In: Creutzfeld W and Pichlmar R, eds. *Liver and Pancreas Transplantation*. Baillières Clin Gastroenterol 1989;3:757-765.

40. Richter GM, Nöldge G, Palmaz JC, Rössle M. The transjugular intrahepatic portosystemic stent-shunt (TIPSS): results of a pilot study. J Cardiovasc Interv Radiol 1990;13:200-207.

41. Barsoum MS, Bolous FI, El-Rooby AA, Rizk-Allah MA, Ibrahim AS. Tamponade and injection sclerotherapy in the managment of bleeding oesophageal varices. Br J Surg 1982;69:76-78.

42. Fischer JE, Bower RH, Atamian S, Weling R. Comparison of distal and proximal splenorenal shunts: a randomized prospective trial. Ann Surg 1981;194:531-544.

43. Soehendra N, Grimm H, Maydeo A, Nam V Ch, Eckmann B, Brückner M. Endoscopic sclerotherapy — personal experience. Hepatogastroenterology 1991;38:220-223.

44. Rösch J, Hanafee WN, Snow H. Transjugular portal venography and radiologic portocaval shunt: an experimental study. Radiology 1969;92:1112-1114.

45. Di Febo G, Siringo M, Vacirca M. Somatostatin (SMS) and urgent sclerotherapy (US) in active oesophageal variceal bleeding. Gastroenterology 1990;98:583.

46. Reichle FA, Fahmy WF, Golsorkhi M. Prospective comparative clinical trial with distal splenorenal and mesocaval shunts. Am J Surg 1979;137:12-21.

47. Paquet KJ, Kalk JF, Koussouris P. Sofortsklerosierung der akuten Oesophagusvarizenblutung während der Notfallendoskopie. Dtsch Med Wochenschr 1986;111:668-671.

Transjugular Intrahepatic Portosystemic Shunt (TIPS) for Bleeding Esophageal Varices in Cirrhosis: Clinical and Portal Hemodynamic Follow-Up

Manuel Maynar[1], Juan Cabrera[2], Elias Gorriz[1], Ricardo Reyes[1],
Rafael Granados[2], Juan Maria Pulido-Duque[1], Pedro Rubio[1]

[1]Vascular and Interventional Radiology Unit, [2]Gastroenterology Unit
Hospital Universitario Nuestra Señora del Pino, Spain

INTRODUCTION

The main advantage of the transjugular intrahepatic portosystemic shunt (TIPS) is the possibility of decompressing the portal venous system without general anaesthesia, thus diminishing operative risk in patients with poor clinical conditions and/or active bleeding (1,2,3). The present prospective study was aimed at investigating the efficacy and safety of elective TIPS procedures and portal hemodynamic behavior over the first year of follow-up.

MATERIALS AND METHODS

The study population was comprised of 51 consecutive cirrhotic patients admitted for esophageal variceal bleeding between May, 1991 and March, 1993. Patients with chronic hepatic encephalopathy; severe acute alcoholic hepatitis; cardiac failure; severe sepsis; or who were terminal were excluded from study entry. All patients provided informed consent. Prior to the TIPS procedure, arterial portography and simultaneous free hepatic venograms were performed.

As previously reported (4), our technique consisted of a right jugular vein approach, 5 Fr Rösch needle (Cook, Bloomington IN), angioplasty in the parenchymal tract, and insertion of the stent (5). In 37 patients, a 10-mm diameter Wallstent™ endoprosthesis (Schneider, Zurich, Switzerland) was deployed, and in 14 cases an 11-mm diameter Strecker™ stent (Boston Scientific Corp., Denmark) was inserted.

All patients were subsequently followed every 3 and 6 months in an outpatient hepatic clinic during the first and second year, respectively.

Selective embolization with absolute alcohol and/or metallic coils of venous tributaries of esophageal varices was the first therapy employed in patients with active bleeding. This latter therapy was also employed when, at any hemodynamic follow-up point, the portacaval post-TIPS gradient (PCPG) remained above 12 mm Hg and variceal filling was observed in the splenoportal venography, in spite of having performed stent dilatation or additional stent placement. Shunt dysfunction was considered when the PCPG showed a greater than 25% increase over previous values and the measured gradient was greater than 12 mm Hg at any time during follow-up.

The baseline clinical characteristics of all patients are summarized in Table 1.

RESULTS

In the present series, a total of 55 TIPS were placed in 51 patients. Four patients required a second procedure, one because of defective deployment of the stent in the parenchymal tract during TIPS placement and the remaining three due to total obstruction observed during follow-up. The mean time of the TIPS procedure was 152.46 ±

Table 1.   Baseline Clinical Characteristics

Sex (male/female)	36/15
Mean ± SD Age (yr)	54 ± 11.2 (range, 14-70)
No. of Patients (%) with:	
Alcoholism	33 (64.7%)
Previous Episodes of GIB	1.73 ± 1 (range, 1-5)
Ascites	16 (31.4%)
Hepatic Encephalopathy	6 (11.5%)
Child-Pugh Class A	25 (49%)
Child-Pugh Class B	13 (25.5%)
Child-Pugh Class C	13 (25.5%)

GIB: Gastrointestinal Bleeding

92.1 min (range, 35-420 min) and the length of hospitalization after TIPS was 5.45 ± 4.61 days (range, 1 to 26 days). The mean follow-up period was 405 ± 215 days (range, 32 to 764 days).

A significant decrease of 21.91 ± 6.27 to 12.8 ± 5 mm Hg was observed in the PCPG immediately after TIPS ($p < 0.0001$). Twelve (23.5%) of the 51 patients had a relapsing bleeding episode. In every rebleeding episode, portal hemodynamic evaluation indicated shunt dysfunction which was treated by means of the previously mentioned endovascular therapies. To date, death secondary to massive rebleeding has occurred in one patient who had laboratory evidence of disseminated intravascular coagulation in spite of having undergone selective embolization of esophageal varices and a second TIPS which was patent at autopsy.

The platelet count was significantly lower among rebleeding patients (86.20 ± 29.97 mm^3) compared to non-rebleeding patients (134.93 ± 59.83 mm^3). Multivariate analysis using the Cox logistic regression model in which all of these variables were entered indicated that none had an independent predictive value of variceal rebleeding during follow-up.

Seven patients (13.7%) have had at least one episode of spontaneous hepatic encephalopathy during follow-up, with two Child-Pugh class C patients developing chronic relapsing encephalopathy.

Nine (17.6%) of the 51 patients died during follow-up. Death was due to a rebleeding episode in one case, hepatic failure in another, and to causes unrelated to the liver disease in six patients (pneumonia in two cases; severe sepsis, hypernephroma, secondary peritonitis, and cerebral stroke in one patient each).

Nineteen patients with shunt dysfunction were submitted to a second hemodynamic evaluation approximately 3 months later and 12 (63.2%) showed repeated shunt dysfunction. In contrast, in a revision of 17 patients with correctly functioning shunts reviewed 6 months later, only 4 (23.5%) showed shunt dysfunction.

DISCUSSION

This high rate of shunt dysfunction stenosis has not been previously published, perhaps due to the fact that our "shunt stenosis" criteria were based on a functional concept, whereas the criteria in other studies have been morphological by means of angiography or Doppler exploration (6). We consider these criteria subjective, and not in agreement with hemodynamic measurement.

Six months after the procedure nearly half of the patients showed a significant increase in PCPG with the theoretical risk of having relapsed bleeding. A high rebleeding rate (23.5%) was observed in our study, with bleeding occurring during early follow-up in most of the cases (i.e., within 6 months). This may be related to an abnormally high PCPG in 45% of the patients after TIPS. No significant differences were observed in mean PCPG, however, among rebleeding and non-rebleeding patients after the procedure. While univariate analysis showed that the platelet count was significantly lower in the rebleeding patients immediately after TIPS, no factor studied was shown to be statistically significant upon multivariate analysis.

The high rate of patients presenting with hemodynamic stenosis during follow-up and the relatively high rate of early rebleeding suggests that portal hemodynamic revision is advisable a few days after the TIPS procedure to determine early parietal hyperplasia. Furthermore, a selective coronary vein embolization during TIPS is a rapid and risk-free maneuver which would avoid these early rebleeding episodes (7).

The efficacy of TIPS in the long-term control of variceal bleeding should be assessed in further follow-up studies; however, the present study shows that shunt patency must be frequently explored to avoid relapse of variceal bleeding. More studies are needed to know the pathogenesis and predisposing factors of stenosis in order to prevent it or to design new stents. Furthermore, randomized trials comparing elective treatment of variceal bleeding with TIPS and currently available pharmacologic, endoscopic, or surgical procedures are necessary.

REFERENCES

1. Rösch J, Hanafee W, Snow H, Barenfus M, Gray R. Transjugular intrahepatic portacaval shunt. Am J Surg 1971;121:588-592.
2. Richter GM, Nöldge G, Palmaz JC, et al. Transjugular intrahepatic portacaval stent shunt: preliminary clinical results. Radiology 1990;174:1027-1030.
3. Ring EJ, Lake JR, Roberts JP, et al. Using transjugular intrahepatic shunts to control variceal bleeding before liver transplantation. Ann Int Med 1992;116:304-309.
4. Maynar M, Cabrera J, Gorriz E, et al. Transjugular intrahepatic portosystemic shunt - early experience with a flexible trocar catheter system. AJR 1993;161:301-306.
5. Pulido-Duque JM, Reyes R, Gorriz E, et al. Intraparenchymal anesthesia infiltration during transjugular intrahepatic portosystemic shunting. Radiology 1992;185:903-904.
6. Longo JM, Bilbao JI, Rousseau HP, et al. Transjugular intrahepatic portosystemic shunt: Evaluation with doppler sonography. Radiology 1993;186:529-534.
7. Coldwell DM, More ADA, Ben-Menachem Y, et al. Bleeding gastroesophageal varices: Gastric vein embolization after partial decompression. Radiology 1991;178:249-251.

PART II

NONVASCULAR STENTS

Pancreatic Duct and Bile Duct

Gastrointestinal Tract

Respiratory Tract

Genitourinary Tract

Percutaneous Placement of Metal-Expandable Stents in the Pancreatic Duct

R.F. Dondelinger[1], P. Magotteaux[2], J.H. Boverie[1]

[1]*Department of Medical Imaging, University Hospital Sart Tilman, Liege, Belgium*
[2]*Department of Medical Imaging, Clinique Saint-Joseph, Liege, Belgium*

INTRODUCTION

Among minimally-invasive diagnostic and therapeutic procedures in the pancreas, the following well-established techniques are regularly used: percutaneous fine needle biopsy; endoscopic or percutaneous insertion of stents in the common bile duct for relief of biliary obstruction caused by pancreatic cancer or pancreatitis; percutaneous chemical neurolysis of the celiac plexus and splanchnic nerves for pain relief from retropancreatic tumor invasion; and endoscopic transmural or percutaneous drainage of pancreatic pseudocysts or abscesses resulting from acute or chronic pancreatitis. Drainage of pancreatic fluid collections can be performed through an external catheter, through a short internal stent which drains into the stomach, or through a gastro- or duodenocystostomy, provided a close contact between the wall of the pancreatic fluid cavity and the stomach or duodenum is present on computed tomography (CT).

Access to the pancreatic ducts is regularly gained by an endoscopic transpapillary approach for completion of various procedures including sphincterotomy of the pancreatic sphincters; endoscopic biopsy inside a sphincterotomy or further inside the pancreatic ducts; sampling of pancreatic fluid for chemical and cytological analyses; endoscopy of the pancreatic duct using small caliber fiber optic or Quartz fiber scopes; balloon dilatation of elective strictures; endoscopic pancreatic lithotripsy and stone extraction; and insertion of plastic pancreatic stents with a variable diameter of 7 Fr to 10 Fr. Recently, the insertion of metal-expandable stents for relief of tight or recoiling stenoses related to chronic pancreatitis, or for treatment of disrupture of the pancreatic ducts due to acute pancreatitis or trauma has been advocated. Other occasional indications for endoscopic pancreatic stenting are a hypertensive pancreatic sphincter, pancreas divisum, or a stenotic minor papilla (1-7). Endoscopic transpapillary access to the pancreatic ducts can fail for several reasons, such as previous gastric or pancreatic surgery; intrathoracic stomach; duodenal diverticula; papillary or peripapillary tumor; esophageal or gastroduodenal obstruction; stones impacted at the level of the papilla; or other anatomical variations.

Endoscopic failures can be avoided by using percutaneous access to the pancreatic duct. Until recently, however, the percutaneous approach was restricted to diagnostic fine needle opacification of the pancreatic ducts (8,9). The dilated pancreatic duct is localized and punctured with a 22-gauge needle under ultrasonography or CT control, contrast medium is injected under fluoroscopic control, and radiographs are taken. Indications for percutaneous pancreatography include pre- or post-operative mapping of the pancreatic ducts in selected patients. The success rate of percutaneous opacification of the pancreatic ducts varies from 80 to 100% when the diameter of the dilated duct equals or exceeds 5 mm.

More invasive percutaneous procedures involving the pancreatic ducts have been only occasionally described due to the fear of severe complications and the technical difficulties inherent with the percutaneous approach.

Percutaneous external drainage of the pancreatic duct was reported in a patient with acute pancreatitis and persistent leakage of pancreatic fluid due to downstream pancreatic obstruction. A drainage catheter was inserted percutaneously with CT guidance by an anterior left lateral approach and external drainage was maintained for 6 months; several catheter exchanges were needed to overcome clogging (10).

Experience with endoscopic or percutaneous insertion of expandable metal stents was gained in the bile ducts for treatment of malignant stenoses and, to a lesser extent, for stenoses of benign origin. Treatment of elective short stenoses of the pancreatic duct related to chronic pancreatitis by endoscopic placement of expandable metal stents is now being evaluated (11).

We have recently described percutaneous placement of metal-expandable stents in the pancreatic ducts and advocate its use when the endoscopic approach is impossible for anatomical reasons or has failed due to conditions such as those listed above (12,13).

PERCUTANEOUS TECHNIQUE

A diagnostic opacification of the pancreatic duct must be obtained before the therapeutic procedure. The patient is sedated and prepared similarly to a percutaneous biliary procedure. A minimal ductal diameter of 3 to 5 mm is required for percutaneous fine needle puncture of the pancreatic duct. Percutaneous puncture can be performed with ultrasonography or CT control. When the pancreatic duct is dilated to 3 mm it is well visualized with ultrasonography, but remains difficult to localize with CT. When calcifications outline the pancreas, percutaneous puncture may be possible under fluoroscopic control. Regardless of the type of imaging guidance used, the number of fine needle passes should remain limited to three or four to avoid complications, although the chronically-inflamed or the tumoral pancreas is less sensitive to needle puncture than normal pancreatic parenchyma. In chronic pancreatitis, the risk of pancreatic fistulization after needle puncture is probably reduced since secretion of pancreatic fluid has decreased. A percutaneous transgastric approach to the pancreatic duct is advisable, allowing placement of a short internal plastic stent between the pancreatic duct and the stomach and obviating the risk of a pancreatic fistula (12). This gastropancreatic stent can be retrieved endoscopically after several weeks or months of function.

The primary disadvantage of the transgastric puncture is that the pancreatic duct is approached in its middle segment and control of its entire length is extremely difficult or not feasible during the same session. The percutaneous access point must be determined on cross-sectional images at the level where a close contact between the pancreas and the posterior wall of the stomach is present. A percutaneous puncture of the pancreatic duct at the level of the pancreatic tail and parallel to the long axis of the pancreas is usually too problematic because a transsplenic, transcolic, or transintestinal approach would be required. The mobility of the pancreatic tail and its posterior orientation also makes this approach more complicated.

Nevertheless, a percutaneous left lateral approach can be performed in selected patients when abundant peri-pancreatic fat planes are present, thus displacing the intestinal structures anteriorly away from the pancreas, or in patients who underwent a splenectomy. The left lateral extragastric approach has the advantage of controlling the entire length of the pancreatic duct, although a temporary pancreatogastric stent cannot be placed at the end of the procedure since the stomach is not punctured. A right lateral transhepatic approach can be used on exceptional occasions when the anterior transgastric or the left lateral puncture was unsuccessful.

A flexible, 22-gauge, Chiba needle is used for the initial percutaneous diagnostic puncture of the pancreatic duct. The skinny needle must be inserted firmly as it can be easily deviated when crossing the gastric walls. When the pancreatic duct is opacified, a second puncture of the pancreatic duct is performed with fluoroscopic control using a 16- or 18-gauge Teflon-sheathed needle. The stomach can be previously distended by air, allowing better localization of the opacified pancreatic duct as well as improved control of the procedure. Biplane fluoroscopy is helpful for three-dimensional orientation, particularly when a left lateral or a right transhepatic approach has been chosen. The Teflon-sheathed needle is directed to the head of the pancreas. Correct positioning of the extremity of the needle inside the pancreatic duct is checked by biplane fluoroscopy without moving the patient. In cases where the Teflon needle has been advanced too far beyond the pancreatic duct, it can be slowly retracted until the extremity is felt to be located in the ductal lumen. Aspiration of pancreatic juice and contrast medium confirms correct needle positioning. A stiff hydrophilic guidewire with a J-curved tip is useful to catheterize the pancreatic duct and papilla. The Teflon sheath is advanced over the guidewire in the duodenum. A stiff 0.035-inch Lunderquist guidewire is then placed inside the Teflon sheath which is retrieved. Semi-rigid 6 Fr to 8 Fr dilators are passed over the Lunderquist guidewire to dilate the percutaneous entry point, gastric walls, and the pancreatic parenchyma. A 7 Fr to 9 Fr working sheath, or a hemostatic valve, can be placed over the Lunderquist guidewire in the pancreatic duct to avoid coiling and curving of other flexible instruments within the stomach during further intrapancreatic introduction. To obtain clear vision for percutaneous pancreatoscopy, irrigation of the pancreatic duct with saline or carbon dioxide is possible through the sidebranch of the hemostatic valve. Contrast medium can also be injected for radiological documentation. When a firm and straight access is established through the working sheath from the percutaneous entry point to the pancreatic duct, the intraductal procedures mentioned above can also be carried

out percutaneously (i.e., balloon dilatation, antegrade sphincterotomy, pancreatoscopy, mechanical lithotripsy, stenting). The percutaneous procedure can also be controlled by peroral duodenoscopy in addition to fluoroscopy, particularly for monitoring correct stent adjustment inside the papilla.

PRELIMINARY RESULTS

Four patients, three male and one female, aged 41 to 81 years (mean, 66.5 years) were treated by percutaneous insertion of a metal-expandable stent in the pancreatic duct. Patient 1 presented with pancreatic cancer without retropancreatic tumor spread but with abdominal pain; patient 2 had a persistent post-traumatic pancreatic fistula which was non-regressive despite endoscopic insertion of a 7 Fr plastic stent. Painful chronic pancreatitis with an elective ductal stricture and dilatation were indicated in patient 3 (Figure 1), and patient 4 presented with a post-operative anastomotic stenosis of the pancreatic duct after a Whipple procedure for benign ampulloma (Figure 2). A Wallstent™ (Medinvent, Lausanne, Switzerland) was used in patients 1, 3, and 4 while patient 2 received two Strecker™ stents (Boston Scientific Corp., Denmark). The stent characteristics as well as the methods employed for placement in each patient are shown in Table 1. The follow-up period in these patients ranged from 2 to 18 months and the clinical outcomes for each patient are shown in Table 2. No complications related to the procedure occurred.

DISCUSSION

Perspectives of Percutaneous Approach to the Pancreatic Ducts

The pancreatic ducts can be approached endoscopically and percutaneously, similar to the techniques developed for the biliary system. Percutaneous access to the pancreatic duct has more inherent technical difficulties

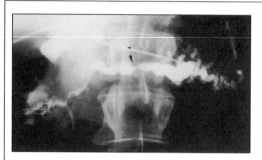

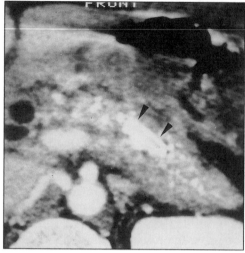

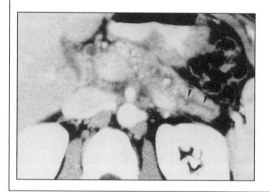

Figure 1. A 41-year-old male presenting with severe abdominal pain related to alcoholic chronic pancreatitis. Endoscopy failed in opacification of the caudal segment of the pancreatic duct. Percutaneous pancreatography confirmed an elective stricture (arrow) in the corporeal segment and upstream dilatation *(top left)*. Previous CT showed calcified chronic pancreatitis and dilatation of the main pancreatic duct (arrows) *(bottom left)*. CT after percutaneous, transhepatic, and transduodenal placement of a "coronary" Wallstent in the pancreatic duct (arrows). The stent is correctly located and displaces a large calcification laterally. No upstream dilatation of the pancreatic duct is visible *(top right)*.

Table 1. Patient and Stent Characteristics

Patient Number	Age/Sex	Percutaneous Approach	Type of Metal Stent	Additional Procedures
1	73/M	Anterior transgastric	1 Wallstent (6 mm, 4 cm)	Percutaneous endoscopy, Biopsy, Pancreatic-gastric 8 Fr plastic stent
2	81/M	Left lateral	2 Strecker (6 mm, 2 cm)	Percutaneous endoscopy
3	41/M	Transhepatic	1 Wallstent (4 mm, 2 cm)	Gallbladder drainage, Pseudocyst drainage
4	71/F	Anterior extragastric	1 Wallstent (10 mm, 3.5 cm)	Cytology, Balloon dilatation

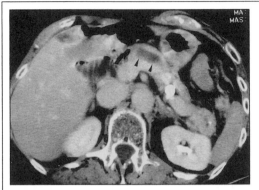
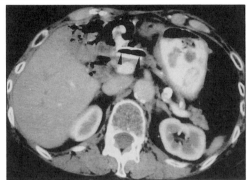
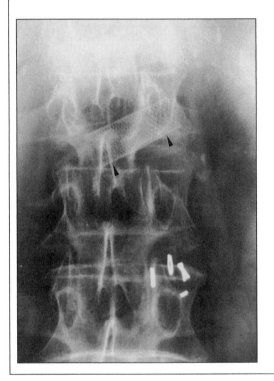

Figure 2. A 71-year-old female who underwent a Whipple procedure for ampulloma. She presented with abdominal pain 6 months after surgery. CT shows severe dilatation of the main pancreatic duct (arrows) above the pancreatic-jejunal anastomosis *(top left)*. Complete dilatation of a 1-cm Wallstent (arrows) placed at the level of the anastomotic stricture by an anterior extragastric approach *(bottom left)*. CT confirms correct stent placement (arrows) and function. No pain *(top right)*.

Table 2. Results Following Percutaneous Stenting of the Pancreatic Duct

Patient Number	Follow-Up Period	Clinical Outcome
1	3 months	Pain decreased until death from pancreatic cancer
2	2 months	Pancreatic fistula closed until death from pneumonia
3	12 months	Pain disappeared until stent obstruction by tissue proliferation
4	18 months	Pain disappeared, stent patent

than percutaneous catheterization of the bile ducts because only one duct is available for puncture. Technical difficulties also include limited dilatation of the pancreatic duct and the deep location of the pancreas in the abdomen. Despite these limitations, percutaneous access to the pancreatic ducts is a minimally-invasive procedure with interesting potential. The transgastric approach creates a communication between the pancreatic duct and the stomach, which has the same effect as the surgical Puestow procedure. This technique can also be used for treatment of communicating pseudocysts.

The combined endoscopic peroral and percutaneous technique used in the bile ducts can also be performed in the pancreatic ducts when endoscopic retrograde catheterization of the papilla has failed. A 5 Fr catheter is inserted percutaneously for antegrade papillary catheterization and gives assistance to the endoscopist. Use of small-sheathed needles provides limited trauma to the stomach and pancreas.

When stenting of the pancreatic ducts with expandable metal stents is considered, a stent diameter of 4 to 6 mm is advisable. In our experience, Wallstents and Strecker stents were placed successfully without technical problems during stent release (12,13). More recently, Gianturco stents have been used with the same ease (14). All types of stents opened correctly and neither secondary migration nor ductal perforation was observed. Video-pancreatoscopy and opacification of the pancreatic duct confirmed optimal opening of the stents. In our experience, however, long-term behavior of expandable metal stents placed in the pancreatic ducts is still unknown. Tissue proliferation through the mesh of the stents can occur in malignant or benign conditions, leading to stent obstruction. Formation of mucus plugs has the same effect. The risk of secondary migration, dislocation, or corrosion of the metal stents must be further evaluated. Changes in secondary pancreatic ducts, consistent with chronic pancreatitis, were observed with temporary plastic stents (15). It

should be assessed if similar changes also occur with metal stents, although they are known to maintain the ostia of collaterals open when placed in arteries, veins, or in the biliary system.

Expandable metal stents placed in the vascular or biliary system are covered by an epithelial layer within several weeks or months. This phenomenon is also expected to occur in the pancreatic duct, which makes removal or exchange of expandable metal stents difficult or impossible. Diathermic tissue ablation, as suggested for cleaning of metal stents placed in the bile ducts, can be applied to metallic pancreatic stents either through the papilla or through the gastropancreatic fistulous orifice or stent (16). There is no need to place the metal stent in a protruded position through the papilla in chronic pancreatitis since the papilla itself is not strictured in this disease.

Failures

Failures of the percutaneous approach to the pancreatic duct are related to a non- or only minimally-dilated cut; intestinal strictures or varices surrounding the pancreas; failure to find a close contact between the stomach and pancreas on cross-sectional images; uncorrectable bleeding tendency; impossible antegrade catheterization of the pancreatic duct with the guidewire; failure to insert catheter due to fibrosis; or an uncooperative patient.

Potential Complications

Potential complications of percutaneous procedures inside the pancreatic ducts include pneumoperitoneum; digestive perforation; bacteremia, septicemia, hematoma, or abscess formation; peritonitis; acute pancreatitis; hemorrhage; pseudo-aneurysm; and vagal shock. When the pancreas is atrophic due to chronic pancreatitis, an acute inflammatory reaction is unlikely to occur.

REFERENCES

1. Fuji T, Amano H, Harima K, et al. Pancreatic sphincterotomy and pancreatic endoprosthesis. Endoscopy 1985;17:69-72.

2. McCarthy J, Geenen JE, Hogan WJ. Preliminary experience with endoscopic stent placement in benign pancreatic diseases. Gastrointest Endosc 1988;34:16-18.

3. Prabhu M, Geenen JE, Hogan WJ. Role of endoscopic stent placement in the treatment of acute recurrent pancreatitis associated with pancreatic divisum: a prospective assessment (abstr). Gastrointest Endosc 1989;35:165.

4. Lehman G, O'Connor G, Troiano F, Benage D. Endoscopic papillotomy and stenting of the minor papilla in pancreas divisum (abstr). Gastrointest Endosc 1989;35:167.

5. Kozarek RA, Patterson DJ, Ball TJ, Traverso LW. Endoscopic placement of pancreatic stents and drains in the management of pancreatitis. Ann Surg 1989;209:261-266.

6. Trondsen E, Rosseland AR, Bakka A. Pancreatic duct prosthesis. Tidsskr Nor Laegeforen 1990;110:1231-1232.

7. Kozarek RA, Ball TJ, Patterson DJ, Freeny PC, Ryan J, Traverso LW. Endoscopic transpapillary therapy for disrupted pancreatic duct and peripancreatis fluid collections. Gastroenterology 1991;100:1362-1370.

8. Ohto M, Karasawa E, Kimura K, et al. Ultrasonically guided percutaneous contrast medium injection and aspiration biopsy using a real-time puncture transducer. Radiology 1980;136:171-176.

9. Haaga JR, Highman LM, Cooperman AV, Owens FJ. Percutaneous CT-guided pancreatography and pseudocystography. AJR 1979;132:829-830.

10. Gobien RP, Stanley JH, Anderson MC, Vujic I. Percutaneous drainage of pancreatic duct for treating acute pancreatitis. AJR 1983;141:795-796.

11. Cremer M, Sugai B, Delhaye M, Deviere J. Expandable pancreatic metal stents (Wallstents) for chronic pancreatitis: first world series (abstr). Gastroenterology 1990;98:A215.

12. Kurdziel JC, Dondelinger RF, Barthelme G. Percutaneous transgastric internal drainage, endoscopy and stenting of the pancreatic duct: a new technique. Eur J Radiol 1991;12:1-3.

13. Dondelinger RF, Kurdziel JC. Percutaneous placement of expandable metal stents in the main pancreatic duct. Sem Intervent Radiol 1991;8:316-320.

14. Mathieson JR, Cooperberg PL, Murray DJ, Dashefsky S, Christensen R, Schmidt N. Pancreatic duct obstruction treated with percutaneous antegrade insertion of a metal stent: report of two cases. Radiology 1992;185;465-468.

15. Kozarek RA. Pancreatic stents can induce ductal changes consistent with chronic pancreatitis. Gastrointest Endosc 1990;36:93-95.

16. Cremer M, Deviere J, Sugai B, Baize M. Expandable biliary metal stents for malignancies: endoscopic insertion and diathermic clearing for tumor ingrowth. Gastrointest Endosc 1990;36:451-457.

Biliary Stenting: Self-Expandable and Balloon-Expandable Stents. Early and Late Results

I.K. Tesdal[1], W. Jaschke[1], C. Düber[2], J. Werhand[3], K.J. Klose[3]

[1]*Institut für Klinische Radiologie, Universitätsklinikum, Mannheim, Germany*
[2]*Institut für Klinische Strahlenkunde, Universitätsklinikum, Mainz, Germany*
[3]*Medizinisches Zentrum für Radiologie, Klinikum der Philipps-Universität, Marburg, Germany*

INTRODUCTION

In selected cases where endoscopic methods fail or cannot be performed, percutaneous transhepatic biliary drainage (PTBD) is an accepted method for biliary decompression, either as a palliation or as a pre-operative treatment (1,2). Most PTBD procedures are performed to place a permanent biliary endoprosthesis. Regardless of whether a percutaneous or endoscopic route has been chosen, the main disadvantage with plastic stents are their high migration and occlusion rates (3,4). Therefore, these stents require frequent replacement (5). The large lumen diameter of metallic stents (up to 30 Fr) theoretically provides a lower occlusion rate, and incorporation of the metallic stent into the bile duct wall makes stent migration virtually impossible. The metallic stents are introduced on a small delivery catheter so that PTBD and stent implantation can be performed in two steps.

Our primary objectives when we began using metallic endoprostheses for the treatment of biliary obstructions were longer patency rates and less reinterventions, as well as reduction in the number of complications. This chapter outlines our experience with Strecker stents and Wallstents to treat patients with malignant and benign biliary obstructions.

MATERIALS AND METHODS

Between February, 1989 and July, 1993, we placed 187 Wallstents™ (Medinvent, Lausanne, Switzerland) in 127 patients and 91 Strecker™ stents (Boston Scientific Corp., Denmark) in 40 patients (86 women and 81 men) with a median age of 66 years (range, 28 to 93 years). The cause of obstructive jaundice and the location of the obstructions are listed in Tables 1 and 2, respectively. Thirty-six patients (21.5%) had previously received biliary surgery. In three patients the stents were introduced via a T-Drainage (Figure 1), while in the other patients the approach was via a peripheral duct in the right (N=130), left (N=4), or both (N=30) liver lobes.

Table 1. Cause of Obstructive Jaundice in 167 Patients

Pancreatic Carcinoma	53	(31.7%)
Biliary Neoplasm		
Duct	40	(24.0%)
Gallbladder	14	(8.4%)
Liver Tumor	3	(1.8%)
Metastases	50	(29.9%)
Benign Obstructions	7	(4.2%)

Table 2. Location of Obstruction Due to Bismuth Classification

Bismuth[a]	No. of Patients (%)
1	22 (13%)
2	27 (16%)
3	18 (11%)
4	32 (19%)
D. Choledochus	68 (41%)

[a] Bismuth 1 and 2: more resp. less than 2 cm from the hepatic bifurcation. Bismuth 3 and 4: reach resp. infiltrate the bifurcation.

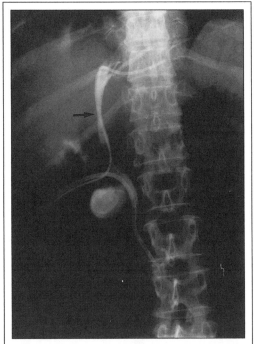

Figure 1. Wallstent introduced via a T-Drainage. Residual stenosis (arrow) immediately after being released.

Intrahepatic abscesses (N=3), bilioms (N=2), local peritonitis (N=1), and intrahepatic hematomas (N=2) were drained. One patient had a cholecystoduodenostomy with partial removal of the Wallstent performed because of a duodenal ulcer caused by the distal stent end. Pulmonary embolism occurred in two patients and there was one episode of acute intestinal bleeding.

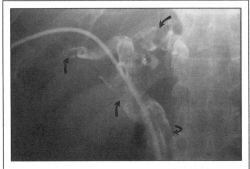

Figure 2. Patient suffering from pancreatic carcinoma. Pulsating arterial bleeding (puncture site) with clots intraductal (arrows). Angiography did not reveal any lesion.

RESULTS

The technical success rate was 94.9%. The procedure was a failure in six patients with Wallstents because the membrane did not roll back sufficiently to release the stents. In the group who received Strecker stents, we were not able to dilate the obstructions in three patients, and therefore the stents could not be deployed. All of these patients (N=9) were treated with plastic stents 2 to 5 days later. Eight patients with Strecker stents (20%) and one patient with a Wallstent (0.8%) (T-stent) had more than 30% residual stenoses.

The 30-day mortality rate was 8.4% (14 of 167), but only one death was related to the procedure (hemobilia with sepsis). Major complications occurred in 18 patients (11.3%). We observed four portal venous and two arterial bleedings; five of these patients had to be treated percutaneously (Figures 2 and 3).

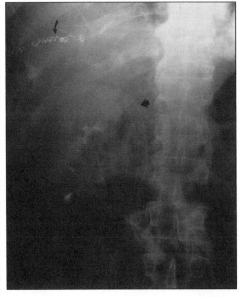

Figure 3. After implantation of a Wallstent (straight arrows) and embolization (curved arrows) of the puncture channel (GAW-coils), the bleeding ceased.

During follow-up, recurrent jaundice occurred in 29.4% of the patients with malignant disease (47 of 160); 19.4% (31 of 160) required a reintervention. The etiology and therapeutic options for recurrent jaundice in patients with malignant obstructions are listed in Table 3. The major causes of reobstruction (Figure 4) were tumor ingrowth (N=17) and tumor overgrowth (N=11). Restenting (N=17) was the most frequently performed treatment for recurrent jaundice.

Table 3. Etiology and Therapeutic Options of Recurrent Jaundice in Patients with Malignant Obstructions

Etiology	No. of Patients (N=47)
Tumor overgrowth distal to stents	11
Tumor ingrowth (invasion)[a]	17
Liver insufficiency	7
Disconnection of stents	2
Sludge	1
Divertikel (juxtapapillär)	1
Unknown	8

Therapeutic Options	No. of Patients (N=31)
Insertion of plastic endoprosthesis	5
PTBD	8
Re-stenting	17
Re-stenting and insertion of plastic endoprosthesis	1
No additional invasive therapy	16

[a] Pancreatic Cancer (N=14)

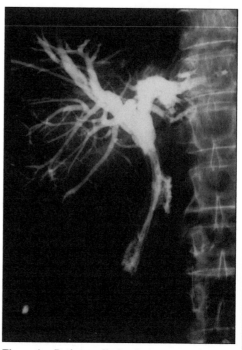

Figure 4. Patient suffering from pancreatic carcinoma. Recurrent jaundice due to tumor ingrowth through the mesh of the Wallstent.

The median stent patency (MSP) was 122 days with a mean survival of 132 days. In patients with carcinoma of the pancreas and gallbladder, the MSP was 107 and 103 days, respectively; the MSP for those with metastases was 95 days. The longest MSP (211 days) was in patients with carcinoma of the bile duct.

Three patients with benign biliary strictures were free of symptoms after 10, 18, and 25 months, respectively. One patient suffered from cholelithiasis after 9 months (Figure 5) and had to be operated on. One patient died after 5 months due to AIDS and two additional patients were lost to follow-up.

DISCUSSION

The use of metallic stents for treatment of bile duct obstruction has recently been reported in the literature (6-14). Most reports are of uncontrolled studies, and the results are contradictory. The early results with Wallstents (9) and Z-stents (6,7) showed occlusion rates of 42 to 50%. These disappointing data were possibly related to some inexperience with the placement technique as

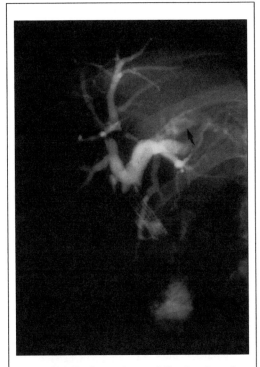

Figure 5. Benign stricture following hepatico-jejunostomy. Occlusion of the Strecker stent (after 9 months) due to cholelithiasis.

well as to the varying spectrum of patients treated (9). More recent studies have cited lower occlusion rates of 15 to 19% (15,16). We observed recurrent jaundice after stenting in 47 patients (29.4%) with malignant obstruction. In seven patients the recurrent jaundice was due to liver insufficiency, while in eight the etiology of the jaundice was unknown. The reobstruction rate in our series can therefore be estimated to be between 20 and 25%. Recently, randomized studies comparing the use of metallic stents and plastic stents in patients with malignant distal and hilar biliary obstructions have demonstrated insignificantly lower stent failure rates in the metallic group (17-20).

The objective of any treatment should be to provide a better quality of life for the patient. The number of reinterventions needed to manage stent-related problems and the rate of complications are important aspects. In our study, 31 patients (19.4%) with malignant disease required reintervention due to recurrent jaundice. It has been reported that up to 40.5 to 41.7% of plastic stents need to be changed (21,22), and randomized studies have shown significantly higher reintervention rates with plastic versus metal stents (18,19).

Endoscopic insertion of plastic stents has been shown to be safer than percutaneous insertion (23). The metallic stents have advantages over plastic stents since they can be introduced on a small delivery catheter (7 Fr). The flexibility of the Wallstent and the Strecker stent makes it possible to deploy them in a curved fashion such as through a T-drainage (Figure 1) and therefore, liver puncture is avoided. Nevertheless, we observed four portal venous and two arterial bleedings (Figures 2 and 3). Since these complications were generally observed during the initial liver puncture and biliary catheterization, they were probably not due to the implantation of the stents.

Approximately 3 to 6% of plastic stents migrate (4,24). Their large inner diameter, coupled with a fixed position after release, make the metallic stents not prone to migration (16,25). On the other hand, the expanding, shortening, and straightening force of the Wallstent makes their behavior somewhat unpredictable. Due to shortening of a transpapillar Wallstent, we observed a mechanically-induced duodenal ulcer in one patient. Ee et al (26) have reported a similar case. A survey of the literature shows lower complication rates with metallic stents compared to plastic stents (10,16-20).

Regardless of cause, patients with benign biliary strictures may be treated with a variety of percutaneous interventional techniques (11,27). Our results with the Strecker stent, albeit in a small number of patients, are encouraging. Besides the known advantages (good radiopacity, no shortening), the Strecker stent can be easily removed, either surgically or with a percutaneous interventional technique (28). One occluded Strecker stent in our series was removed without any anatomical or technical difficulties (Figure 5).

CONCLUSIONS

Compared to plastic endoprostheses, metallic stents offer definite advantages concerning implantation technique, patency rate, number of reinterventions, and complications. The rate of recurrent jaundice requiring intervention (about 20%) is still disappointingly high, and will need to be reduced through further improvement of the metallic stents.

REFERENCES

1. Hoevels J, Lunderquist A, Ihse I. Perkutane transhepatische Intubation der Gallengänge zur kombinierten inneren und äußeren Drainage bei extraheptischer Cholestase. Röfö 1978;129:533.
2. Ring EJ. Radiologic approach to malignant biliary obstruction: review and commentary. Cardiovasc Intervent Radiol 1990;13:217-222.
3. Huibregtse K. *Endoscopic Biliary and Pancreatic Drainage.* Stuttgart: Georg Thieme Verlag; 1988.
4. Mueller PR, Ferrucci JT, Teplick SK, et al. Biliary stent endoprosthesis: analysis of complications in 113 patients. Radiology 1985;156:637-639.
5. Cotton PB. Management of malignant bile duct obstruction. J Gastroenterol Hepatol 1990;Suppl 1:63-67.
6. Coons HG. Self-expanding stainless steel biliary stents. Radiology 1989;170:979-983.
7. Irving JD, Adam A, Dick R, Dondelinger RF, Lunderquist A, Roche A. Gianturco expandable metallic biliary stents: results of a European clinical trial. Radiology 1989;172:321-326.
8. Lammer J, Klein GE, Kleinert R, Hausegger K, Einspieler R. Obstructive jaundice: use of expandable metal endoprostheses for biliary drainage. Radiology 1990;177:789-792.
9. Gillams A, Dick R, Dooley JS, Wallsten H, El-Din A. Self-expandable stainless steel braided endoprosthesis for biliary strictures. Radiology 1990;174:137-140.
10. Adam A, Chetty N, Roddie M, Yeung E, Benjamin IS. Self-expandable stainless steel endoprostheses for treatment of malignant bile duct obstruction. AJR 1991;156:321-325.
11. Jaschke W, Klose KJ, Strecker EP. A new balloon-expandable tantalum stent (Strecker-stent) for the biliary system: preliminary experience. Cardiovasc Intervent Radiol 1992;15:356-359.
12. Gordon RL, Ring EJ, Laberge JM, Doherty MM. Malignant biliary obstruction: treatment with expandable metallic stents — follow-up of 50 consecutive patients. Radiology 1992;182:697-701.
13. Salomonowitz EK, Antonucci F, Heer M, Stuckmann G, Egloff B, Zollikofer CL. Biliary obstruction: treatment with self-expanding metal prostheses. JVIR 1992;3:365-370.
14. Huibregtse K, Carr-Locke DL, Cremer M, et al. Biliary stent occlusion: a problem solved with self-expanding metal stents? Endoscopy 1992;24:391-394.
15. Lee MJ, Dawson SL, Mueller PR, Krebs T, Saini S, Hahn PF. Palliation of malignant bile duct obstruction with metallic biliary endoprostheses: technique, results, and complications. JVIR 1992;3:665-671.
16. Stoker J, Lameris JS. Complications of percutaneously inserted biliary Wallstents. JVIR 1993;4:767-772.
17. Davids PHP, Groen AK, Rauws EAJ, Tytgat GNJ, Huibregtse K. Randomized trial of self-expanding metal stents versus polyethylene stents for distal malignant biliary obstruction. Lancet 1992;340:1488-1492.
18. Knyrim K, Wagner H-J, Pausch J, Vakil N. A prospective, randomized, controlled trial of metal stents for malignant obstruction of the common bile duct. Endoscopy 1993;25:207-212.
19. Wagner H-J, Knyrim K, Vakil N, Klose KJ. Plastic endoprostheses versus metal stents in the palliative treatment of malignant hilar biliary obstruction. A prospective and randomized trial. Endoscopy 1993;25:213-218.
20. Hausegger KA, Wilding R, Flueckiger F, Thurnher S, Winkelbauer F, Lammer J. Plastic versus expandable metal biliary endoprostheses: final report of a randomized trial (abstr) RSNA 1993;307.

21. Polydorou AA, Chisholm EM, Romanus AA, et al. A comparison of right versus left hepatic duct endoprosthesis insertion in malignant hilar biliary obstruction. Endoscopy 1989;21:266-271.

22. Schlieper M. Ergebnisse der perkutanen transhepatische Gallengangsdrainage bei der Therapie des Verschlußikterus. Inauguraldissertation, Fakultät für Klinische Medizin Mannheim, Universität Heidelberg 1991.

23. Speer AG, Cotton PB, Macrae KD. Endoscopic management of malignant biliary obstruction: Stents of 10 French gauge are preferable to stents of 8 French Gauge. Gastrointes Endosc 1988;34:412-417.

24. Lammer J, Neumayer K. Biliary drainage endoprostheses: experience with 201 placements. Radiology 1986;159:625-629.

25. Lee MJ, Dawson SL, Mueller PR, et al. Percutaneous management of hilar biliary malignancies with metallic endoprostheses: results, technical problems and causes of failure. Radiographics 1993;13:1249-1263.

26. Ee H, Laurence BH. Haemorrhage due to erosion of a metal biliary stent through the duodenal wall. Endoscopy 1992;24:431-432.

27. Lammer J, Deu E. Percutaneous management of benign biliary strictures. In: Kadir S, ed. *Current Practice of Interventional Radiology*. Philadelphia: Decker, Inc.; 1991; 550-553.

28. Liermann D, Zegelmann M, Kollath J, Satter P. Möglichkeiten zur Bergung fehlplazierter oder verschlossener metallischer Endoprothesen. In: Kollath J and Liermann D, eds. *Stents II*. Konstanz: Schnetztor-Verlag; 1992; 139-150.

Transjejunal Stent Implantation

Jürgen Triller[1], Walter Schweizer[2], Leslie H. Blumgart[2]

[1]*Institute of Diagnostic Radiology and* [2]*Clinic of Visceral and Transplant Surgery*
Bern University, Bern, Switzerland

INTRODUCTION

We classify benign biliary strictures according to Bismuth with slight modifications (Figure 1) (1). Most biliary strictures, especially Types 1 and 2, can be successfully surgically treated by establishing a mucosa-to-mucosa anastomosis between the common bile duct and a jejunal loop. At specialist centers, definitive healing can be anticipated in more than 90% of all cases (2).

Complicated intra- and extrahepatic obstructions of the biliary ducts tend to cause recurrent strictures and cholangitis, and even a good surgical technique is unable to prevent recurrence in all cases (2). Interventional radiologic and endoscopic techniques alone are difficult, have a high complication rate, and are frequently impracticable for technical reasons (3-6). To prevent the patient from undergoing repeated surgery, access for any necessary subsequent intervention can be established during the initial procedure subject to radiological supervision, particularly if the patient exhibits one or more of the risk factors defined in Table 1. (1,2). The method discussed below can combine the advantages of surgical and interventional radiology in cases of complicated benign and malignant biliary duct strictures.

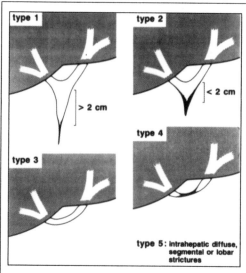

Figure 1. Classification of biliary strictures (Types 1-4, Bismuth).

Table 1. Risk Factors[a]

- High biliary obstruction (Types III, IV, V)
- Segmental or diffuse biliary strictures atrophy/hypertrophy complex
- Multiple previous operative interventions, portal hypertension, intrapheptic concrements, or debris
- Recurrent cholangitis and jaundice
- Restricted hepatic function, fibrosis, cirrhosis
- External and/or internal biliary fistula

[a] Patients with three or more risk factors were considered candidates for combined procedure.

METHODS

After clarification with percutaneous transhepatic cholangiography (PTC) or endoscopic retrograde cholangiopancreatography (ERCP), sonography, and CT scans, the indication for operative and subsequent interventional/radiological procedures was determined at a multidisciplinary consultation between gastroenterologists, radiologists, and surgeons.

After appropriate preparation of the patient (general and nutritional status), the biliodigestive anastomosis was executed using a 70-cm long Roux-Y loop. In those patients with complicated benign biliary stricture it was naturally impossible to perform a perfect mucosa-to-mucosa anastomosis above the stricture as is the standard procedure. Accordingly, an ideal an anastomosis as possible was attempted, and subsequently a blind Roux-Y loop end was directed to the abdominal wall (Figure 2). The loop was not executed as a stoma but was only affixed to the parietal peritoneum of the abdominal wall, initially leaving a silicone drain *in situ* near the anastomosis (1).

Any additional interventional surgery in the post-operative phase (cholangiography, lavage, stone extraction, dilatation, stent implantation) in the area of the intrahepatic biliary ducts and the anastomosis could be executed via that access. Access to the biliary ducts in the post-operative phase was either directly via the established drain or later after direct puncture of the jejunal loop affixed to the abdominal wall and super-selective catheterization of the anastomosis (1,7-9).

Patients with curatively resectable biliary duct tumors, but with a high risk of anastomosis stricture, or patients with non-resectable tumors received either a hepaticojejunostomy or a Segment III bypass with the blind end of the loop diverted to the abdominal wall. Interventional surgery on the biliary ducts was then performed via that access.

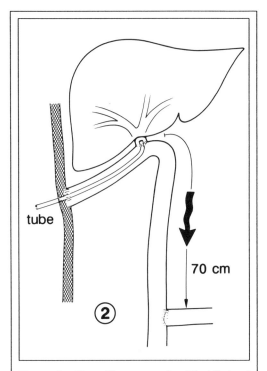

Figure 2.   Roux-Y reconstruction. The blind end is affixed to the abdominal wall and access secured by a silicone drain.

After the appropriate x-ray examinations or necessary radiological intervention, the intraoperatively established drain was left in the Roux-Y loop near the anastomosis in the jejunum for 3 to 6 months for control purposes and ultimately removed after a final follow-up examination, usually combined with hepato-iodida-scintigraphy. Should there be a further stricture at a later date, the Roux-Y loop can again be radiologically punctured and depicted at the old site with ultrasound, and any necessary radiological intervention performed through that access.

Prior to stent implantation, a cholangiography was performed via the silicone drain placed with the tip above the biliodigestive anastomosis. Under a local anaesthetic, the silicone drain was then exchanged in standard technique and a 7 Fr sheath inserted in the jejunal loop after securing the access route to the liver. Finally, a 7 Fr balloon catheter (balloon length 4 cm, diameter 10 mm) was used to dilate the stenotic segment. After retraction of the balloon catheter, the stent mounted on the tip of the insertion catheter was placed in the stenosis using the guidewire and released using a standard technique (Wallstent™; Schneider, Zurich, Switzerland) (10). As a rule, biliary stents with a diameter of 10 mm and a length of 3.5 to 7 cm were selected. Stent release was immediately followed by additional dilatation of the endoprosthesis and angiographic monitoring.

PATIENTS

Between 1987 and 1992, 30 patients were treated for a complicated benign or malignant biliary stricture using a combined surgical/interventional/radiological method. Eleven cases involved a stricture following cholecystectomy, two involved echinococcosis of the liver, two involved sclerosing cholangitis, and three involved complicated congenital (N=2) or post-operative stricture following liver resection (N=1). A self-expanding metal endoprosthesis was implanted in two cases of balloon-resistant stenosis. Twelve cases involved patients with a proximal cholangiocarcinoma. Curative surgery was initially planned in 10 cases. Owing to inoperability, however, a palliative Segment III bypass was established. A metal endoprosthesis was implanted percutaneously near the hilus postoperatively via a jejunal loop diverted to the abdominal wall. In two cases with curatively resectable cholangiocarcinoma but with the risk of an anastomosis stricture, a hepaticojejunostomy was established and a blind jejunal loop affixed to the abdominal wall. In the event of recurrence, a stent was inserted via that access.

RESULTS

In all patients with complicated benign stricture, the cholangiogram could easily be performed post-operatively as planned to show the anastomosis and biliary ducts. In three patients, small residual concrements could be expelled by repeated lavage. In six cases an anastomosis was dilated using a balloon catheter and in five cases, stones could be extracted from the intrahepatic biliary ducts by radiological intervention. Two patients with recurrent and balloon-resistant stricture received a self-expandable metal endoprosthesis (Figure 3).

After an average follow-up period of 12 months, eight patients have had no clinical complaints, one patient still exhibits a slight increase in alkaline phosphatase despite clinical well-being, and one patient continues to suffer from mild bouts of cholangitis. One patient with *Echinococcus alveolaris* exhibits significant clinical improvement although the underlying disease cannot, of course, be cured.

An endoprosthesis was implanted in 10 patients with malignant stricture. In eight cases an endoprosthesis was placed either in the bifurcation or in the proximal part of the hepatocholedochus duct via the palliatively established Segment III bypass (Figure 4). The average follow-up period was 12 months. Stents remained patent until the time of patient death (mean, 6 months).

DISCUSSION

The combined surgical/interventional/radiological procedure was developed primarily for the treatment of patients with a high biliary stricture (Types III, IV, and V), where certain risk factors were involved which prevented reconstruction of the biliary ducts and the treatment of additional secondary complications (intrahepatic calculus, strictures) by surgical means alone (1,2,7,8). The operative procedure involved restoration of normal bile flow, while creating percutaneous access to the biliodigestive anastomosis and the intrahepatic biliary ducts. In the postoperative phase, this access can then be used to perform any necessary further intervention (flushing out detritus, stone extraction, dilatation, stent implantation) with classic

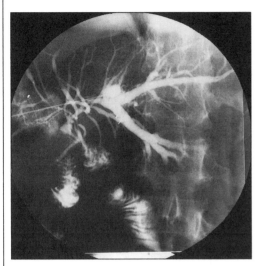
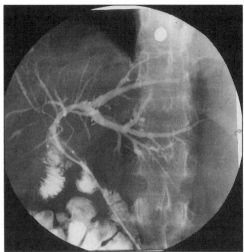
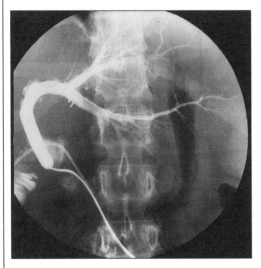
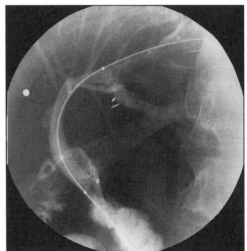

Figure 3. Stent implantation in a case of a recurrent benign stricture. PTC. Status after Roux-Y reconstruction. Anastomosis stricture, atrophy of the right liver lobe, hypertrophy of the left lobe *(top left)*. Percutaneous, transperitoneal puncture of the blind end of the diverted jejunal loop. Probing of left biliary duct system *(top right)*. Balloon dilatation of the stricture *(bottom left)*. Stent implantation *(bottom right)*.

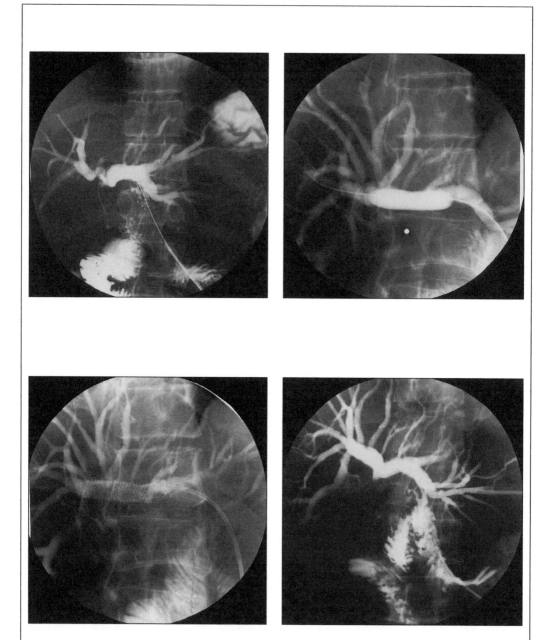

Figure 4.   Stent implantation in a case of a malignant stricture (non-resectable Klatskin tumor). Status after establishment of a Segment III bypass. Cholangiography via an inserted silicone drain. Stenosis in the area of the bifurcation with encroachment on the right hepatic duct *(top left)*. Balloon dilatation *(top right)*. Stent implantation *(bottom left)*. Control cholangiogram. Sufficient drainage of the right liver lobe via the stent into the left lobe. Patent Segment III bypass with good drainage of the contrast medium out of the left liver lobe *(bottom right)*.

radiological techniques. The respective operations can be performed after introduction of appropriate catheter systems via an intraoperatively-established silicone drain.

Should there be any subsequent biliary obstruction as a consequence of anastomosis stricture, this technique can save the patient from further surgery. All catheter procedures can be performed via the jejunal loop affixed to the abdominal wall. The majority of cases involve anastomosis stricture, and balloon dilatation is generally performed. Where there is benign biliary stricture, implantation of a biliary stent is indicated in exceptional cases if a balloon-resistant stricture continues in recurrent stenoses.

A similar technique was developed on the basis of this experience for the palliative treatment of patients with a malignant, high-lying tumor in the biliary duct. Candidates for this technique are patients in whom a hilar biliary duct tumor (Klatskin tumor) has been radically resected but who have a high risk of anastomosis stricture. This technique is suitable for patients where no curative surgical intervention is possible and palliative drainage of the biliary duct is therefore established in the form of a Segment III bypass. The bypass can be modified such that the blind end of the jejunal loop anastomosed with Segment III is affixed to the abdominal wall and access to the liver hilus is secured via an intraoperatively-established silicone drain. During the post-operative phase this access route can be used to insert a stent in the liver hilus, allowing both the right and left-hand liver lobes to be drained via the Segment III bypass. An additional advantage of this technique is that sufficient biliary duct drainage of the obstructed right liver lobe reduces the risk of cholangitis and thus improves the long-term quality of life for the patient. This combined surgical/interventional/radiological procedure saves the patient from otherwise necessary transhepatic biliary duct intervention which involves a substantially higher risk of complications.

REFERENCES

1. Schweizer WP, Matthews JB, Baer HU, et al. Combined surgical and interventional radiological approach for complex benign biliary tract obstruction. Br J Surg 1991;78:559-563.

2. Blumgart LH. Benign biliary stricture. In: Blumgart LH, ed. *Surgery of the Liver and Biliary Tract*. Edinburgh: Churchill Livingstone; 1988;721-752.

3. Blumgart LH. Hilar and intrahepatic biliary-enteric anastomosis. In: Blumgart LH, ed. *Surgery of the Liver and Biliary Tract*. Edinburgh: Churchill Livingstone; 1988;899-913.

4. Martin EC, Karlson KB, Fankuchen El, Mattern RF, Casarella WJ. Percutaneous transhepatic dilation of intrahepatic biliary strictures. AJR 1980;135:837-840.

5. Moore Jr AV, Illescas FF, Mills SR, et al. Percutaneous dilation of benign biliary strictures. Radiology 1987;163:625-628.

6. Mueller PR, Van Sonnenberg E, Ferrucci JT. Percutaneous biliary drainage: technical and catheter-related problems in 200 procedures. AJR 1982;138:17-23.

7. Barker EM, Winkler M. Permanent access hepaticojejunostomy. Br J Surg 1984;71:188-191.

8. Gibson RN, Adam A, Czerniak A, et al. Benign biliary strictures: a proposed combined surgical and radiological management. Aust NZ J Surg 1987;57:361-368.

9. Russel E, Yrizarry JM, Huber JS, et al. Percutaneous transjejunal biliary dilatation: alternate management for benign strictures. Radiology 1986;159:209-214.

10. Triller J, Looser Ch, Schweizer W, Blumgart LH. Erste Erfahrungen mit einer selbstexpandierenden Endoprothese (Wallstent) zur pallitiven Behandlung der biliären Obstruktion. In: Kollath J and Liermann D, eds. *Stents*. Konstanz: Schnetztor Verlag; 1990;106-111.

Use of Original, Modified, and Spiral Z-Stents in the Biliary System

Hideo Uchida[1], Tetsuya Yoshioka[1], Munehiro Maeda[1], Hiroshi Sakaguchi[1],
Hitoshi Yoshimura[1], Hajime Ohishi[1], Sohjirou Morita[2], Hiroya Saitoh[3], Yutaka Morita[4]

[1]*Departments of Radiology and Oncoradiology, Nara Medical University, Japan*
[2]*Department of Radiology, Kochi Municipal Central Hospital, Japan*
[3]*Department of Radiology, Asahikawa Kosei Hospital, Japan*
[4]*Department of Radiation Technology, College of Medical Technology,*
Hokkaido University, Japan

The clinical use of expandable metallic biliary endoprostheses (EMBE) using original, modified, and spiral Z-stents in the treatment of patients with unresectable malignant biliary obstruction was evaluated. Original and modified Z-stents were placed in 164 patients who ranged in age from 45 to 88 years (mean, 71 years). Eighty-nine patients had bile duct cancer, in 61 of whom radiotherapy, including intracavitary irradiation, was performed before EMBE. The overall external tube-free rate was 89% and there was no significant difference between patients who received radiation (RT group) versus those who did not (non-RT group). The 1, 2, and 3-year survival rates in the RT group were 54%, 20%, and 9%, respectively; these were higher than the respective rates in the non-RT group (12%, 0%, 0%, respectively). Intrahepatic EMBE was carried out in 26 cases with hilar to intrahepatic bile duct invasion, of which 19 cases had bile duct cancer. The external tube-free rate was 81% in all patients and 89% in patients with bile duct cancer. The average follow-up was 209 days (range, 9 to 712 days). Of the 164 cases who underwent EMBE, 36 (22%) developed reobstruction. In 18 of these 36 cases (50%), the reobstruction was caused by tumor growth into the stent; 15 cases (42%) again became tube-free after further management. Spiral Z-stents were placed in 38 cases with biliary obstruction and showed several advantages over the original and modified Z-stents such as greater flexibility and uniformity.

INTRODUCTION

Most patients with obstructive jaundice due to malignant tumors are not candidates for resection due to their advanced state. The recent introduction of expandable metallic biliary endoprostheses (EMBE) has markedly improved the therapy options for patients with unresectable advanced malignant biliary obstruction and has contributed to an improvement of quality of life for these patients. There are several issues which need to be resolved with this procedure, however, including the prevention of reobstruction of EMBE caused by tumor ingrowth into the stents, intrahepatic biliary stenting for cases with hilar to intrahepatic biliary obstruction, and the management of obstruction after EMBE. We discuss here the use of modified and spiral Z-stents in the biliary system, focusing on four topics: biliary stenting for malignant biliary obstruction including the role of radiotherapy; intrahepatic biliary stenting; management of reobstruction after biliary stenting; and the efficacy of biliary spiral Z-stents.

MATERIALS AND METHODS

In April, 1987, we began using the original and modified Gianturco™ expandable metallic zigzag stents (Z-stents) (Cook,

Bloomington IN). These were placed in 174 patients, including 164 with malignant biliary obstruction and 10 with benign biliary obstruction. Causes and methods of management for obstruction were analyzed.

Two years ago, the spiral Z-stent was introduced for EMBE. This stent, which was developed by Maeda et al, has been used in 38 patients with biliary obstruction. The efficacy of these newer stents in EMBE was evaluated in comparison with the original and modified Z-stents. Biliary spiral Z-stents were made of a single wire (0.009- to 0.010-inch) bent in a zigzag pattern with legs of alternating length, 10 mm and 12 mm. Leg bends were connected with a nylon monofilament suture to form a tube. The Wallstent™ (Medinvent, Lausanne, Switzerland) and Strecker™ (Boston Scientific Corp., Denmark) stent were used in three and seven cases, respectively.

RESULTS

Patients

One-hundred and sixty-four patients ranging in age from 45 to 88 years (mean, 71 years) with malignant biliary obstruction were treated with the original or modified Z-stents. Eighty-nine of these patients had biliary obstruction due to bile duct cancer; in 60 of these patients radiotherapy (RT), including external RT (Ext-RT) and intracavitary RT (Int-RT), was performed prior to EMBE. The average irradiation dose was 30 Gy each for Ext-RT and Int-RT. Int-RT was performed using cobalt 60 or iridium 192 and most recently, with Au-198 as the source of the Int-RT. Intrahepatic EMBE for malignant biliary obstruction was performed for 26 cases with hilar to intrahepatic bile duct invasion, of which 19 had bile duct cancer. Eighteen of these cases underwent EMBE into the right second biliary branch, namely the segmental branch. One case of EMBE was performed in the left bile duct. Sixteen patients received RT before EMBE; three underwent combined therapy with intraarterial chemoinfusion and RT. Of

the 164 cases with malignant obstruction undergoing EMBE, 36 (22%) developed reobstruction.

EMBE and Radiotherapy

In 140 of the 164 patients (84.5%), external drainage tubes could be removed following therapy. After EMBE, respective 6-month and 1-year patency rates were 78% and 63% in patients who received RT and 59% and 0% in patients who did not receive RT. After becoming tube-free following stenting, survival rates for all patients with bile duct cancer were 32% at 1 year, 13% at 2 years, and 2% at 3 years, with corresponding rates in the RT and non-RT groups of 54%, 20%, and 9% and 12%, 0%, and 0%, respectively. The 50% survival period was 216 days in all patients, while it was 413 days in the RT group and 177 days in the non-RT group.

Intrahepatic EMBE

The initial success rate of intrahepatic EMBE for the 26 patients with hilar to intrahepatic bile duct invasion was 100%. Figure 1 displays cholangiograms and a radiograph obtained before and after intrahepatic EMBE in a 68-year-old man. Reobstruction occurred in five patients (19.2%), with an average time to blockage of the EMBE of 148 days (range, 40 to 286 days). The tube-free rate was 81% overall and 89% for the 19 patients with bile duct cancer. The 30-day mortality rate was 7.7%. The average length of follow-up was 209 days (range, 9 to 712 days) in 25 patients, and 22 patients died after an average of 200 days. The three survivors have been alive for an average of 274 days (range, 169 to 416 days).

Management of Reobstructed EMBE

In 18 of the 36 cases with reobstructed EMBE, the reobstruction was caused by tumor growth into the stent. Cholangiograms from a 71-year-old man with an obstructed EMBE are shown in Figure 2. The other causes of reobstruction were sludge inside the stent

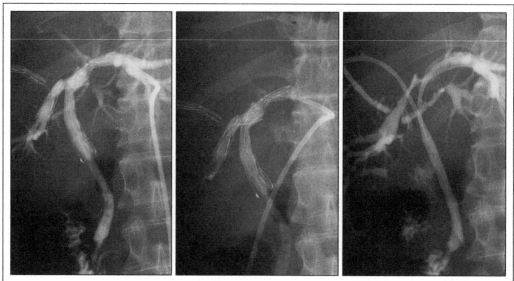

Figure 1. A 68-year-old man with bile duct cancer treated by intrahepatic EMBE using an original Z-stent. Cholangiogram obtained simultaneously through the two internal-external drainage catheters *(left)*. The external drainage catheter shows obstruction of the right anterior and posterior hepatic ducts, the left hepatic duct, and the hepatic bifurcation. Plain radiograph obtained immediately after EMBE *(middle)* showing the multiple stents which are inserted into the right anterior and posterior hepatic ducts, the left hepatic duct, and the common bile duct. Cholangiogram obtained 7 days later *(right)* demonstrating passage of contrast medium from the stented intrahepatic ducts through the common bile duct into the duodenum.

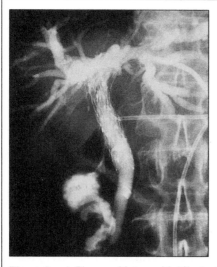
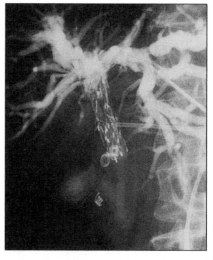

Figure 2. A 71-year-old man with bile duct cancer treated by re-stenting inside a previously obstructed EMBE. Cholangiogram obtained through the external drainage catheter showing obstruction of the previous EMBE which was inserted into the bile duct 2 1/2 years earlier *(left)*. Cholangiogram obtained after insertion of the original Z-stent inside the previous EMBE showing good patency of the stents *(right)*.

(N=11), lymph node enlargement (N=1), and unknown (N=6). Of the reobstructed cases, 15 (42%) again became tube-free following further management, of which PTC drainage was the most common. Fourteen of the 15 cases were successfully managed by insertion of stents inside a previous EMBE and the remaining case was treated with a plastic endoprosthesis.

Spiral Z-Stents

The spiral Z-stents advanced easily through a 7 Fr inner diameter catheter with a coaxial safety guidewire as well as through a 5.5 Fr catheter without the use of a guidewire (Figure 3). Modified Z-stents required an 8.5 Fr catheter; it was not always easy to deliver four or more body-connected modified stents through a sharply curved biliary tract. All but one spiral Z-stent relieved the obstructions immediately after placement and the drainage tubes could be removed in a few days. The spiral Z-stent conformed to the curve of the bile duct more smoothly than did the modified Z-stent. Figure 4 displays cholangiograms from a 44-year-old woman with biliary obstruction who received a spiral Z-stent.

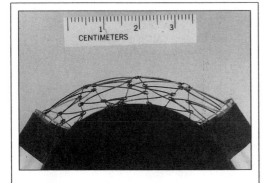

Figure 3. Evaluation of the spiral Z-stent flexibility. Flexibility was evaluated by the degree of deformation of the stent pushed against different curves of a cylindrical surface.

DISCUSSION

The vast majority of malignant tumors with complicated biliary obstruction are too advanced at diagnosis for radical surgery. External radiation or intraoperative irradiation has not proved very effective. Compared with external irradiation, intracavitary irradiation has the potential to deliver a higher local dose. In our initial experience prior to introducing radiation as a pre-stenting therapy, EMBE was occluded due to tumor ingrowth inside the stent within a short period of time after stenting. To prevent tumor invasion into the bile duct through the stent mesh after stenting, we introduced intracavitary radiation (Int-RT) in addition to ordinary external radiation (RT) before EMBE. To evaluate the efficacy of EMBE combined with RT, including Int-RT, in the management of bile duct cancer, we compared the therapeutic results such as the removal rate of the external drainage catheter, reobstruction rate after stenting, and survival rate between patients in the RT group and those in the non-RT group. Although intracavitary irradiation was performed at Nara Medical University with a cobalt 60 source which necessitated a 14 Fr conduit with a diameter of 0.035 inches, iridium 192, which could be placed in a much smaller catheter, was used at another institution. We have recently started to use Au-198 as a smaller source because it can be easily introduced through a smaller catheter.

Original and modified Z-stents were useful in the management of malignant biliary obstruction; radiotherapy before EMBE appeared to prevent tumor ingrowth into the stent in some cases. EMBE combined with radiotherapy, including Int-RT, appears to be effective for inoperable bile duct cancer and to play a useful role in improving patient's quality of life, including the prolongation of survival. When intrahepatic EMBE for malignant biliary obstruction involving the intrahepatic bile ducts was evaluated, the success rate was high and the procedure was not

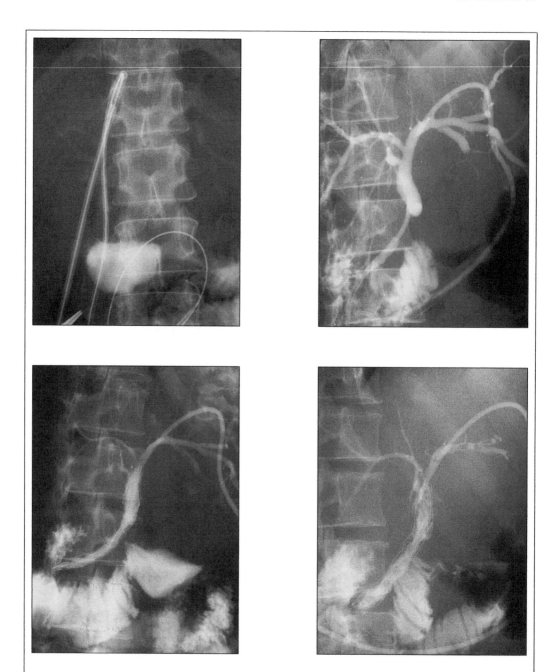

Figure 4.   A 44-year-old woman with biliary obstruction due to lymph node metastases from colon cancer. The external drainage catheter introduced into the hepatic duct with a sharply curved angle *(top left)*. Right anterior oblique cholangiogram obtained through the external-internal drainage catheter revealed obstruction of the common bile duct. The drainage catheter shows the acute angle at the inserted portion into the liver *(top right)*. Cholangiogram obtained immediately after easy insertion of spiral Z-stent through the sharply curved introducer showed good passage of contrast medium inside the stent *(bottom left)*. Cholangiogram obtained 1 week after EMBE *(bottom right)* demonstrating further dilatation of the stent diameter relative to 1 week earlier, with good stent patency.

technically difficult. Our results suggest that intrahepatic EMBE using Z-stents offers effective palliation in patients with malignant biliary obstructions involving intrahepatic multiple ducts.

Obstruction of EMBE was encountered after biliary stenting due to such causes as tumor growth or sludge inside the stents. Management of obstruction after biliary stenting is very important and in about 40% of reobstructed cases, a tube-free state was again obtained after re-stenting. As many of the biliary reobstructions were due to tumor ingrowth, the use of a Z-stent or soft stent contributes to recanalization of the biliary obstruction.

When the newly developed spiral Z-stent was compared with the original and modified Z-stent in EMBE, several advantages were noted. Specifically, spiral Z-stents offered uniform expansile force which eliminated the tendency for dislodgment and enhanced stent stability. The ratio of the useful diameter to the compressed size of the stent was also somewhat better for the spiral Z-stent compared to the modified Z-stent. Additionally, spiral Z-stents can also be delivered through somewhat smaller catheters and conform more smoothly to the curve of the bile ducts.

CONCLUSIONS

In conclusion, original, modified, and spiral Z-stents are useful in the management of biliary obstruction. Stenting combined with radiation therapy, including intracavitary irradiation, appears to be effective for inoperable bile duct cancer. Intrahepatic biliary stenting is very useful for the management of unresectable malignant biliary obstruction involving the intrahepatic bile ducts. Spiral Z-stents were easy to deliver and reliably dilated the biliary obstruction; moreover, they offered several advantages compared to original and modified Z-stents.

RECOMMENDED READING

Coons HG. Self-expandable stainless steel biliary stents. Radiology 1989;170:979-983.

Yoshioka T, Sakaguchi H, Yoshimura H, et al. Expandable metallic biliary endoprosthesis: preliminary clinical evaluation. Radiology 1990; 177:253-257.

Yoshimura H, Sakaguchi H, Yoshioka T, et al. Afterloading intracavitary irradiation and expandable stent for malignant biliary obstruction. Radiation Med 1989;7:36-41.

Maeda M, Timmermans HA, Uchida BT, Uchida H, Keller FS, Rösch J. In vitro comparison of the spiral Z-stent and the Gianturco Z-stent. JVIR 1992;3:565-569.

Nitinol Self-Expandable Strecker Stents in Biliary Obstruction: Clinical Results

Mario Bezzi and Plinio Rossi

Department of Radiology, III Cattedra, University "La Sapienza", Rome, Italy

The clinical efficacy of a new metallic stent for the management of biliary obstruction was investigated in a clinical study. The self-expandable stent was made of a nickel-titanium alloy which has a mesh-like structure similar to the design of the Strecker stent and is 10 mm in diameter and 6 cm in length. From February, 1991 to February, 1994, 37 stents were placed in 21 patients with obstructive jaundice due to cholangiocarcinoma (N=6), pancreatic carcinoma (N=7), lymph node metastasis to the liver hilum (N=5), gallbladder carcinoma (N=2), and intraductal papillary mucosal hyperplasia (N=1). The obstruction was located in the common duct in 17 patients and at the hilar confluence in 4 patients. Stent placement was successful in 20 of the 21 patients. In one patient, stent dislodgment into the duodenum occurred and the patient was excluded from follow-up. There were no other procedure-related complications or deaths within 30 days following the procedure. Of the remaining 20 patients, 3 (15%) are still alive after an average of 6.5 months and 17 (85%) have died after a mean survival of 7.6 months (range, 2 to 17 months). Three patients had a stent obstruction, two of whom underwent repeated interventions (15% obstruction rate; 10% reintervention rate). Adequate palliation until death was obtained in 83% of patients. Average stent patency was at least 7.5 months. The new nitinol Strecker stent has technical and physical properties that make it adequate to reestablish bile flow in obstructive jaundice; its efficacy and patency rates were adequate in our patient population.

INTRODUCTION

Malignant obstruction of the bile ducts may be managed by transhepatic or endoscopic drainage with excellent clinical results and indwelling endoprostheses provide adequate bile flow (1-3). The major problems associated with plastic endoprostheses are dislocation and obstruction due to bile encrustation which necessitate a new drainage procedure.

An optimal stent for permanent palliation of patients with neoplastic obstructive jaundice has not been found as yet. It had been originally hoped that metallic stents would occlude and migrate less frequently than plastic endoprostheses due to their larger lumen and to the fact that the metallic mesh is embedded into the biliary mucosa. This hypothesis prompted clinical investigations and within the last 5 years, several reports on the use of various metallic stents have been pub-

lished with encouraging, but not definitive, results (4-7).

To increase the clinical efficacy of metallic stents, a new self-expandable stent has been developed based on the design of the balloon-expandable Strecker stent (8). We report our clinical experience with this new device in patients with neoplastic obstruction of the bile ducts.

MATERIALS AND METHODS

The self-expandable stents are made of a 0.13-mm nickel-titanium alloy wire (Elastalloy™, Boston Scientific Corp., Denmark); the mesh design, with looped ends, is similar to the tantalum Strecker™ stent (Boston Scientific Corp., Denmark) (8). When expanded, the stents are 10 mm in diameter and 6 cm in length (a stent prototype, 8 mm in diameter and 4 cm in length, was used in the first 10 patients [9]). The Strecker design is flexible for introduction through tortuous strictures; its soft-looped ends should cause no injury to the ductal or bowel mucosa. The radiopacity of the nickel-titanium alloy wire under fluoroscopy is low and is similar to that of the stainless steel Wallstent™ (Medinvent, Lausanne, Switzerland). The 10 Fr introducing system is made of a shaft and an outer plastic sheath which holds the stent in place (Figure 1); the device can be directly placed transhepatically over a guidewire. Stent release is obtained by withdrawing the sheath; the constrained stent is shortened by approximately 35% as it expands. Shortening and low radiopacity may render positioning difficult, however. In order to enhance precision during release, there are three radiopaque markers on the shaft (Figure 1). The middle marker indicates where the proximal stent end will be after expansion, while the distal marker indicates the distal end of the unexpanded and expanded stent. To avoid stent shortening from both sides, the distal portion is maintained in place by six stabilization wires which anchor the metallic mesh while the sheath is withdrawn. In this way, shortening takes place only from the proximal side and is more predictable. After release, the prongs slide easily out of the distal loops of the stent.

From February, 1991 to February, 1994, 37 stents were placed in 21 patients who presented with biliary obstruction (8 men and 13 women; mean age, 66 years; range, 39 to 83 years). Jaundice was due to pancreatic carcinoma (N=7) (Figure 2), cholangiocarcinoma (N=6), metastatic lymph nodes to the liver hilum (N=5), gallbladder carcinoma (N=2), and intraductal papillary hyperplasia in a patient with a benign biliary stricture previously treated with "Z" stents (10). The strictures were located at the hilar confluence in four patients (one of which had a hepato-jejunostomy), in the middle common bile duct (CBD) in eight patients, and in the lower

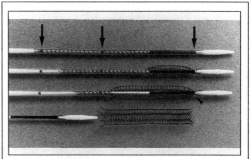

Figure 1. The stent and its delivery system. The constrained stent *(top)* is held onto the shaft by a plastic sheath; the arrows indicate the three radiopaque markers. While the sheath is withdrawn *(middle)*, one can clearly see that the stent shortens from its proximal portion, while the distal end is kept in position by six nitinol stabilization wires *(arrowhead)*. After complete sheath withdrawal, the nitinol Elastalloy Strecker stent *(bottom)* is fully expanded.

CBD in nine patients. Serum bilirubin levels ranged from 8 to 24 mg/dL.

All patients first underwent percutaneous biliary drainage followed by stent insertion approximately 5 days later. Strictures were dilated before stent placement in most cases. The endoprostheses were positioned after the stenosis so that the stent covered the normal duct above and below the obstruction in order to prevent restenosis due to tumor growth; more than one stent was often necessary to achieve such "overstenting". In the four patients with hilar obstruction, two stents could be placed side-by-side in a "Y" configuration since the good outward force prevented stent collapse. After the procedure, a 5 Fr catheter was left through the stent or above it for 1 to 3 days and was used for flushing and allowing access to the biliary tree. The stents usually reached their final diameter after 1 to 3 days.

Follow-up evaluations were based on clinical records, laboratory tests, and phone interviews with the patients. Imaging investigations were undertaken when patients developed symptoms of recurrent jaundice or cholangitis. One patient was not included in the follow-up (see below). Seventeen patients

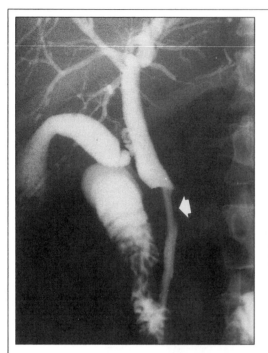
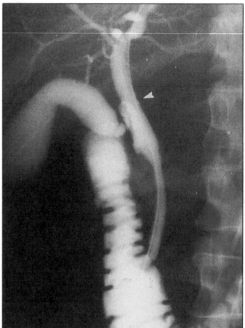
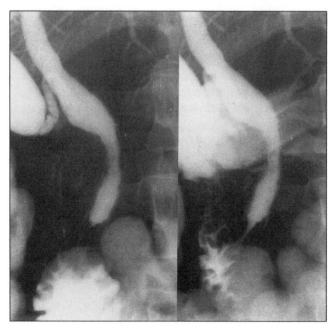

Figure 2.   Cholangiograms obtained in a 59-year-old man with biopsy-proven pancreatic carcinoma. After biliary drainage, injection of contrast material demonstrates a short stricture involving the lower third of the CBD (arrow) *(top left)*. A 6-cm stent was placed to dilate the stricture: the cranial margin of the stent is well above the obstruction lesion (arrowhead) *(top right)*. After 24 hours the stent was expanded: the close-up view shows that the function of the papilla was maintained *(bottom center)*. The patient is alive at 3 months without recurrence of jaundice.

were followed until death (follow-up, 2 to 17 months). The three patients who are still alive had a follow-up of 15, 3, and 1 months, respectively.

RESULTS

Technique and Complications

Placement of the metal endoprostheses was successful in 20 of 21 patients (95%); in one patient, two 4-cm stents were displaced into the duodenum after correct release in an attempt to place a catheter through them. The patient was eventually treated by insertion of a Carey-Coons endoprosthesis (Boston Scientific Corp., Watertown MA). In two other patients, difficulties were caused by friction inside the sheath due to an angled transhepatic tract; two stents did not release and were exchanged with new ones which were correctly released. These problems have been eliminated by changes in the delivery system.

Other than the above mentioned displacement, there were no complications related to stent insertion. Transient intraductal bleeding was observed in two patients in whom the stent was dilated. In an additional two patients, partial stent obstruction was seen prior to removal of the catheter and was considered to be due to fibrin deposition; consequently, the stents were cleaned with balloon catheters. There were no deaths (procedure-related or otherwise) within the first 30 days after the procedure and late stent migration did not occur. There was one episode of late cholangitis (5%) 2 months after the procedure which responded to treatment with intravenous antibiotics.

Patient Survival and Stent Patency

The one patient with stent dislodgment is not included in the follow-up. Of the remaining 20 patients, 3 (15%) are still alive and 17 (85%) have died after a mean survival of 7.6 months (range, 2 to 17 months). Serum bilirubin levels returned to below 2 mg/dL in all patients after stent insertion. Jaundice recurred in 3 of the 17 patients who died; this occurred after 2.5 months in one patient with gastric carcinoma and liver metastases but the cause was not investigated. In the other two patients, both with pancreatic carcinoma, jaundice presented after 8 and 15 months, respectively, and was due to stent occlusion. In both cases, percutaneous cholangioscopy demonstrated tumor growth through the metallic mesh causing only narrowing of the lumen; obstruction had been caused mainly by debris. The stent was recanalized in both patients and a drainage catheter was left in place. Overall, recurrent jaundice was seen in 3 of 20 patients (15%) while the reintervention rate was 10%. The three patients who are still alive have not displayed signs of stent obstruction. During follow-up, five patients had surgery for small bowel obstruction due to peritoneal spread of malignancy; none of them required manipulation of the biliary drainage during surgery.

DISCUSSION

The major problems associated with plastic endoprostheses are occlusion, migration, and late cholangitis. In three large series, occlusion occurred in 6 to 23% of patients, migration in 3 to 6%, and late cholangitis in up to 20% of patients (1,2,11). The use of metallic stents in the treatment of biliary obstruction has been prompted by the need to overcome these problems.

Metallic biliary endoprostheses present several potential advantages when compared to plastic stents. In the expanded state their lumen is 20 to 30 times greater; in addition, the surface exposed to bile encrustation is minimal. Both of these features should diminish the risk of occlusion and late cholangitis. Finally, the metal embeds into the ductal mucosa which will eventually cover the stent, thus making late migration very unlikely.

The purpose of our trial was to test a new metallic stent on a limited number of patients in order to evaluate its clinical efficacy and technical properties. The stent (Strecker Elastalloy stent) originates directly from the design of the tantalum Strecker stent (8). In order to make it self-expandable, the wire mesh is made of nitinol, a nickel-titanium alloy with a high percentage of titanium which gives the stent remarkable flexibility, elasticity, and radial outward force. The original balloon-expandable Strecker stent does not have enough force to stent rigid strictures which recoil after dilation (12). For the same reason, patients with stenoses involving the hepatic ducts cannot be treated with two of these stents since the first one could collapse when the second one is dilated. In our study, the nitinol stents had the necessary expanding force to be used in tight stenoses or to be placed in a "Y" configuration when needed.

The metallic mesh of the Elastalloy stent is poorly radiopaque and high-resolution fluoroscopy is needed for placement. In some instances (mainly in obese patients), it is difficult to see the stent and one has to rely on the markers placed on the delivery system. As with other self-expandable stents, shortening after placement is the rule. When the constraining sheath is removed, the distal end of the nitinol stent is held in place by six prongs and therefore the stent can shorten only from the proximal portion when the sheath has been completely withdrawn (Figure 1). This feature and the presence of the three markers should be used to predict the final position of the stent after shortening.

An important aspect of the stent design is the presence of looped ends. This compares favorably with the other stent widely employed in the biliary tree, the Wallstent, which has sharp wires on both ends. Although rare, these sharp wires may cause CBD ulceration (5), duodenal ulcerations when the stent is placed across the papilla (5), and bleeding from the bowel mucosa in hepatojejunostomy. The looped ends of the nitinol stent enhanced safety and did not cause any of these erosive complications in our series. The introducer system of the Strecker Elastalloy stent is 10 Fr

in diameter and a potential disadvantage as compared with the Wallstent whose introducer is 7 Fr in diameter.

Besides technical characteristics and safety, other important aspects in the evaluation of any new biliary drainage device include efficacy of palliation, frequency of delayed complications, and cost.

Assessment of the mean patency of any stent type is difficult since many patients die before their stents have been in place long enough to become obstructed (survival is usually less than 6 months). The number of patients with documented occlusion in our series is too small to be of any significance. Jaundice recurred in 3 of 20 patients (15%), however, and only two had cholangiographically-documented obstruction which was followed by stent recanalization. The average patency in these two patients was 8.5 months, with a reintervention rate of 10% for the whole series.

From a clinical view point, the stents were effective. The average survival of the 20 patients was 7.6 months, which is higher than the survival reported in most series (5,6). Notably, 83% of these patients had adequate palliation from jaundice during their life without need for further interventions. Therefore, we can say that the average patency of this new stent type is at least 7.5 months. This value compares favorably with the values reported in the two largest series with plastic endoprostheses (2,11). Lammer et al observed a patency rate of 26 weeks (2), while Dick et al reported 4.3 months of average patency (11).

Results with the Wallstent, another self-expandable metallic stent, have been published. Gordon et al observed an occlusion rate of 24% and an average patency of 6.7 months (13) and Adam et al (6) reported an occlusion rate of only 7%. The median survival of patients in this latter series, however, was 3.5 months (6). An occlusion rate of 14% in a group of patients with a median survival of 3.2 to 4.3 months was reported by Lameris and colleagues (5); Salomonowitz et al reported an occlusion rate of 17.5% in a group of 80 patients with an average survival of 5.6 months (14). In our multi-institutional experience, the obstruction rate was 17.7% in 197 patients with an average patency of 5.9 months (7). It must be noted that higher obstruction rates were seen in studies with longer average survival, i.e., 5.8 months in Gordon's study (13) and 5.6 months in our series (7) and Salomonowitz's study (14). The above mentioned results compare favorably with the results of the present series (average patient survival 7.6 months; 15% obstruction rate; patency, 7 to 8.5 months).

The cause of occlusion in the two patients who underwent cholangioscopy was a combination of partial tumor growth through the stent and bile encrustation. In our experience, this is also the most common cause of obstruction with other stent types (7). No obstruction from only tumor overgrowth was observed which is probably because we routinely tried to obtain an "overstenting" of the lesion.

Once placed, all metallic stents anchor to the ductal wall. Migration is very unlikely and was not seen in our series. In addition, only one case of late cholangitis was observed which resolved with antibiotics. These two aspects represent a specific advantage of metallic stents as compared to plastic stents which have a migration rate ranging from 3 to 6% (1,2,11) and may cause late cholangitis in up to 20% (2) or 36% (15) of cases.

The Strecker Elastalloy stent will certainly be more expensive than the plastic endoprostheses. In the long-term, however, there are factors that may balance the initial cost. Longer patency and decreased incidence of cholangitis should reduce the need for hospital readmission and shorten the length of hospital stay in case of reintervention (15,16). Moreover, the "one-step" insertion with the 10 Fr introducer could result in a reduced hospital stay for the first procedure.

A limitation of our work is the small number of patients treated. These preliminary results, however, document that the new stents have technical and physical properties that make them adequate to be used in the occluded biliary tree. They are easy and safe to use and did not cause any short-term or long-term complications.

REFERENCES

1. Mueller PR, Ferrucci Jr JT, Teplick SK, et al. Biliary stent endoprosthesis: analysis of complications in 113 patients. Radiology 1985;156:637-639.
2. Lammer J, Neumayer K. Biliary drainage endoprostheses: experience with 201 placements. Radiology 1986;159:625-629.
3. McLean GK, Burke DR. Role of endoprostheses in the management of malignant biliary obstruction. Radiology 1989;170:961-967.
4. Lammer J, Klein GE, Kleinert R, Hausegger K, Einspieler R. Obstructive jaundice: use of expandable metal endoprosthesis for biliary drainage. Radiology 1990;177:789-792.
5. Lameris JS, Stoker J, Nijs HGT, et al. Malignant biliary obstruction: percutaneous use of self-expandable stents. Radiology 1991;179:703-707.
6. Adam A, Chetty N, Roddie M, Yeung E, Benjamin IS. Self-expandable stainless steel endoprostheses for treatment of malignant bile duct obstruction. AJR 1991;156:321-325.
7. Rossi P, Bezzi M, Rossi M, et al. Metallic stents in malignant biliary obstruction: results of a multicenter European study of 240 patients. JVIR 1994;5:279-285.
8. Strecker EP, Berg G, Schneider B, Freudenberg N, Weber H, Wolf RD. A new vascular balloon-expandable prosthesis: experimental studies and first clinical results. J Intervent Radiol 1988;3:59-62.
9. Bezzi M, Orsi F, Salvatori FM, Maccioni F, Rossi P. Self-expandable nitinol stent for the management of biliary obstruction: long-term clinical results. JVIR 1994;5:287-293.
10. Rossi P, Bezzi M, Salvatori FM, Maccioni F, Porcaro M. Recurrent benign biliary strictures: management with self-expanding metallic stents. Radiology 1990;175:661-665.
11. Dick BW, Gordon RL, LaBerge JM, Doherty M, Ring EJ. Percutaneous transhepatic placement of biliary endoprostheses: results in 100 consecutive patients. JVIR 1990;1:97-100.

12. Jaschke W, Klose KJ, Strecker EP. A new balloon-expandable tantalum stent (Strecker stent) for the biliary system: preliminary experience. Cardiovasc Intervent Radiol 1992;15:356-359.

13. Gordon RL, Ring EJ, LaBerge JM, Doherty MM. Malignant biliary obstruction: treatment with expandable metallic stents. Follow-up of 50 consecutive patients. Radiology 1992;182:697-701.

14. Salomonowitz EK, Adams A, Antonucci F, Stuckmann G, Zollikofer CL. Malignant biliary obstruction: treatment with self-expandable stainless steel endoprosthesis. Cardiovasc Intervent Radiol 1992;15:351-355.

15. Knyrim K, Wagner HJ, Pausch J, Vakil N. A prospective, randomized, controlled trial of metal stents for malignant obstruction of the common bile duct. Endoscopy 1993;25:207-212.

16. Wagner HJ, Knyrim K, Vakil N, Klose KJ. Plastic endoprostheses versus metal stents in the palliative treatment of malignant hilar biliary obstruction. A prospective randomized trial. Endoscopy 1993;25:213-218.

Expandable Metallic Biliary Endoprostheses Combined with Radiotherapy in the Management of Bile Duct Carcinoma

Yutaka Morita[1], Hiroya Saitoh[2], Tadashi Kamada[3],
Testuya Yoshioka[4], Hideo Uchida[4], Sohjiroh Morita[5]

[1]Department of Radiation Technology, College of Medical Technology,
Hokkaido University, Japan
[2]Department of Radiology, Asahikawa Kosei Hospital, Japan
[3]Department of Radiology, Hokkaido University, Japan
[4]Department of Radiology, Nara Medical University, Japan
[5]Department of Radiology, Kochi Municipal Central Hospital, Japan

INTRODUCTION

Self-expandable biliary endoprostheses (EMBE) are accepted alternatives to surgical treatment for malignant obstructive jaundice. In general, EMBE is contraindicated in patients with malignant biliary obstruction because intraluminal tumors invade the struts of the stent. EMBE combined with radiotherapy, however, may be an alternative therapy to control the stenosis of the bile duct in patients with malignant biliary obstruction.

We report the results of a multicenter study of EMBE combined with radiotherapy in the management of bile duct carcinoma.

PATIENT CHARACTERISTICS

Eighty-nine cases of biliary obstruction caused by bile duct carcinoma were treated by EMBE; 61 were treated with radiotherapy (RT group) while the remaining 28 cases were treated without radiotherapy (non-RT group). Patients were comprised of 58 men and 31 women who ranged in age from 48 to 88 years (mean, 71 years). The tumor locations were classified as intrahepatic, hilar, extrahepatic, and all. In the RT group, external irradiation of ~20 to 60 Gy was performed in seven cases, intraluminal irradiation of 30 Gy was performed in one case, and both external and intraluminal irradiation of ~60 to 90 Gy were performed in the remaining cases (N=53).

The types of stents placed in the bile duct were hand-made original Gianturco™ stents (Cook, Bloomington IN) (N=65), Z-stents (N=20), and other stents (N=4).

RESULTS

The RT and non-RT groups were compared with respect to removal rate of the external bile duct tube, reobstruction rate, and survival rate. The tumor removal rate was 90.2% and 85.7% in the RT and non-RT groups, respectively, with an overall removal rate of 88.8%. After removal of the external bile duct, the reobstruction rate was 35.4% in the RT group and 29.2% in the non-RT group. The total reobstruction rate was 32.9%. As seen in Figure 1, the 1-, 2-, and 3-year survival rates were 54.1%, 20.4%, and 8.7% in the RT group and 12.4%, 0%, and 0% in the non-RT group, respectively. The time to 50% survival was also longer in the RT group (413 days) compared to the non-RT group (177 days).

DISCUSSION

From the large number of papers available on the efficacy of stenting for biliary obstruction (e.g., 1-4), a negative opinion has emerged that stent placement is able to enlarge stenosis but does not cure the underlying cancer.

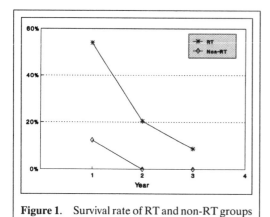

Figure 1. Survival rate of RT and non-RT groups

The final goal of treatment for unresectable biliary obstruction is to control tumor growth and internal drainage of the biliary obstruction. Malignant biliary obstruction caused by extrahepatic bile duct carcinoma is one of the rare diseases in which radiotherapy is effective. At present, we consider EMBE combined with radiotherapy to be the most suitable treatment for unresectable bile duct carcinoma. Radical treatment of extrahepatic bile duct carcinoma is not considered possible due to its particular local invasion and anatomical specificity. It is possible to control tumor growth, however, by expanding along the choledochal wall with intraluminal radiotherapy combined with external radiotherapy (5).

Radiotherapy alone, however, does not provide enough dilation at the obstructive region; patients therefore often require long-term hospitalization. To improve the quality of life of these patients, stent placement after radiotherapy should be adopted for continuous dilation.

The tumor removal rate after EMBE combined with radiotherapy in our study was 90.2%. These results are relatively similar to other reports, although the reobstruction rate after removal of the external bile duct in the RT group (35.4%) was higher than in other reports (~16 to 17.5%) (3,4). In our series the causes of reobstruction were recurrence of tumor (42.1%), debris (36.8%), and reactive edema (5.3%); all were considered to be affected by irradiation. These results suggest the difficulty in controlling tumor growth by radiotherapy and necessity for appropriate timing and a suitable area of stent placement.

The 1-, 2-, and 3-year survival rates in the RT group were 54.1%, 20.4%, and 8.7%, respectively, which are much higher than the previous reports. It had been predicted that the survival rate of the RT group would be higher than that of the non-RT group (12.4%, 0%, 0%). On the other hand, the reported survival rates with radiotherapy alone after 1, 2, and 3 years are 46.7%, 20.0%, and 6.7%, respectively (5). Thus, the survival rate in patients treated with radiotherapy and EMBE (RT group) is somewhat higher than that previously reported for patients treated with radiation alone. This small difference results in a better quality of life for patients in the RT group.

CONCLUSIONS

EMBE combined with radiotherapy for bile duct carcinoma is a useful method of controlling tumor growth and jaundice. To obtain good results, however, the following criteria should be satisfied:

- Stenting should be performed within 1 month of radiotherapy.
- The area of stenting should be as limited as possible.
- The dose of irradiation should be approximately 70 to 90 Gy.
- Both external and intraluminal radiotherapy should be used.

REFERENCES

1. Rossi P, Bezzi M, Salvatori FM, et al. Recurrent benign biliary stricture: management with self-expanding metallic stents. Radiology 1990;175:661-665.
2. Lee MJ, Dawson SL, Mueller PR, et al. Palliation of malignant bile duct obstruction with metallic biliary endoprostheses: tech-

nique, results and complications. JVIR 1992;3:665-671.

3. Salomonowitz EK, Antonucci F, Heer M, et al. Biliary obstruction: treatment with self-expanding metal prostheses. JVIR 1992;3:365-370.

4. Coons H. Metallic stents for the treatment of biliary obstruction: a report of 100 cases. Cardiovasc Intervent Radiol 1992;15:367-374.

5. Kamada T. Intraluminal radiotherapy for the bile duct carcinoma. In: *Progress Series of Imaging Medicine (IV)*. Tokyo: Nakayama-shoten; 1993;61-75.

Esophageal Nitinol Stents: Long-Term Results

Wojciech Cwikiel

Department of Diagnostic Radiology, University Hospital, Lund, Sweden

INTRODUCTION

Dysphagia is the most significant problem for patients with esophageal strictures. Preliminary results following treatment of dysphagia by insertion of self-expanding nitinol Strecker stents were first presented at the 'International Stent Symposium' held in Frankfurt in 1991. Long-term results following placement of these stents are presented below and are based on the treatment of 70 patients with significant dysphagia, with a follow-up period of up to 26 months.

PATIENT CHARACTERISTICS

Forty-four males and 21 females, ranging in age from 21 to 92 years (mean, 70.2 years), were treated for malignant esophageal strictures. The strictures were caused by primary squamous cell carcinoma (N=30), primary adenocarcinoma (N=19), recurrent anastomotic carcinoma (N=9), and mediastinal tumors (N=7). Prior to stent placement, 32 patients were repeatedly treated by endoscopic laser therapy and 13 by combined radiotherapy and chemotherapy.

Five patients (two males and three females) between the ages of 13 and 82 years were also treated by insertion of nitinol stents for benign strictures. The strictures were secondary to reflux esophagitis in two patients and to ingestion of alkali in the other three patients. Repeated dilatation had incomplete and short-lasting effects, and none of the strictures could be dilated to the maximum angioplasty balloon diameter (12 mm) before stent insertion.

MATERIALS AND TECHNIQUE

Self-expanding nitinol Strecker™ stents (Boston Scientific Corp., Denmark; also called Elastalloy™ stents) are knitted of a 0.15-mm nitinol wire. Flexible in the long axis, fully expanded stents measure 18 mm in diameter, with the proximal end flared into a 5-mm long collar with a 20-mm diameter. The delivery system includes a 95-cm long (2-mm OD) Teflon catheter with a distal olive-shaped widening and a soft 4-cm long tip (to simplify insertion), and a covering sheath. To minimize the diameter of the stent at insertion, it is stretched, compressed, and encased in gelatin. Thus, in the delivery device, 10- and 15-cm long stents are stretched to 14 and 19 cm, respectively. The 60-cm long (8-mm OD), proximally-tapered, Teflon sheath covering prevents contact of the stent with fluid inside the esophagus during insertion. The delivery system with the stent is introduced over a 0.038-inch guidewire. When in position, the sheath covering the stent is quickly removed, and the stent expands immediately after dissolution of the gelatin, generally within 2 to 4 minutes.

Before stent insertion, extension of the strictures was evaluated by radiography. Topical anaesthesia in the form of spray and gel lidocaine was administered, and when necessary, a mild sedative (i.e., diazepam) was added intravenously. Under fluoroscopic guidance, a 5 to 8 Fr feeding tube and a 0.035- to 0.038-inch guidewire were jointly manipulated through the stricture. In patients with tortuous or hard strictures, an Amplatz superstiff™ guidewire (Boston Scientific Corp., Watertown MA) was left in place. Dilatation of the stricture, using a 10- to 12-mm angioplasty balloon introduced over the guidewire, was performed to facilitate placement of the stent. The delivery system containing the stent was subsequently advanced over a guidewire into the stricture. When the stent had been released in an adequate position, it was further expanded with a balloon catheter to attach the stent to the esophageal wall. When necessary, additional stents were positioned partially into the first stent to include the whole stricture. All patients were examined with an esophagography after 24 hours. If the stent was not fully expanded, further fluoroscopic or endoscopic follow-up examinations were performed at intervals of 5 to 7 days until the stent was adequately expanded. Only liquids and a diet of soft foods were advisable during stent expansion. Following complete expansion, a regular diet was allowed and carbonated drinks after meals were recommended.

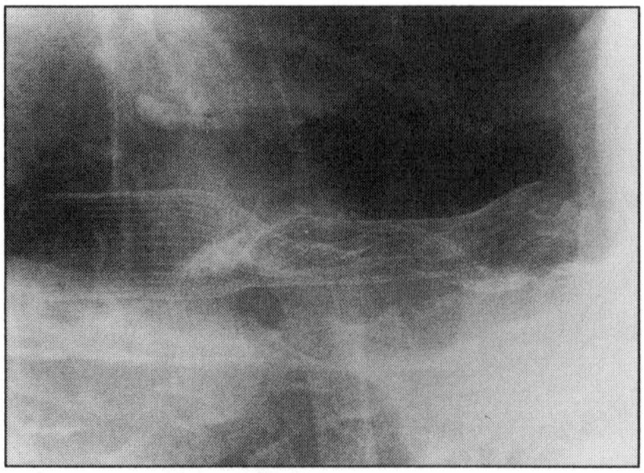

Figure 1. Twisted esophageal stent. Patient was treated pre-operatively and the stent subsequently removed by surgery.

RESULTS

Malignant Strictures

Successful stent placement was achieved in all patients. Placement of two coaxial stents was necessary in six patients, with all other patients receiving a single stent. During delivery, one coaxial stent was fixed in large tumor masses involving the stomach and left misplaced. Twelve stents could be dilated directly to the maximum stent diameter and 21 other stents self-expanded within 24 hours after insertion. Twenty-nine stents completely self-expanded following 2 to 21 days, while the three remaining stents were incompletely expanded due to twisting inside the stricture. Two of these stents had to be partially removed using endoscopy. The third twisted stent was surgically removed (Figure 1).

Substantial reduction of dysphagia was noted in all patients, in most within 24 hours. Stent migration occurred in one patient with recurrent cancer in an esophagojejunal anastomosis. The stent passed through the gastrointestinal tract 1.5 months after insertion without causing any serious symptoms. Tumor ingrowth through the stent mesh was seen at endoscopy in nine patients 4 to 11 months after stent insertion. Tumor overgrowth necessitated secondary intervention in two patients 6 and 18 months after insertion, respectively. One patient developed

a new (benign) stricture at the upper edge of the stent after 18 months of treatment (Figure 2). This patient also had ingrowth of the tumor into the lower portion of the stent and two additional stents were inserted. An unclear inward bend in the stent (Figure 3) has been observed in two patients 12 and 18 months after stent insertion, respectively. Three patients developed esophagorespiratory fistulas through the stent mesh; two received coated Gianturco stents with good effect, while the third died before insertion of a coated stent could be performed.

Sixty-one of the patients treated for malignant strictures died 0.2 to 16.5 months (mean, 3.8 months) after stent insertion. Eighty percent of these patients received a normal diet following stent expansion, 13% were allowed soft foods, and 7% were allowed liquids only. At the end of the study, four patients with esophageal carcinoma were alive 10 to 26 months (mean, 14.7 months) after stent insertion. All of these patients are receiving a normal diet.

Benign Strictures

In patients treated for benign strictures, all of the stents self-expanded to their maximum diameter within 2 to 14 days, with a reduction in dysphagia noted. During a fol-

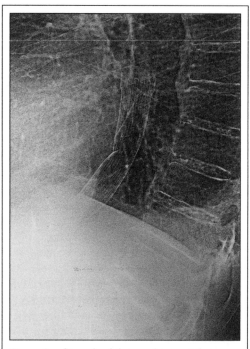

Figure 2. Stenosis of the esophagus at the upper part of the stent developed after 18 months.

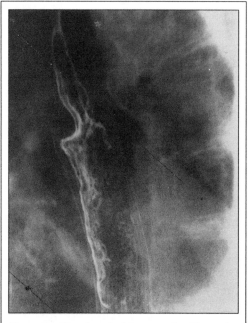

Figure 3. "Breakage" of the stent after 12 months, possibly due to weariness of material.

low-up period of up to 20 months, three patients developed new stenoses at the stent edges. In two of these patients, additional treatment of these stenoses was required.

DISCUSSION

Metallic expandable stents offer new options in the treatment of esophageal strictures and insertion is easy and safe. All treated patients were able to receive an oral diet following stent placement, with the majority able to return to a normal diet. The subsequent complete self-expansion of the majority of the nitinol stents demonstrates that the radial expansive force of the stent is sufficient for successive dilatation of both benign and malignant esophageal strictures to the maximum stent diameter. Such a gradual dilatation probably reduces the traumatic injury to the esophageal wall, which in turn diminishes the risk of rupture. Ingrowth of tumor through the stent wall was observed in several cases, but the majority of patients with malignant esophageal strictures die before the stent is occluded. Coating of the stents may prevent tumor ingrowth and, more importantly, be able to close an esophagorespiratory fistula. There is a risk, however, that coated stents may become less adherent to the esophageal wall resulting in migration.

The number of patients treated for benign strictures is few. Due to development of new stenoses at the stent edges in these patients, stent insertion may be advisable only as pre-operative nutritional support or in selected elderly patients. Self-expanding stents are, however, recommended for palliative treatment in patients with malignant esophageal strictures.

RECOMMENDED READING

Bethge N, Knyrim K, Wagner HJ, Starck E, Pausch J, Kleist DV. Self-expanding metal stents for palliation of malignant esophageal obstruction — a pilot study of eight patients. Endoscopy 1992;24:411-415.

Cwikiel W, Stridbeck H, Tranberg K-G, et al. Malignant esophageal strictures: treatment with self-expanding nitinol stent. Radiology 1993;187:661-665.

Cwikiel W, Willén R, Stridbeck H, Lillo-Gill R, Staël von Holstein Ch. A new self-expanding stent in the treatment of benign esophageal strictures: experimental study in pigs and presentation of clinical cases. Radiology 1993;187:667-671.

Do YS, Song HY, Lee BH, et al. Esophago-respiratory fistula associated with esophageal cancer: palliation with a modified Gianturco stent tube. Radiology 1993;187:673-677.

Domschke W, Foerster EC, Matek W, Rödl W. Self-expanding mesh stent for esophageal cancer stenosis. Endoscopy 1990;22:134-136.

Frimberger E. Expanding spiral — a new type of prosthesis for the palliative treatment of malignant esophageal stenoses. Endoscopy 1983;15:213-214.

Knyrim K, Wagner HJ, Bethge R, Keymling M, Vakil N. A controlled trial of an expansile metal stent for palliation of esophageal obstruction due to inoperable cancer. N Engl J Med 1993;329:1302-1307.

Kozarek RA, Ball TJ, Pattersson DJ. Metallic self-expanding stent application in the upper gastrointestinal tract: caveats and concerns. Gastrointest Endosc 1992;38:1-6.

Lindberg GC, Cwikiel W, Ivancev K, Lundstedt Ch, Stridbeck H, Tranberg K-G. Laser therapy and insertion of Wallstents for palliative treatment of esophageal carcinoma. Acta Radiol 1991;32:345-348.

Neuhaus H. Metal esophageal stents. Sem Intervent Radiol 1991;8:305-310.

Neuhaus H, Hoffmann W, Dittler HJ, Niedermeyer HP, Classen M. Implantation of self-expanding esophageal metal stents for palliation of malignant dysphagia. Endoscopy 1992;24:405-410.

Schaer J, Katon RM, Ivancev K, Uchida B, Rösch J, Binmoeller K. Treatment of malignant esophageal obstruction with silicone-coated metallic self-expanding stents. Gastrointest Endosc 1992;38:7-11.

Song HY, Choi KC, Cho BH, Ahn DS, Kim KS. Esophagogastric neoplasms: palliation with a modified Gianturco stent. Radiology 1991;180:349-354.

Song HY, Choi KC, Kwon HC, Yang DH, Cho BH, Lee ST. Esophageal strictures: treatment with a new design of modified Gianturco stent. Radiology 1992;184:729-734.

Silicone-Covered Self-Expandable Z-Stents in the Treatment of Malignant Esophageal Obstructions and Esophagorespiratory Fistulas

Josef Rösch, Richard R. Saxon, Robert E. Barton, Barry T. Uchida, Frederick S. Keller

Dotter Interventional Institute, Oregon Health Sciences University, Portland, OR USA

Silicone-covered self-expandable Gianturco-Rösch type Z-stents (GRZ stents) were used for the treatment of 43 patients with malignant esophageal obstructions and 10 patients with esophagorespiratory fistulas. In all patients, fluoroscopically-guided stent placement was well tolerated. Immediate relief of dysphagia was achieved in 95% of patients with malignant obstructions and was sustained in 80% with an average follow-up of 3.2 months (range, 1 week to 10 months). In patients with esophagorespiratory fistulas, aspiration was completely relieved in 70% while it was partially relieved in the remaining 30%. No complications occurred during stent placement. Later complications including stent migration, membrane disruption, food impaction, esophageal perforation, or hemorrhage occurred mainly in 66% of the 9 patients who received the early stent design. With the current stent design, occurrence of these complications was limited to 16% of 44 patients. The covered GRZ stents are an effective and relatively safe means of palliating patients with severe malignant esophageal obstructions and esophagorespiratory fistulas.

INTRODUCTION

Severe dysphagia and esophagorespiratory fistulas secondary to advanced malignancies of the esophagus, lung, or mediastinum are difficult to treat. Repeated laser ablations and placement of rigid prostheses are usually used for the treatment of dysphagia. The treatment of repeated aspiration symptoms has mostly consisted of supportive care with percutaneous gastrostomy placement and esophageal intubation. Expandable metallic stents have recently been introduced with good success for the treatment of malignant obstructions (1-10). We report our results in the treatment of 53 patients with malignant esophageal obstructions and esophagorespiratory fistulas using silicone-covered Gianturco-Rösch type expandable Z-stents (GRZ stents).

PATIENTS

From July, 1990 to September, 1993, 43 patients with malignant esophageal obstruc-

tions and 10 patients with esophagorespiratory fistulas were treated with GRZ stent placement. Of these 43 patients, 38 were male; ages ranged from 19 to 90 years (mean, 68.3 years). None of the patients were considered candidates for surgery and the majority were treated on an outpatient basis.

Malignant esophageal obstruction was caused by either adenocarcinoma (N=27), squamous cell carcinoma (N=10), or metastases (N=6). The location of the obstruction was in the proximal esophagus (N=1), middle esophagus (N=12), and distal esophagus (N=30). Eleven patients had previously undergone surgical resection and had recurrent disease. Thirty-eight (88%) patients had dysphagia refractory to other modes of therapy. In all patients dysphagia consisted of an inability to swallow both solids and liquids (grade 3) or an inability to swallow even saliva (grade 4). Five patients received stents as their initial treatment.

The esophagorespiratory fistulas were related to esophageal squamous cell carcinoma

(N=2), pulmonary adenocarcinoma (N=4), laryngeal carcinoma (N=2), mediastinal lymphoma (N=1), and surgically-treated Castleman's disease (N=1). All patients had midesophageal fistulas to either the trachea or bronchus with severe aspiration of both liquids and solids. Only 6 of these 10 patients had a clearly demonstrated esophageal obstruction together with the fistula. No prior therapy was attempted in any of these fistulas patients.

STENTS

The silicone-covered GRZ stents were handmade in our research laboratory from 0.018-inch stainless steel wire bent in a zigzag fashion to form 2-cm long segments (Figure 1). Four to seven segments were connected with sutures to form a stent 8 to 14 cm in length. A silicone cover was placed over the stents to prevent tumor ingrowth and to close the fistulas. All stents had barbs on the central bodies to "anchor" them within the tumor. The original stent design used in the first nine patients was 15-mm in diameter, was placed through a 18 Fr delivery system, and for 2 patients, had an antireflux valve caudally. Due to problems with this design, however, the stent was modified. The antireflux valve was removed, the stent diameter was increased to 18 mm, and the proximal stent body was flared to a diameter of 25 mm. In addition, the silicone covering was generally reinforced and folded at the ends of the stent to prevent perforation, and the barbs on the external surface of the stent were extended and curved in an attempt to prevent migration. These changes led to our current stent design, which we have placed through a 30 Fr delivery system in 44 patients.

TECHNIQUE

All patients with malignant obstructions as well as esophagorespiratory fistulas underwent a preliminary barium esophagogram to

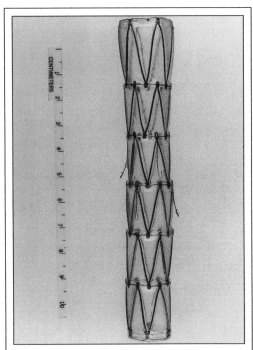

Figure 1. A 12-cm long, silicone-covered esophageal, Gianturco-Rösch self-expandable Z-stent.

determine the extent of the lesion and its location. Stents were individually designed for each patient based on the esophagogram. Endoscopy was also performed to evaluate tumor morphology and to determine its location relative to the larynx. Esophageal strictures were predilated to 10 to 12 mm under either fluoroscopic or endoscopic guidance. Stents were subsequently placed under fluoroscopic guidance in the interventional angiographic suite using light sedation. A 5.5 Fr angiographic catheter was first passed through the stenosis using a Bentsen guidewire which was then exchanged for a 0.038-inch Amplatz superstiff™ wire (Boston Scientific Corp., Watertown MA). Stents were front-loaded into a 30 Fr delivery system and passed over the guidewire across the lesion. Contrast medium injected through the sideport of the delivery system helped to properly position the stent across the lesion. The stent was then deployed by holding it in position with a pusher and by withdrawing the outer sheath. All patients underwent a follow-up esophagogram and most also had endoscopic examination immediately after stent placement. When possible, patients were also evaluated by barium esophagogram 2 and 6 months after placement. Endoscopy was repeated when clinically indicated. Clinical assessment was performed at monthly intervals until death or until the time of this paper submission. Most patients with distal esophageal lesions in which the stent extended across the gastroesophageal junction received histamine H_2-receptor antagonists.

RESULTS

Stent placement was successful and well tolerated in all 53 patients. Follow-up endoscopic and radiologic evaluations confirmed the improvement in esophageal luminal diameter in patients with esophageal obstructions, and good fistula coverage in patients with esophagorespiratory fistulas.

In malignant esophageal obstructions, immediate clinical improvement was achieved in 41 patients (95%). In 15 patients, dysphagia completely disappeared (see Figures 2 and 3) and in 26 its grade was lowered from 3 or 4 to 1 (i.e., some dysphagia to normal solids). Of the two patients who did not respond, one also had severe neurogenic esophageal motility disorder due to tumor invasion while the other died one week after stent placement secondary to metastatic disease. Relief of dysphagia without other interventions was sustained in 33 patients (80%) (range, 1 week

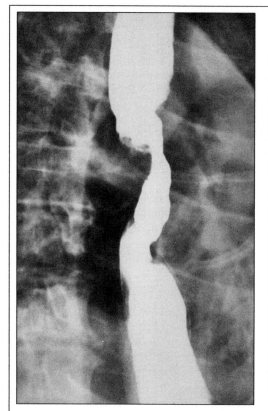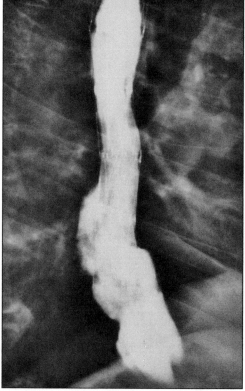

Figure 2. Obstruction of the middle esophagus due to adenocarcinoma in a 62-year-old man treated with GRZ stent placement. The patient had sustained dysphagia relief until his death 2 months later. Barium esophagogram showing a 7-cm long obstruction of the middle esophagus *(left)*. Barium esophagogram immediately after stent placement exhibiting relief of obstruction with good lumen of the esophagus *(right)*.

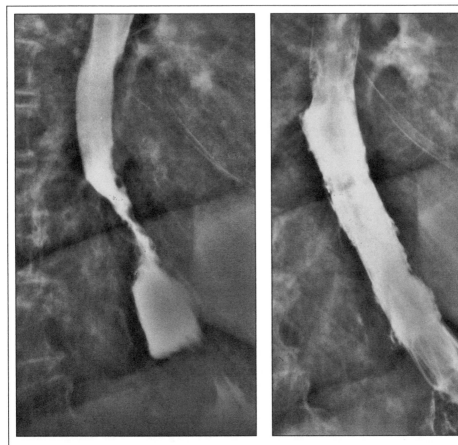

Figure 3.   Obstruction of the distal esophagus due to adenocarcinoma in an 83-year-old man treated with GRZ stent placement. The patient had sustained dysphagia relief until his death 10 months later. Barium esophagogram showing a 3-cm long obstruction of the distal esophagus *(left)*. Barium esophagogram one week after stent placement *(right)* exhibiting relief of obstruction with good lumen of the esophagus.

to 10 months; mean, 3.2 months). Recurrent dysphagia in eight patients was caused by stent migration (N=3), tumor in- or overgrowth (N=3), and food impaction (N=2). Five of these patients were successfully treated by interventional food desimpaction or new stent placement for an overall clinical success rate of 88%.

In the 10 patients with esophagorespiratory fistulas, immediate complete relief of aspiration symptoms was achieved in seven (70%) which lasted until their deaths from 1 to 11 months (mean, 4.2 months) after stent placement (see Figure 4). The three other patients (30%) had a partial response, experiencing relief to soft solids, but having residual aspiration symptoms to liquids. Barium esophagogram revealed leakage around the stent in two of these patients and a membrane disruption in the other. Despite additional stent placement, aspiration symptoms to liquids did not completely disappear. Two of these patients died 1 and 9 months after stent placement, respectively, while the remaining patient is still alive 9.5 months after placement.

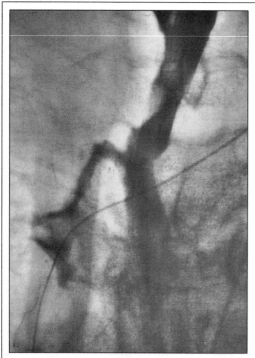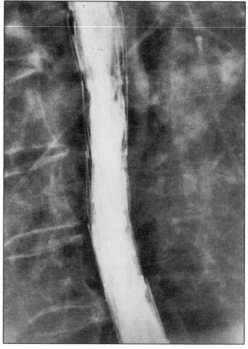

Figure 4.   Esophagotracheal fistula due to esophageal squamous cell carcinoma in a 68-year-old man treated with GRZ stent placement. The patient had sustained complete relief of his aspiration until his death 11 months later. Barium esophagogram showing a 6-mm wide fistula between the esophagus and trachea and mild esophageal narrowing *(left)*. Barium esophagogram 2 months after stent placement *(right)* showing good diameter of the esophagus and no fistula filling.

COMPLICATIONS

At the time of stent placement no serious complications occurred. Several patients complained of discomfort and chest pain during predilation of the obstruction and after stent placement. This disappeared in about 2 to 3 hours, and in only two patients did pain persist requiring long-term analgesics.

Later complications occurred in six patients (66%) with the early stent design and in seven patients (16%) with the present stent design. Two patients with the early stent design had food impaction and two had membrane disruption. These were not observed with the new stent design. Stent migration into the stomach was encountered in four patients, in two with the old design (22%) and in two with the present stent (5%). Migration has occurred only in patients with distal esophageal obstructions involving the gastroesophageal junction where stents extended into the gastric fundus. Adjunctive chemotherapy in one of these patients may have contributed to the stent migration by decreasing the degree of stenosis. Two patients passed their migrated stents, one was removed endoscopically, and one remained in the stomach without sequelae.

Severe delayed complications developed in four patients, which consisted of esophageal perforation in one patient and hemorrhage in the remaining three. Perforation developed in one patient with the early stent design 2 months after stent placement and the patient subsequently died of sepsis. At autopsy, the perforation was found at the distal end of the stent within tumor tissue and it was not clear whether the perforation was secondary to stent trauma or from tumor degeneration. With use of the new stent we do not know of other cases of esophageal perforation although autopsies were not routinely obtained when patients died. Of the three patients with hemorrhage, two died. One patient with a large upper esophageal squamous cell carcinoma developed severe hemorrhage 2 weeks after stent placement. Endoscopy revealed active bleeding around the stent. No autopsy was performed to determine if bleeding was due to erosion of the tumor or the stent into a large artery leading to exsanguination. Stent-related mortality in our series of 53 patients was 5.6% (3/53).

DISCUSSION

Silicone-covered self-expanding GRZ stents are an efficacious means of palliating esophageal obstructions as well as esophagorespiratory fistulas. Despite the selection of patients who had often failed with other forms of therapy, a sustained relief of dysphagia was achieved in 88% (38 of 43) of patients. In patients with the fistulas, a sustained complete relief of aspiration symptoms was achieved in 70% (7 of 10) of patients and partial relief in 30% (3 of 10). The silicone-covered GRZ stents used were made in our research laboratory. The GRZ esophageal stents now made by Cook (Europe) are of a similar design as our stents, but are covered by polyethylene which facilitates both loading into the delivery sheath and subsequent delivery. We have used these stents in two of our more recent patients with very satisfactory results.

Another Z-stent modification for esophageal application was introduced in Korea by Dr. Song (7). Its individual stent segments are connected with metallic struts. This stent does not have barbs, both of its ends are widened to prevent migration, and it is covered by silicone. It has been used in more than 100 patients with malignant esophageal obstructions and several patients with esophagorespiratory fistulas (2,8). Rates of placement success, palliation efficacy, and complication occurrence with this double-barreled Z-stent are similar to our series. The only notable difference is a higher occurrence of persistent chest pain (11%) and an occasional upward migration (2%) with the double-barreled Z-stent (8).

Two other types of self-expandable non-covered stents have also been used for treatment of malignant esophageal obstructions — a Wallstent made of stainless steel alloy and the nitinol Strecker stent. Both stent types are very flexible, easy to place, and their early treatment results are similar to those with the covered Z-stents (1,3,4,6). Later on, however, they exhibit a higher rate of dysphagia recurrence due to tumor ingrowth through the uncovered stent wall (1,3,9). Placement of another stent or laser ablations of the ingrowing tumor have been successfully used for the dysphagia recurrence with these stents.

In general, the expandable metallic stents are a preferable means for palliation of malignant esophageal obstructions and esophago-respiratory fistulas and have several advantages over laser treatment and rigid endoprosthesis placement. In comparison with the Nd:YAG laser treatment, the expandable stents are less expensive, can be used in submucosal lesions, and with the covered Z-stents, one treatment is usually sufficient for long-term palliation (10). Compared with rigid endoprostheses, expandable stents are free of complications during their placement, particularly of esophageal perforation, and they exhibit a lower rate of late complications such as stent obstruction and migration (10).

CONCLUSION

Covered GRZ stents are an effective and relatively safe means of palliating patients with severe malignant esophageal obstructions and esophagorespiratory fistulas.

REFERENCES

1. Cwikiel W, Stridbeck H, Tranberg KG, et al. Malignant esophageal strictures: treatment with a self-expanding Nitinol stent. Radiology 1993;187:661-665.
2. Do YS, Song HY, Lee BH, et al. Esophagorespiratory fistula associated with esophageal cancer: treatment with a Gianturco stent tube. Radiology 1993; 187:673-677.
3. Ivancev K. Metallic expandable stents in the treatment of malignant esophageal obstructions. Presented at the Annual Meeting of Western Angiographic and Interventional Society, Portland, Oregon, September 30, 1993.
4. Knyrim K, Wagner HJ, Bethge N, Keymling M, Vakil N. A controlled trial of an expansible metal stent for palliation of esophageal obstruction due to inoperable cancer. N Engl J Med 1993;327:1302-1307.
5. Lindberg CG, Cwikiel W, Ivancev K, Lundstedt C, Stridbeck H, Tranberg KG. Laser therapy and insertion of Wallstents for palliative treatment of esophageal carcinoma. Acta Radiologica 1991;32:345-348.
6. Maynar M, Rivero L, Pulido-Duque JM, et al. Treatment of malignant dysphagia with the Strecker stent: preliminary results. Presented at the Annual Meeting of Western Angiographic and Interventional Society, Portland, Oregon, September 30, 1993.
7. Song HY, Choi KC, Kwon HC, Yang DH, Cho BH, Lee ST. Esophageal strictures: treatment with a new design of modified Gianturco stent. Radiology 1992;184:729-734.
8. Song HS. Expandable esophageal metallic stents: Experiences in 104 patients. Presented at the Annual Meeting of Western Angiographic and Interventional society, Portland, Oregon, September 30, 1993.
9. Wagner HJ, Knyrim K, Bethge N, Starck E, et al. Palliativtherapie der malignen ösophagusobstruktion mit selbstexpandierenden metallendoprothesen. Dtsch med Wschr 1992;117:248-255.
10. Wu WC, Katon RM, Saxon RR, et al. Silicone-covered self-expanding metallic stents for the palliation of malignant esophageal obstruction and esophagorespiratory fistulas: experience in 32 patients and a review of the literature. Gastrointest Endosc, in press.

Endoprostheses in the Treatment of Esophageal Stenoses

D. Liermann[1], M. Jung[2], V. Paolucci[3]

Departments of [1]Radiology, [2]Internal Medicine, and [3]General and Abdominal Surgery
J.W. Goethe University Hospital, Frankfurt am Main, Germany

INTRODUCTION

Stenosis or occlusions within the gastrointestinal tract can have completely different causes depending on the particular section of the tract affected. In the esophagus, stenoses from tumors play an essential role (1-3). Constrictions of a non-malignant genesis can be caused by congenital deformities, such as the aorta ring, or by an acquired change, such as impressions produced by esophageal varices. Rarer cases consist of lengthy cicatrized stenoses caused by alkali or acid burn, or stenoses occurring as part of a systemic disease, such as sclerodermatitis, or resulting from ulcerative cicatrization arising from reflux disease (3-6). In the stomach, ulcerative or tumorous diseases clearly dominate stenoses in the antrum and pylorus, as well as in the fundus (7-12). As far as the duodenum is concerned, with the exception of the pylorus, stenoses are mainly caused by external stenotic tumorous processes from the pancreas or porta of the liver with obstruction of the lumen (13,14). Inflammatory diseases are a more common cause of stenosis in the small intestine just as tumorous diseases are more rare (10,15-27). In the large intestine, in addition to various large intestinal tumors, inflammatory changes, such as ulcerative colitis or diverticulitis, play a role (20,27-31). In the small pelvis, a number of external tumors infiltrating the sigma or rectum can be responsible for stenoses or occlusions (22,24,29,32-34).

The use of non-surgical methods for removing stenoses or occlusions is mainly restricted to the esophagus through to the duodenum, as it is not possible to reach the lower regions orally using normal methods (10,34-39). Rectal methods of non-surgical therapy are restricted to the transition from ileus to cecum at the most, but as a rule only to the sigma. Of the various causes of stenosis listed above, only compression caused by malignant tumors or cicatrized strictures has been considered suitable up to now for non-surgical methods, with all other indications treated by surgery or possibly endoscopic methods (1-3,5,8,9,12,40-44). The latter include the use of both laser and balloon dilatation to remove stenoses in the esophagus and pylorus (41,45-49). In the esophagus in particular, the final possible choice for inoperable tumors affecting the mediastinum is the use of the Celestin tube (2,41,50,51). It is well known that this is a complicated method which, as a rule, must be performed under anaesthesia. The risk of perforations in the tumor should also not be underestimated, nor should the possibility of iatrogenic creation of fistulas in the tracheobronchial system or in the mediastinum with consecutive mediastinitis (50,52).

Although it was a relatively late development, interest grew in the possibility of using metal endoprostheses in such processes, avoiding the need for anaesthesia along with the risk of perforation. For a long time, one problem in using endoprostheses in these hollow organs was the insufficient diameter of the endoprosthesis. The only type used was the Gianturco Z-stent; however, in widely bifurcated branches it concealed the risk of rapid growth through the filaments and carried the risk of easy dislocation (53,54). The current form of a Wallstent endoprosthesis which expands to at least 16 mm, or the nitinol endoprosthesis with a diameter of up to 18 mm, has gradually expanded the range of endoprosthesis applications in the esophagus for the treatment for tumorous stenoses. The purpose of this experimental study was to determine whether Wallstents or nitinol stents were capable of maintaining an esophageal lumen in the tumorous area, and to evaluate problems inherent with the use of endoprostheses in this region.

MATERIALS AND METHODS

The indication for stent implantation can only be given following detailed diagnosis by means of endoscopy, contrast medium in the esophagus, CT, and histology, together with consideration of alternative processes such as surgery or bougienage. As a rule, the stent should be implanted under full anaesthesia with endoscopic and x-ray control. Patients who have fulfilled these requirements are monitored by radiologic or endoscopic control or both, during which the stenosis is probed, a guidewire is inserted, and the corresponding stenosis is carefully dilatated up to the required diameter (at least 10 mm) using a balloon. After dilatation, the corresponding stent system is positioned at the particular height of the esophageal section and the stent is deployed.

The tantalum endoprosthesis is easily visible by x-ray and is easy to position. This stent is woven from a single tantalum wire. The individual loops can be shifted horizontally and longitudinally to each other, giving the stent extreme flexibility. The diameter of the tantalum wire for the reinforced esophageal stent ranges from 0.15 to 0.2 mm. Various types of tantalum endoprostheses are available for implantation. The stent is fixed at its ends to the balloon with approximately 1-cm long silicone sleeves to avoid unintentional dislocation while being positioned. The balloon is insufflated by means of a pressure injection to release the endoprosthesis. The balloon expands initially in its middle sec-

tions and presses the prosthesis against the vascular wall or against the lumen being treated. The ends of the balloon are expanded by further insufflation. During this phase, the silicone sleeves are rolled back, completely releasing the expanding stent.

Endoprostheses of the nitinol type (Boston Scientific Corp., Denmark) available for implantation consist of a mesh similar to the woven Strecker™ stent (Boston Scientific Corp., Denmark). In contrast to the tantalum endoprosthesis, however, the material consists of an alloy of nickel and titanium, whose special properties are a so-called memory function and pseudoelasticity, together with great rigidity. Endoprostheses are available for use in the gastrointestinal tract with a diameter of 18 mm when expanded, and in lengths ranging from 10 to 15 cm. The 18-mm stent for use in the gastrointestinal tract is not only safeguarded by means of a sheath membrane, but because of the strong expansion forces, it is fixed on the implant system by gelatin. This dissolves after the addition of water, releasing the stent. The implant system cannot be removed until the gelatin has dissolved and the stent has been fully expanded. This stent tends to shorten considerably according to its expansion (Figure 1).

The Wallstent™ (Medinvent, Lausanne, Switzerland) is a self-expanding endoprosthesis made of stainless steel which combines rigidity with flexibility due to the metal's spring-like characteristics and restoring forces. The endoprosthesis is arranged in a mesh with interlinked filaments that lie parallel to each other when the stent is folded up, but stand up when the stent expands giving it its typical appearance. This endoprosthesis can be used in varying lengths between 4 and 10 cm at diameters of up to 16 mm and even 20 mm. The wire in the larger stents is between 0.12 and 0.17 mm thick. When deploying the stent, the space between both membranes of the implant system must first be evacuated as far as possible by syringe and then filled with contrast medium at a pressure of 3.5 atm until a small drop of contrast medium is

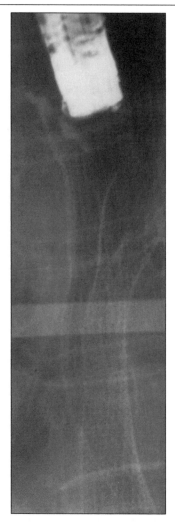 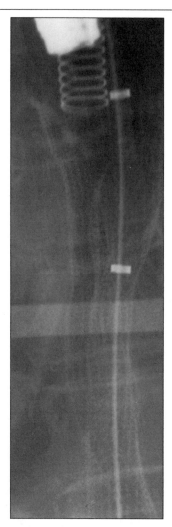

Figure 1. Illustration of a released nitinol stent in the esophagus which has not yet expanded in all sections.

visible in the tip of the catheter. Then and only then is the space filled sufficiently to avoid any friction between the membrane and catheter. The pressure in the membrane space is reduced again. The catheter-stent tandem prepared in this way is inserted through a sheath and along a 0.035-inch guidewire. The endoprosthesis shortens on deployment and is positioned in the stenosis in such a way that the stenosis will be fully covered upon stent expansion. When the endoprosthesis has been correctly positioned, contrast medium is again injected into the membrane space for separation of the sheath membrane. The sheath membrane is then released by means of a pressure injection of up to 4 atm, and a handle on the proximal end of the catheter is pulled back along the guide rod. Care is required here to ensure that the stent which is located at the end of the guide rod is held unchanged in the same position and does not become dislocated. After being deployed, the stent expands to a maximum diameter of 16 mm (20 mm); during this process, it typically shortens in length from 4 to 10 cm. In the event of malpositioning, before complete expansion and before the sheath film is withdrawn back from the caudal end of the stent, it is possible to either remove the stent or to position it again along the return route. Repositioning of the partially deployed stent distal of its current position, however, is not possible. Once the retaining foil has been withdrawn back beyond the caudal end of the stent, the stent is fully deployed and can no longer be manipulated by the implant system.

Deployment and regular positioning of the stent is followed by x-ray or endoscopic control. The patient is subjected to further follow-up examinations after 1 week, then monthly or possibly at 6-month intervals, or whenever there is a complaint. If required, revision is possible using a laser or to remove impaction from the stent.

INDICATIONS

The indication for application of one or all of the stent types described above is restricted initially to malignant compression in the esophagus. In a second phase, we intend to expand this indication to include benign esophageal stenoses. A further indication will emerge for the rectum or sigma in cases of local inoperability. Where malignant processes are concerned, there is no age restriction for any of the indications. For benign processes, the patients should have reached their fifth decade of life. Use of the nitinol stent should be ruled out in the case of severe nickel allergies because of the nickel component of the stent alloy. The process is used as a rival method to implantation of the Celestin tube. Patients should be informed of all alternatives, including induced feeding methods by means of a gastrostomy.

Contraindications to stent implantation, which were only available to us in non-coated form, were esophagotracheal fistulas and long stenoses caused by acid and alkali burns.

PATIENT POPULATION

We have treated 40 patients to date (18 female, 22 male) aged between 45 and 81 years (mean, 62 years). The ratio of malignant to benign stenosis was 30 to 10. Twenty-two patients suffered from esophageal carcinoma and eight from mediastinal tumors. All cases of malignant genesis were hindered by local inoperability. The length of the tumor stenoses varied between 3 and 12 cm. All patients were in a poor state of general health because of the prevailing nutritional problems. Of the 40 patients, 67.5% were treated with nitinol stents, 22.5% with Wallstents, and 10% with the tantalum stent. The stents were positioned using joint endoscopic-radiologic teamwork. Isolated cases will be described as examples of the general procedure.

A 56-year-old male patient suffered from a severe esophageal stenosis at the bifurcation covering a length of 6 cm. Following an endoscopic examination after taking the appropriate contrast media, the level of the stenosis was located by screening, marked by means of a metal strip, and a Wallstent was deployed (Figure 2). There were no problems in delivering the stent. Although we had observed the location marking exactly, the control examination revealed that during the shortening process of the stent, the stent had been dislocated within the stenotic area. In doing so, part of the self-expanding stent had been forced under the lower edge of the stenosis, where it remained in an unfolded but relatively compressed state. This condition was revealed by the clearly constricted position of the diamond shapes. In the stent's cranial section, which still covered the whole stenotic section through to the upper edge of the stenosis, the diamond shapes were extended and the stent was narrower in its lumen. The self-expansion forces had not expanded the stenosis properly, but these forces had resulted in partial migration of the stent out of the stenosis in a downwards direction. Although the results were not optimal, the

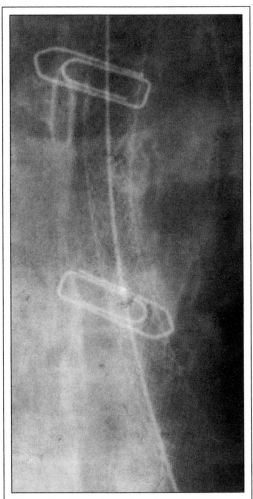

Figure 2. Illustration of a released Wallstent in the esophagus.

ing the release phase of the stent (Figure 3). It took 5 minutes before the stent was released to such an extent that the implant set could be withdrawn without problems because the esophagus was straight here. Irritation resulted from the stent remaining compressed in part of its cranial section so that proper radial expansion was not possible. A PTA attempt did not change anything. After 3 days, a control revealed a correctly expanded stent, suggesting that this type of stent takes several days for full expansion. The stent remained open and expanded in the right position for approximately 3 months, allowing the patient to take food properly. The lumen was not constricted by the tumor, but did get obstructed by impacted food, which had to be removed twice in the 3-month period. The patient had no subjective complaints.

RESULTS

Evaluation of the results for all cases indicated a clear improvement of the clinical situation in 20%. Seventy percent of patients were able to proceed with unlimited food intake. Removal of the stents because of malpositioning or functional stenosis was necessary in 10% of the cases. The mean survival time following stent implantation covered periods ranging from 15 days to 8 months (mean, 5 months).

Figure 4 summarizes the results observed with all three stent types. Complications included dislocation and/or migration in approximately 20% of the cases. Migrations occurred in 30% of all nitinol stents and 50% of all Wallstents, whereas the tantalum stent revealed no cases of migration. This also applies to stent shortening, which occurred only with nitinol stents and Wallstents. Deformation occurred in 30% of all nitinol stents, 50% of all Wallstents, and 100% of all tantalum stents. Complete expansion had taken place for 80% of the nitinol stents, 60% of the Wallstents, and none of the tantalum stents.

passage of food was still possible. The follow-up period only lasted for one week, as the patient died from other complications of his tumor. Permission for an autopsy was not given.

A second patient, a 64-year-old woman, had inoperable esophageal carcinoma resulting in a stenosis approximately 8-cm long in the middle third of the esophagus. Here again, following preliminary checks and marking the stenosis location on the skin, the relatively rigid implant set was inserted and the nitinol stent delivered under endoscopic and radiologic control. Difficulties were met dur-

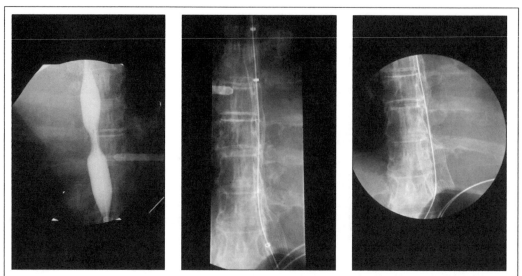

Figure 3. Evidence of an extensive, inoperable esophageal carcinoma with severe stenosis in the middle third *(left)*. After release of the nitinol endoprosthesis, the prosthesis is not fully expanded *(middle)*. Even 3 days after deployment, the stent has not unwound properly because of the lack of space in the tumor *(right)*. This is avoided with the new nitinol stent.

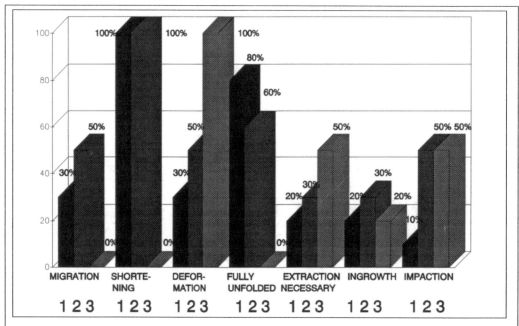

Figure 4. Comparison of the three implanted stent types in the esophagus. The number of patients implanted with each stent was: nitinol (N=27), Wallstent (N=9), tantalum (N=4). Key: 1 = nitinol stent; 2 = Wallstent; 3 = tantalum stent.

Food impaction (with endoscopic revision) occurred in 45% of all cases (10% for nitinol stents, 50% for Wallstents and tantalum stents). Ingrowth of granulation and tumor tissue with the possibility of laser revision occurred in 35% of the cases (20% for nitinol and tantalum stents, 30% for Wallstents). Restenosis caused by stent compression occurred only where tantalum stents had been used. Stent extraction was necessary for 20% of the nitinol stents, 30% of the Wallstents, and 50% of the tantalum stents.

DISCUSSION

With the exception of the Gianturco endoprosthesis which has a large lumen as required for stent implantation in the esophagus, prototypes from other manufacturers have only been recently available. The classic Gianturco stent has the unpleasant tendency of being rapidly dislocated. Particularly in hard stenoses, it slips out and then expands in a funnel shape, making it unsuitable for implantation in the esophagus because of its mechanical stresses and strains (55). Only recently has it been possible to fix modifications of the Gianturco-Rösch stent more permanently in the stenosis, thus achieving acceptable results (24,54). The Wallstent in its current shape with a diameter of 16 mm when expanded was originally intended for use in venous vessels. Its lumen appears to be relatively narrow for a stent to be installed in the esophagus. The fact that it slipped out of the stenotic area, displacing stent components into healthy tissue, appears to be a fault which will occur regardless of diameter. The development of longer stents with larger diameters which can be fixed above and below the stenosis at the same time is needed. Although the clinical results were satisfactory, implantation of this type of endoprosthesis cannot be recommended until these problems are addressed. A new type of this stent was made available to us until towards the end of this study. This new version has a length of more than 10 cm with a diameter between 20 and 22 mm. Problems caused by migration and impaction because of the small diameter should therefore be eliminated or reduced. At the same time, improvements in a completely new implant system for the stent should be able to remedy the problem of malpositioning with the resulting need for stent extraction. In contrast to implantations in the trachea, the Wallstent can be extracted from the esophagus without causing major injuries.

The positive aspects of the tantalum stent are its good positioning properties and the fact that it can be easily extracted without causing injuries. This stent, however, has a number of negative attributes, such as deformability, necessary extractions, and food impaction, and it cannot be recommended for routine use.

Application of the nitinol stent requires a certain degree of experience with this kind of endoprosthesis in order to avoid problems. As expected, the diameter of the implant set which is nearly 9 mm for an endoprosthesis expanding to 18 mm is not to be underestimated, and certainly causes problems for a patient who is only under sedation. In addition, the relative rigidity of the implant set is a disturbing factor. Consideration must also be given to the problem of the stent mesh snaring in the back of the guide rod during implantation. In some cases, extreme difficulties have been encountered in sections of the esophagus having only very slight curves. This therapy can only be recommended when the manufacturer has satisfied demands for introduction of a conical shape for the back of the guide rod. The prototypes which we had modified ourselves, disconnecting the tip before withdrawing the set through the deployed stent, are not particularly well-suited for routine use. A further problem occurred not infrequently in narrow stenoses, where the stent did not expand adequately after being deployed and following dissolution of the gelatin, and had to be removed because of the practical occlusion of the esophagus. This problem was caused by the way in which the stent was folded and fixed, practically wound around the implant system. If the stent could not unwind properly in a relatively narrow stenosis, problems were then inevitable. Both faults have been virtually eliminated in the new type made available to us toward the end of the study. First, the back of the guide rod had been formed in a conical shape, and second, the stent was not wound around the applicator.

In contrast to the most frequently used method of splinting inoperable esophageal stenoses using the Celestin tube, the use of endoprostheses appears far less risky and traumatic for the patient (2,41,49). At the moment, it should only be considered as a palliative approach to replace surgery. Wherever there is a chance for a cure, surgery must be given priority. Without any doubt, further problems are created with the use of stents by the need to treat impaction in cases of unrestricted food intake and thus, where applicable, the diet should be restricted.

REFERENCES

1. Berdal P. Die Verätzungsfolgen in der Speiseröhre und deren Behandlung. HNO 1973;21:264-267.

2. Dzieniszewski GP, Gamstatter G, Klotter HJ, Rothmund M. Palliative surgical therapy of incurable esophageal cancer by stomach bypass and endotube. Zentralbl Chir 1981;109:1550.

3. Hegemann G, Gall F. Diagnose und Behandlung instrumenteller Oesophagusverletzungen. Thoraxchir vasku Chir 1967;15:233-240.

4. Blum AL, Siewert R. Pathogenese, Diagnostik und konservative Therapie der Refluxkrankheit. In: Siewert R, Blum AL, Waldeck F, eds. *Funktionsstörungen in der Speiseröhre.* Berlin: Springer; 1976.

5. Peiper HJ, Siewert R. Chirurgische Erkrankungen der Speiseröhre. In: Zenker R, Deutscher F, Schink W, eds. *Chirugie der Gegenwart.* München: Urban & Schwarzenberg; 1974.

6. Siewert R, Blum AL, Waldeck F. Funktionsstörungen der Speiseröhre. Berlin: Springer; 1976.

7. Benjamin SB, Cattau EL, Glass RL. Balloon dilatation of the pylorus: therapy for gastric outlet obstruction. Gastrointest Endosc 1982;28:253.

8. Holle F. Spezielle Magenchirurgie. Berlin: Springer; 1968.

9. Martini GA. Erkrankungen des Magens und Zwölffingerdarms. In: Buchborn E, Jahrmärker H, Karl HJ, et al, eds. *Therapie innerer Krankheiten.* Berlin: Springer; 1974.

10. Mc Lean GK, Burke DR, Meranze SG. Interventional radiologic treatment of enteric strictures. In: Castaneda-Zuniga WR and Tadavarthy SM, eds. *Interventional Radiology.* Baltimore: Williams & Wilkins; 1992;1238-1253.

11. Pichlmayr R, Büttner D. Reintervention bei Carcinomen von Oesophagus, Cardia und Magen. Langenbecks Arch Klin Chir 1976;342:227-235.

12. Pichlmyr R, van Alste E. Die totale Gastrektomie als Regeloperation beim operablen Magencarcinom. Langenbecks Arch Klin Chir, 1977;345:595.

13. Kern E. Pankreaschirurgie. In: Zenker R, Deucher F, Schink W, eds. *Chirugie der Gegenwart.* München: Urban & Schwarzenberg; 1974.

14. Starzl TE, Todo S, Tzakis A, et al. Abdominal organ cluster transplantation for the treatment of upper abdominal malignancies. Ann Surg 1989;210:374-386.

15. Carron DB, Douglas AP. Steatorrhoea in vascular insufficiency of the small intestine. Quart J Med 1965;34:331.

16. Dollinger HC, Malabsorption - Zur Klinik und Therapie der Resorptionsstörungen. Z Allg Med 1972;35:1624-1632.

17. Fahrländer H. Klinik und Verlaufsformen der ulzerösen Colitis. In: Kremer K and Kevelitz H, eds. *Colitis Ulcerosa.* Stuttgart: Thieme; 1977.

18. Friedel W, Möslein G, Jaeger K, Herfarth C, Propping P. Familiäre adenomatöse Polyposis. Paradigma einer therapierbaren genetischen Krankheit. Dtsch Ärzteblatt 1991;88:1261-1276.

19. Goebell H, Dollinger H. Dünndarm. In: Lindenschmidt Th.O, ed.*Pathophysiologische*

Grundlagen der Chirugie. Stuttgart: Thieme; 1975.

20. Herfarth Ch, Ewe K. Die chirurgische Behandlung des Morbus Crohn. Multicenter Crohnstudie II. Chirurg 1977;48:569-576.

21. Herfarth CH, Stern J. *Colitis Ulcerosa, Adenomatosis coli.* Berlin: Springer; 1990.

22. Kewenter J, Kock NG, Myrvold H, Phillipson B. The continent ileostomy. In: Kremer K and Kevelietz H, eds. *Colitis Ulcerosa.* Stuttgart: Thieme; 1977.

23. Kock NG. Continent ileostoma. Prog Surg 1973;12:180-201.

24. Pichlmaier H. Eingriffe am Dickdarm, Mastdarm und Anus. In: Zenker R, Berchtold R, Hammelmann H, eds. *Allgemeine und Spezielle Chirurgische Operationslehre Bd VII.I: Die Eingiffe in der Bauchhöhle.* Berlin: Springer; 1975.

25. Spiro HM. *Clinical Gastroenterology.* London: Collier Mc Millan; 1970.

26. Tilson MD. Carcinoid syndrome. Surg Clin N Am 1974 2:409-423.

27. Wenckert A, Kristensen M, Eklund AE, et al. The long-term prophylactic effect of salazosulphapyridine in primarily resected patients with Crohn's disease. A controlled double-blind trial. Scand J Gastroent 1976;11(Suppl):38,93.

28. Fallier-Becker P, Betz E, Wolburg-Buchholz K, Fotev Z. Fibromuscular proliferates induced *in vitro* using a trans-filter culture system. Res Exp Med 1991;11-25.

29. Goligher JC. *Surgery of the Anus, Rectum and Colon.* London: Baillier & Tindall; 1976.

30. v. Herbay A. Pathologische Anatomie von Colitis ulcerosa und familiärer Adenomatosis coli. In: Herfarth Ch and Stern J, eds. *Colitis Ulcerosa, Adenomatosis coli.* Berlin: Springer; 1990;49-62.

31. Lennard-Jones JE. Medical management of colitis. In: Kremer K and Kevelietz H, eds. *Colitis Ulcerosa.* Stuttgart: Thieme; 1977.

32. Day DW, Morson BC. The adenoma-carcinoma sequence. In: Morson BC, ed. *The Pathology of Colorectal Cancer. Major Problems in Pathology.* Philadelphia: WB Saunders; 1982;58-71.

33. Junghanns K, Arnold K. Anus praeter Fiebel. Stuttgart: Fischer; 1974.

34. Lux G, Lux E. Kolonoskopische Polypektomie-Karzinomprophylaxe. In:

Demling L and Ottenjahn R, eds. *Endoskopische Polypektomie im Gastrintestinaltrakt.* Stuttgart: Thieme; 1973.

35. Castaneda-Zuniga WR, Gomes A, Weens C, Ketchum D, Amplatz K. Transluminal angioplasty in the treatment of abdominal angina. Röfo 1982;137:330-332.

36. Kippfmüllert K. Vorraussetzungen zur endoskopischen Ösophagektomie. Langenbecks Arch Chir Suppl, Kongressbericht 1991;424-429.

37. Lewis D, Waye J. Total small bowel enteroscopy. Gastrointest Endosc 1987;33:435-438.

38. Manger T, Winkler H. Erfahrungen in der intraluminalen Dünndarmschienung. Zentralbl Chir 1990;ll5:749-755.

39. Schreiber HW, Effenberger TH. Chirugische Lapraskopie. — minimal-invasive Chirurgie. Langenbecks Arch Chir 1991;376:65-66.

40. Kirschner MB. Ein neues Verfahren der Oesophagoplastie. Arch Klin Chir 1920; 114:606.

41. Lishman AH, Dellipiani AW, Devlin HP. The insertion of oesophagogastric tubes in malignant esophageal strictures: endoscopy or surgery? Br J Surg 1980;67:257.

42. Mannell AP, Becker PJ, Nissenbaum M. Bypass surgery for unresectable oesophageal cancer: early and late results in 124 cases. Br J Surg 1988;75:283.

43. Ong GB, Lam KH, Wong J, Lim TK. Jejunal oesophagoplasty for carcinoma of the oesophagus. Jpn J Surg 1980;10:15.

44. Siewert JR. Wert klinischer und experimenteller Ergebnisse für die Praxis in der Oesophaguschirurgie. Langenbecks Arch Chir Suppl, Kongressbericht 1991;282-287.

45. Kelling G. Über die Besichtigung der Speiseröhre und des Magens mit biegsamen Instrumenten. Verh Dt Naturf Ärzte 1901;II:73.

46. Kollath J, Starck E, Paolucci V. Dilation of esophageal stenosis by balloon catheter. J Cardiovasc Interv Radiol 1984;153:31.

47. Loizou LA, Crigg D, Atkinsaon M, Robertson C, Brown SG. A prospective comparison of laser therapy and intubation in endoscopic palliation of malignant dysphagia. Gastroenterology 1991;100 1303-1310.

48. Mellow MH, Pinkas H. Endoscopic therapy for esophageal carcinoma with Nd:YAG

laser: prospective evaluation of efficacy, complications and survival. Gastrointest Endosc 1984;30:334-339.

49. Paolucci V, Henne T, Schmidt Matthiesen A. Endoskopisch palliatve Tubus — und Lasertherapie bei fortgeschrittenem Carcinom von Oesophagus und Cardia. Chirurg 1990;61:43-48.

50. Martini N, Goodner TJ, Di Angielo GJ, Beatti EJ. Tracheooesophageal fistula due to cancer. J Thorac Cardiovasc Surg 1970;59:319.

51. Maynar M, Rösch J. Treatment of malignant esophageal obstruction with silicone-coated metallic self-expanding stents. In: Kollath J and Liermann D, eds. *Stents II*. Konstanz: Schnetztor Verlag; 1992; 252-259.

52. Hajek M. Rekonstruktive Operationen bei Trachealstenosen und erworbenen Tracheo-Oesophagealfisteln. Z Erkr Atmungsorgane 1986;166:116-118.

53. Charnsangavej C, Carrasco CH, Wright KC, Richli S, Wallace S, Gianturco C. A new expandable metallic stent for dilatation of stenotic tubular structures: Experimental and clinical evaluation. Houston Med J 1987;3:41-51.

54. Rösch J, Putnam JSE, Uchida BT. Modified Gianturco expandable wire stents in experimental and clinical use. Ann Radiol 1988;31:100-103.

55. Rauber K, Franke C, Rau WS, Syed-Ali A. Venendurchwanderung bei Gianturco-Wallace-Stents. Zentralblatt d Radiol — Radiology 1990;141:293.

Digestive Duct Stenting: Report of Primary Cases

Ren-Jie Yang, Xiang-Dong Wang, Shi-Wen Song, Jun Hung,
Hong-zhi Chang, Geng-Nian Liu

Institute of Interventional Biology, Beijing Medical University, Beijing, China

A Dacron knit fabric-covered modified Gianturco metallic stent was placed in seven patients as palliative treatment for esophageal carcinoma. The body of the stent was 18- or 12-mm in diameter and the end portions were 22-mm in diameter. They were connected at obtuse angles to keep the stent from migrating. In addition to esophageal cancer, four patients also had esophagorespiratory fistulas. All patients were treated by means of fluoroscopically-guided peroral intubation of the stent. Due to severe dyspnea, stents were first placed in the trachea and then the esophagus in one patient. All stents were successfully placed without technical failure. Clinical symptoms of aspiration were relieved in all patients with esophagorespiratory fistulas and the food intake capacity of all patients was improved. Four patients died between 3 and 20 weeks after stent placement (mean, 8.2 weeks) while three patients are currently alive with patent stents for 12 to 24 weeks (mean patency, 14 weeks). Dacron knit fabric-covered stents are safe and effective for the palliative treatment of esophageal carcinoma.

INTRODUCTION

Esophagogastric carcinoma causes progressive dysphagia, and approximately 60% of patients are unlikely candidates for surgery due to extensive tumor infiltration (1-3). Morbidity and mortality of esophageal carcinoma in China are quite high (4-6). In the late stages of this disease, a patient's ability to swallow generally diminishes; tumor infiltration into the surrounding tissue causes severe complications with esophagorespiratory fistula.

Many types of prostheses have been considered for palliative intubation but as of yet, none have achieved popularity (3,7-10). Recently, Song et al (11-13) have reported on the palliative treatment of esophagogastric carcinoma with covered metallic stents. Our primary experience with a dacron knit-covered metallic stent in seven patients having esophagogastric carcinoma is reported herein.

MATERIALS AND METHODS

Patients

Seven male patients who ranged in age from 49 to 88 years (mean, 65.8 years) were treated in this study (Table 1). All patients had esophageal cancer and suffered from dysphagia. Four patients also had a esophagorespiratory fistula associated with their cancer. All patients were treated with peroral intubation of a Dacron knit fabric-covered modified Gianturco™ metallic stent (Cook, Bloomington IN) under fluoroscopic control. Due to severe dyspnea, a stent was first placed in the trachea and then the esophagus in one patient.

Stent Design

We improved the modified retrievable Gianturco stent (14-16) by wrapping it with Dacron knit fabric. The stent wire was 0.4-mm in diameter and the length of each single body of the stent was 20 mm. The diameter of the stent was 18 mm (12 mm in diameter for anastomosis sites). The proximal and distal portions were wider (22 mm in diameter) than the body (18 mm in diameter) and were connected at obtuse angles to keep the stent from migrating upward or downward. A Dacron knit fabric was wrapped around the outside of all stents to inhibit tumor growth

Table 1. Clinical Characteristics

| No./Age/Sex | Previous Treatment | Stricture | | | Fistula | Food Intake Capacity |
		Location	Length (cm)	Minimum Diameter (mm)		
1/65/M	Radiation	Middle	12	Occlusion	Yes	None
2/70/M	Surgery	Middle	3	3	No	None
3/59/M	Radiation	Upper	6	2	Yes	None
4/88/M	Chemo-therapy	Lower	4	3	No	None
5/49/M	Radiation	Middle	8	Occlusion	Yes	None
6/60/M	Surgery	Middle	12	5	Yes	None
7/70/M	Surgery	Lower	4	2	No	None

into the stent (Figure 1). The delivery set consisted of a long sheath and a Teflon rod pusher.

TECHNIQUE

A small amount of liquid contrast or barium-enhanced fluoroscopy was used to identify the length of the stricture or location of the fistula. Oropharyngeal anaesthesia was routinely performed by means of an aerosol spray (1% lidocaine); sedation was not used. A suction tube was useful in removing saliva

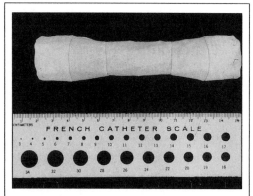

Figure 1. Dacron knit fabric-covered modified Gianturco metallic stent.

during the entire procedure (13). A 0.035- or 0.038-inch, 260-cm long guidewire with a rotational handle was used; this was convenient when changing the wire advance direction. After the guidewire was advanced across the stricture portion and into the stomach, a balloon catheter (7 Fr, 12-mm diameter) was passed through the guidewire and the stricture was dilated. The following stenting procedure was used: (1) the stent was compressed and put in the distal end of the introducing tube; (2) the balloon was then inflated and the introducing tube was moved along the guidewire until beyond the stricture portion, about 2 cm; (3) the balloon was deflated, holding the pusher, and withdrawn into the introducing tube followed by stent placement; and (4) esophagograms were obtained immediately after stent insertion.

To evaluate the improvement in food intake capacity after stent placement, the following scale was used: no foods, liquid only, soft foods, most foods, and all foods (i.e., normal).

RESULTS

All stents were successfully placed and there were no technical failures or esophageal perforations. After stent placement, esophagograms immediately displayed that all strictures were opened and all esophagorespiratory fistulas were successfully occluded (Table 2; Figures 2-4). Five patients felt dull chest pain which disappeared within 1 week in three patients. The remaining two patients required analgesic medication to control their pain. Two patients felt a foreign body-like feeling after stenting but did not require treatment.

Most patients could not swallow before stenting. After the procedure, food intake capacity was improved in all patients. One patient resumed eating normally, one patient was able to eat most food, and the remaining patients could eat soft food. Clinical symptoms of aspiration were relieved in all patients with esophagorespiratory fistulas and less severe pulmonary symptoms were noted during follow-up. Stent migration occurred in only one patient (Table 2, case no. 3). A Wilson-Cook stent was first placed in the trachea and due to severe dyspnea, was then placed in the esophageal tract. On follow-up, the stent tube had migrated slightly downward (see Figure 3). Tumor overgrowth was seen in the distal edge of the stent in one patient after 1 month (case no. 1) and therefore another stent was placed with a slight overlap at the ends (see Figure 2). Three of the seven patients are still alive with patent stents. One patient died of metastases while three died as a result of their general debilitated condition.

DISCUSSION

In China, the morbidity and mortality of esophageal carcinoma are very high (5,6,14). In late stage patients who cannot eat or drink, esophagorespiratory fistula may develop due to carcinoma which has infiltrated the surrounding tissue. The tumor protrudes into the trachea and causes dyspnea, aspiration, and pneumonia which are devastating and can be life-threatening. Resection of the carcinoma in these patients is impossible, and mortality following bypass surgery is high (1-3). Palliative treatment in such patients includes restoration of their ability to swallow and prevention of aspiration because of esophagorespiratory fistula.

The self-expandable stainless steel stent was devised by Dr. Gianturco in 1985 (17). Many interventional radiologists have reported both their experimental studies and clinical applications using the Gianturco stent in vessels (18-20), the biliary duct, and the tracheobronchial tree (21-24). In 1991, Song et al first described the use of silicone-covered Gianturco stents in esophageal strictures (13).

Table 2. Clinical Results Before and After Stent Placement

Case No.	Diameter of Narrowest Point (mm)		Food Intake Capacity	
	Before	After	Before	After
1	Occlusion	18	None	Soft
2	3	12	None	All
3	2	12	None	Most
4	3	12	None	Soft
5	Occlusion	18	None	Soft
6	5	18	None	Soft
7	2	12	None	Soft

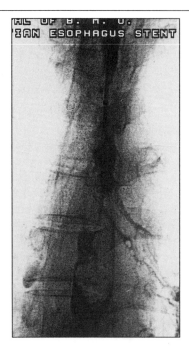
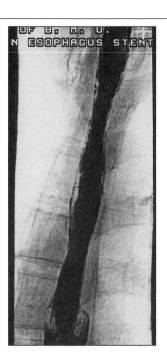
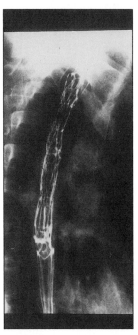
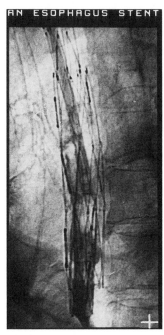

Figure 2. Patient No 1, a 65-year-old man. Esophagogram *(upper left)* shows total obstruction of the middle esophagus by carcinoma and an esophagorespiratory fistula. Esophagogram obtained immediately after stent placement *(upper right)* shows good patency; the fistula is occluded. One month later, the stent is still patent; distal end shows tumor overgrowth *(bottom left)*. Esophagogram obtained immediately after second stent placement shows good patency *(bottom right)*.

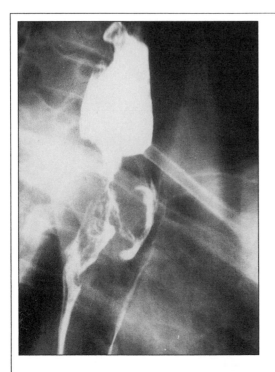

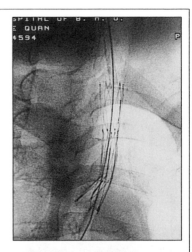

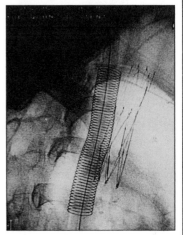

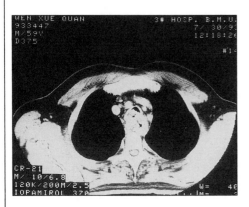

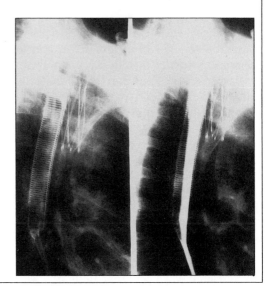

Figure 3. Patient No. 3, a 59-year-old man. On esophagogram, the upper thoracic esophagus shows irregular narrowing and infiltrated tumor shadow *(upper left)*. Barium contrast through the fistula into the trachea. CT scan *(bottom left)* shows an esophagorespiratory fistula with the tumor protruding into the trachea. In order to relieve dysphagia, a stent was placed in the trachea *(upper right)*, and then a thick Wallstent tube (Wilson-Cook) was placed *(middle right)*. On follow-up, the esophageal stent shows good patency and a slight downward migration can be seen *(bottom right)*.

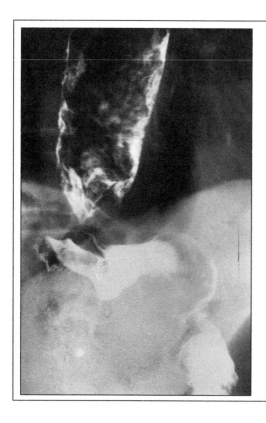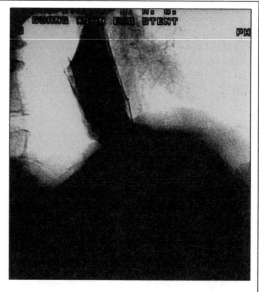

Figure 4. Patient No. 7, a 70-year-old man. Esophagogram shows severe narrowing of anastomotic site *(left)*. After stent placement *(right)*, a good flow of contrast is seen.

In our studies, we wrapped the dacron knit fabric material on a Gianturco metallic stent to inhibit tumor growth into the stent lumen. Our preliminary experience suggests that the Dacron knit fabric-covered stent has obvious advantages. First, the construction of the stent is based on the modified retrievable Gianturco stent (14-16) and therefore can be relocated. Secondly, there is less friction with the dacron covering compared to the silicone rubber-covered stent, making intubation easier. Finally, the proximal and distal portions are connected at obtuse angles with the body stent (see Figure 1) which not only keeps the stent from migrating, but causes less injury to the esophagus. This design has no reflux occurrence and can relieve the dysphagia caused by stubborn stricture.

CONCLUSIONS

In conclusion, the Dacron knit fabric-covered modified Gianturco stent is a safe and effective palliative treatment for esophageal carcinoma and represents a good method for improving patients' quality of life. Additional cases and a long-term study are needed to support and verify these conclusions.

REFERENCES

1. Saunders NR. The celestin tube in the palliation of carcinoma of the esophagus and cardia. Br J Surg 1979;66:419-421.
2. Earlam R, Cunha-Melo JR. Oesophageal squamous carcinoma. 1. A critical review of surgery. Br J Surg 1980;67:381-390.
3. Valbuena J. Endoscopic palliative treatment of esophageal and cardial cancer: a new antireflux prosthesis. A study of 40 cases. Cancer 1984;53:993-998.
4. Jun-li yao. *Research Progress of Esophageal Cancer*. First Edition. China: People's Publishing House; 1986;274-301.
5. Waterhous JAH, et al. *Cancer Incidence in Five Continents*. Volume 3, IARC Scientific Publications No. 15, 1976.

6. Whelan SL, et al. *Patterns of Cancer in Five Continents*. World Health Organization. IARC Scientific Publication No. 102, 1990.

7. den Hartog Jager FC, Bartelsman JF, Tytgat GN. Palliative treatment of obstructing esophagogastric malignancy by endoscopic positioning of a plastic prosthesis. Gastroenterology 1979;77:1008-1014.

8. Lishman AH, Dellipiani AW, Delvlin HB. The insertion of oesophagogastric tubes in malignant oesophageal strictures: endoscopy or surgery? Br J Surg 1980;67:257-259.

9. Sarr MG, Harper PH. Peroral pulsion intubation of malignant esophageal strictures using a fiberoptic technique. Am Surg 1984;50:437-440.

10. Haynes JW, Miller PR, Steiger Z. Celestin tube use: radiographic manifestations of associated complications. Radiology 1984;150:41-44.

11. Song HY, Chung JY, Han YM, et al. Expandable esophageal metallic stents coated with silicone rubber: an experimental study in rabbits. J Korean Rad Soc 1990;26:829-834.

12. Song HY, Choi KC, Cho BH, et al. Esophagogastric neoplasms: palliation with a modified Gianturco stent. Radiology 1991;180:349-354.

13. Song HY, Choi KC, Kwon HC, et al. Esophageal strictures: treatment with a new design of modified Gianturco stent. Radiology 1992;184:729-734.

14. Yang RJ, Yamada R, Sato M, et al. A new device: the retrievable metallic expandable stent. Nippon Act Radial 1990;50(2):s146.

15. Yang RJ, Yamada R, Sato M, et al. A study of new retrievable expandable metallic stent. Nippon Act Radial 1991;51:970-972.

16. Yang RJ. Development of retrievable expandable metallic stent: experimental studies and clinical applications. J Wakayama Med, Japan 1992;43:241-255.

17. Wright KC, Wallace S, Charnsangavej C, Carrasco CH, Gianturco C. Percutaneous endovascular stents: an experimental evaluation. Radiology 1985;156:69-72.

18. Duprat G Jr, Wright KC, Charnsangavej C, Wallace S, Gianturco C. Self-expanding metallic stents for small vessels: an experimental evaluation. Radiology 1987;162:469-472.

19. Yoshioka T, Weight K, Wallace S, et al. Self-expandable endovascular graft: an experimental study in dogs. AJR 1988;151:673-676.

20. Furui S, Sawada S, Irie T, et al. Hepatic inferior vena cava obstruction: treatment of two types with Gianturco expandable metallic stents. Radiology 1990;176:665-670.

21. Wallace MJ, Charnsangavej C, Ogawa K, et al. Tracheobronchial tree: expandable metallic stents used in experimental and clinical applications. Radiology 1986;158:309-312.

22. Carrasco CH, Wallace S, Charnsangavej C, et al. Expandable biliary endoprostheses: an experimental study. AJR 1985;145:1279-1281.

23. Rossi P, Bezzi M, Salvatori FM. Recurrent benign biliary stricture: management with self-expandable metallic stents. Radiology 1990;175:661-665.

24. Irving JD, Adam A, Dick R. Gianturco expandable metallic biliary stents: results of a European clinical trial. Radiology 1989;172:321-326.

Flexible Metal-Mesh Stents in the Colorectum

K.E. Grund

University Clinics, Tübingen, Germany

INTRODUCTION

Despite the current enthusiasm with stenting in most parts of the human body, the colorectum does not appear to be an ideal or preferred localization for stent placement. Only a few reports exist in the literature concerning this topic.

The most common treatment for colorectal cancer is a colostomy which can seriously affect a patient's quality of life. Alternatives to this treatment are laser therapy (critical to perform) or cryosurgery (limited in access and indication).

Despite prevailing skepticism, our favorable experiences with stenting in the upper gastrointestinal tract encouraged us to attempt this procedure in the colorectum.

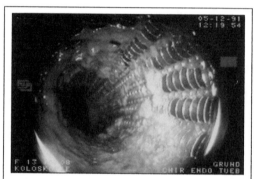

Figure 1. Deployed stent *in situ* in the rectosigmoid (diameter: 18 mm)

MATERIALS AND METHODS

A highly flexible, self-expanding nitinol stent with a luminal diameter of 18 mm after deployment (Ultraflex™, Boston Scientific Corp., Denmark) was used for the palliative treatment of colorectal cancer (Figure 1).

Nineteen stents were implanted in 16 patients (Table 1). The tumors mainly originated from the colorectum and the prostate, as well as from anastomotic recurrences. One-half of the patients were considered to be problematic cases due to length, highgrade stenosis, or kinking. Some tumors were situated high in the sigmoid colon whereas others were situated very low in the anorectum.

Due to highgrade stenoses, pre-treatment with the newly developed Argon-Plasma-Coagulation (APC) was necessary in the majority of patients.

Table 1. Patients and Tumor Characteristics

Patients	
Male/Female	9/5
Mean Age (Range) (years)	73 (41-90)
Origin of Tumor (No. of Patients)	
Colorectum	11
Prostate	2
Anastomotic Recurrence	3
Tumor Dimension	
Average Length (Range) (cm)	7 (3-12)
Average Free Lumen (Range) (mm)	7 (3-12)
Average Margin (Range)	
Upper (cm)	15 (8-31)
Lower (cm)	7 (3-25)

RESULTS

All stents were placed successfully and most (N=9) opened immediately. All stents were deployed after 5 days. The best control of implantation proved to be a combination of endoscopy and fluoroscopy.

Technical and functional success was evident in approximately 80% of the patients during the follow-up period of 16 to 42 weeks (Table 2). Evacuation improved significantly as indicated by a decrease in evacuation scores and thorough clinical evaluations. There were no or only mild complaints following stent placement and all stents remained open during the follow-up period. There were, however, problems with primary and secondary dislocations, fracture of stent wires, and with the introducer and material (Table 3).

In contrast to esophageal stenting, the rate of tumor ingrowth was relatively low, and all tumor ingrowth was effectively treated with APC. No bleeding, perforation, or other complications were noted.

Advantages of this form of palliative treatment of colorectal tumors include:

• Good evacuation function due to the wide luminal diameter (18 mm).

• Good tolerance and comfort for the patient due to the high flexibility of the stent.

• Unproblematic implantation (no general anaesthesia, outpatient procedure).

• Possibility of removing the stent endoscopically if necessary (not feasible with other types of metal stents).

The main disadvantages of this treatment are the necessity for pre- or post-treatment as well as the high cost of the device.

Unsolved problems remain with the stent design because it was primarily derived from that used in the esophagus. Adaptations should incorporate considerations of colorectal anatomy with regards to diameter (it should be about 25 to 30 mm), funnels (at the correct side and with special shapes), and different grades of elasticity of the whole stent. Tailor-made stents may be necessary for individual cases. Coating does not appear to be as critical in these stents compared to those used in the esophagus but should be considered to prevent tumor ingrowth (Table 3).

Table 2. Results Following Stent Implantation[a]

Technical Success	16/19 implantations
Functional Success	15/19 implantations
Follow-Up Period	Mean: 16 weeks
	Range: 2-42 weeks
Control Endoscopies	Mean: 2 times
	Range: 0-11
Evacuation Score[b]	
Before Stenting	Mean: 4
	Range: 3-5
After Stenting	Mean: 2
	Range: 1-3
Complaints	
None	12/16 patients
Mild	4/16 patients
Severe	0/16 patients

[a] All stents open during follow-up period.
[b] Scores could range from 0 to 4 (best to worst).

Table 3. Problems in the Clinical Series

Problem	Occurrence Rate
Primary dislocation	3/19 implantations
Secondary dislocation	2/19 implantations
Fracture of stent wire or mesh	2/19 implantations
Temporary problems with introducer and material	1/19 implantations
Tumor ingrowth	3/16 patients

CONCLUSIONS

Despite our previous skepticism, colorectal stenting offers effective, long-lasting palliation of colorectal cancer with a low complication rate and good tolerance for patients. The main benefit for patients appears to be the avoidance of a colostomy.

A definitive critical analysis of colorectal stenting as a new therapeutic modality is not yet possible; we must first have stents adapted to the colorectal anatomy (only prototypes are now available) and experience with more patients. Our preliminary results with colorectal stenting, however, are encouraging.

Stenting of the Central Airways

H.D. Becker[1], B. Wagner[1], D. Liermann[2], S. Urhoj[3], S. Mechmann[3]

[1]Departments of Internal Medicine/Oncology and Endoscopy,
Thoraxklinik der LVA Baden, Heidelberg, Germany
[2]Department of Radiology, J.W. Goethe University Hospital, Frankfurt am Main, Germany
[3]BSC Medintechnik GmbH, Hilden, Germany

INTRODUCTION

Considerable progress has been made in the field of tracheobronchial stenting since the Second International Stent Symposium held in Frankfurt in 1991. This is reflected by the introduction of new devices and a steady increase in the number of stent applications. Some of the problems previously described (1) were widely recognized by others, and different approaches have been taken to overcome these. An ideal stent for which most of the problems of tracheobronchial stenting have been solved may soon be available, possibly resulting in this procedure becoming routine in the near future. Comparatively recent therapeutic procedures such as the Nd:YAG laser and brachytherapy have become much less frequently used at our institution following the introduction of tracheobronchial stenting. The number of stent procedures has risen steadily from 10 and 15 in 1989 and 1990 to 42 in 1991, 59 in 1992, and up to 131 in 1993.

INDICATIONS AND GENERAL ANATOMICAL, FUNCTIONAL, AND TECHNICAL CONSIDERATIONS

All causes of stenosis of the central airways may now be treated by stenting provided that surgical repair, which is still the preferred method, poses some risk for the patient. In our series of 257 procedures in 125 patients up to December, 1993, the ratio of malignant to benign causes has been 6:4. In tumors, compression (26%) and stenosis due to endoluminal tumor growth (21%) have been equally frequent. Of the benign causes, a combined injury of granulomatous scar formation and chondromalacia due to intubation trauma, prolonged ventilation, or tracheostomy was much more frequent (23%) than isolated scars (11%) or tracheobronchomalacia (7%). Concomitant involvement of the esophagus, either by compression or esophagotracheal fistula, was comparatively frequent (12%) and required additional stenting.

The complex anatomical and functional structures of the tracheobronchial tree have been a major obstacle to endobronchial stenting. For the sake of safe ventilation, the physiological bends and ramifications of the airways may not be disturbed. The elasticity of the tracheobronchial wall due to the combination of flexible and rigid structures provides stability during the considerable changes in length and diameter which occur under widely varying intrathoracic pressures (which can reach well over 300 Torr) (2). Maintenance of the airways also is essential for ventilation and clearance of secretions. The ideal stent should mimic these properties as closely as possible and should stay safely fixed once in position (3,4). On the other hand, a stent should be easily removable in the event of complications. It should also be resistant to further treatment, such as lasers or irradiation. In addition, introduction of the stent should be easily performed and ventilation should not be compromised during implantation.

CURRENT STENT SYSTEMS

Stents of Plastic Material and Composites

In general there are two types of tracheobronchial stents: plastic tubes and metallic stents. Of the plastic stents, the Dumon stent is the most widely used and consists of a silicone tube of varying lengths and diameters with external protrusions for fixation (5). Usually providing patent airways, it has some disadvantages regarding function and implantation technique. As the airflow inside the stent is slower, obliteration by secretions is comparatively frequent (6). In smaller bronchi, the inner diameter of the appropriate stent is very small due to the thickness of the plastic material, thus leaving very little lumen for ventilation and clearance of secretions. Stenting of the subglottic area and of very short stenoses is not recommended since fixation in this region and type of stenosis are not very safe. Implantation is only possible by use of a special rigid introducing bronchoscope under general anaesthesia. The recommended technique of blind introduction under fluoroscopic control has been felt to be awkward by some and the implantor system is comparatively expensive. Several modifications have been proposed, including use of a routine bronchoscope either by folding the prosthesis into the scope itself or by loading it partially onto the bronchoscope and optic. We have constructed a simple pusher with a conically-shaped end through which ventilation can be provided while the stent is safely placed under visual control (7).

Due to their geometry, Dumon stents frequently become obliterated by sticky secretions, especially during the first time after application. Freitag, therefore, developed an advanced type of silicone prosthesis, the dynamic stent, in which the ventral part is enforced by metallic bands for stabilization while the dorsal part is elastic, similar to the membranous wall of the airways. Narrowing of the airway diameter during coughing is thus provided which results in a higher velocity of the air flow and better mucus clearance. Fixation is achieved by branching of the distal end of the prosthesis into both main bronchi. Isolated stenosis of one main bronchus or of the higher parts of the trachea up to the subglottic region are not indicated for this type of stent

because a considerable part of the unaffected airways would also be covered by the stent (6).

Metallic Stents

The thickness of the wall as compared to the diameter is negligible in metallic stents. There are basically two types of metallic stents: expandable and self-expanding systems. The expandable systems, mainly the Palmaz stent and the Strecker stent, are meshworks cut from a stainless steel tube or knitted from tantalum wire (8-10). Being compressed onto a balloon, they are introduced into the tracheobronchial tree after prior dilatation of the stenosis; once set in place, they become expanded by inflation of the introducer balloon. Fixation to the tracheobronchial wall is achieved by the expanding pressure. After some time these stents may become totally embedded into the bronchial wall since the mucosa protrudes through the gaps (11). In excessive inflammatory granuloma or exophytic tumor growth, complete internal occlusion may cause life-threatening symptoms of restenosis. There is no resistance inside the airways to the considerable intrathoracic pressures in the thoracic cavity in contrast to other organs such as the barely compressible content of the blood vessels. Thus, the stent may collapse under constant strain. This is especially true for the Strecker stent, but can also occur with the Palmaz stent. If this occurs, it may be difficult, if not impossible, to remove the stent from the airways once it has been fully integrated into the bronchial wall. Therefore, we do not recommend the application of these stents in the central airways (1).

Self-expanding devices derive their expanding force either by their geometric configuration or by a so-called memory effect of special alloys. Stents of the former type include the Gianturco stent and the Wallstent. The Gianturco stent is constructed of a very rigid steel wire arranged in a crown using a zigzag configuration. Once released from its compressed form by retraction of a retaining sheath from the introducer on which it is mounted, the stent unfolds to its utmost pre-set diameter. As the expanding pressure is concentrated on a very small surface area, especially at the pointed ends, perforation of the bronchial wall has been common, result-ing in tracheobronchial fistula or fatal hemorrhage due to erosion of the pulmonary artery. The Gianturco stent is fixed by hooks at the pointed ends and cannot be readily re-moved in case of complications. Moreover, the gaps between the wires are very large and early reocclusion by prolapsing tumor is com-paratively frequent. In our opinion, this re-stricts its use only to extrinsic tumor compres-sion (1). To our knowledge there have been no reports of long-term experiences with a coated system in the airways (12). The Wallstent, a much tighter meshwork also made of stainless steel filaments that are arranged in a spiral pattern, conveys its expanding force onto a considerably higher surface area. There-fore, despite its pointed edges, perforation does not typically occur. Granuloma ingrowth and tumor occlusion do occur, however, and removal of the stent may also be difficult and can only be achieved by destruction of the stent and extraction of the single filaments (13).

The most recent development in stenting of the central airways is the nitinol prosthesis. Nitinol is a binary alloy of nickel and tita-nium, the physical properties of which were detected at the Naval Ordinance Laborato-ries (NOL) in Maryland (USA). After me-chanical deformation, a wire made of this material regains its preset configuration at temperatures above 20°C (14). For the con-struction of endoprostheses, the wires are knit to meshworks. In our experience these stents diminish their diameter during respira-tory and coughing maneuvers in a physiologi-cal manner and do not convey unphysiological high pressures to the bronchial wall during re-expansion. Our most extensive experience in tracheobronchial stenting is with this sys-tem.

RESULTS

During the period from 1989 to 1993 we placed 257 stents in 125 patients suffering from ventilation problems of the central air-ways. Their ages ranged from 2 to > 80 years. The indications for stenting in our patients have been described above. Stents were placed in the laryngeal region (N=31), the trachea (N=141), the main bronchi on both sides equally (N=64), and on the lobar level, mostly for treatment of stenoses of anastomosis after sleeve resections (N=21). The stents used were Dumon stents (N=38), Strecker™ stents (N=36) (Boston Scientific Corp., Denmark), nitinol stents (N=166), and stents of various other kinds (N=17). We have observed pa-tients for up to 3½ years after stent place-ment, the longest of which has been in those with benign lesions. Due to additional inter-ventions such as endoluminal brachytherapy or photodynamic laser therapy, even some patients with malignant disease have survived for a few years after stent placement.

In preparation of stent placement for widening of the central airway stenosis, vari-ous procedures to open the lumen should be performed, such as dilatation by balloon or a rigid bronchoscope, or mechanical debridement by forceps or laser ablation. The lumen should become as close to the physi-ological diameter as possible. These proce-dures allow almost complete expansion and good function of the stent immediately after insertion. In the case of necrosis, particularly if there is additional involvement of the adja-cent esophageal wall, extensive damage must be avoided since there is a high risk of an esophagotracheal fistula occurring, especially if further radiotherapy is considered. For safe fixation, the diameter of the chosen stent should be similar to the physiological dimen-sions and the largest possible stent should be introduced without use of excessive force. In our opinion, stenting of the central airways for exact placement and the prevention of complications should always be performed under visual control by the endoscope. The appropriate length may be measured by the difference of the external length of the bronchoscope being placed with its tip at the distal and proximal end of the stenosis, respectively. The diameter is judged from the diameter of the largest bronchoscope that can be passed after dilatation or from inserting an opened biopsy forceps and comparing the distance of the tips of its branches to the stenosis. Once these procedures have been performed the stent may be inserted.

The Dumon stent allowed for stability and safe placement; however, several disadvantages including secretion retention, difficulties in such areas as the larynx, the bifurcation, smaller bronchi and in kinking due to external compression or following surgical resections occurred (Figure 1). We do not

have any further experience with the Freitag dynamic stent since it has only been recently developed. It is reported to be superior to the Dumon stent, however, with regard to mucus clearing, but from its construction it has the similar limitations of application (10). As an alternative to the Dumon stent, we tried the expandable Strecker tantalum stent. We soon recognized, however, that this stent could not withstand the strain of chronic pressure changes, especially in the larger central airways. In our 36 procedures with this stent, we observed several complications, even life-threatening, due to collapse and almost complete occlusion by ingrowing tissue. Therefore, we have stopped using this stent type (Figure 2). We were also forced to remove the much stronger Palmaz stents due to collapse, even after several had been inserted telescopically for increased stability (1). Although the Wallstent is re-expanding and more stable, it has been described as being very difficult to remove. Thus, we began using the nitinol-type prosthesis and it is with this stent that we have gained the most experience.

The nitinol stent has been used in angiology and gastroenterology. For the latter application in esophageal stenoses, it is available as the Ultraflex prosthesis, which is compressed and glued to the introducer by

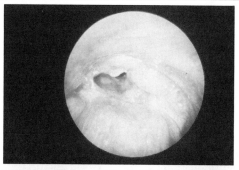

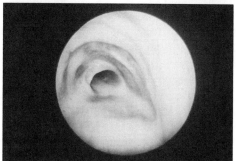

Figure 1. Stenosis at the site of an anastomosis between the trachea and left main bronchus after right pneumonectomy and carinal resection *(top)*. The stenosis is due to scar formation and excessive granuloma after partial dehiscence of the suture. Stenting of the stenosis by Dumon stent *(bottom)*. Due to the bend of the airways the stent is tilting towards the tracheal wall causing retention of secretions.

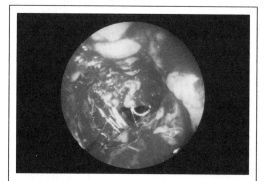

Figure 2. Total collapse of an almost completely incorporated tracheal Strecker stent, placed for the treatment of benign stenosis of the lower trachea after tracheotomy. Further damage and occlusion occurred after the endoscopist attempted an extraction instead of a dilatation procedure. Extensive tracheal resection had to be performed.

gelatin that dissolves in a moist environment for release of the stent. It obviously could not be used in this way for the central airways. We began inserting the nitinol prosthesis by folding it around the optic inside the rigid bronchoscope. Release was achieved by withdrawing the bronchoscope while keeping the prosthesis in place by a biopsy forceps. We felt that there should be a system by which stenting of the central airways is possible using the flexible bronchoscope under local anaesthesia for less complicated procedures. Thus, a new introducing device was constructed in which the stent was compressed down to 3 mm and fixed on an introducer by a thread. The stent became released under visual control by pulling the retaining thread (Figure 3). In more than 30 procedures, this "crochet" system has proven to be very effective and will hopefully be commercially available by the end of 1994. As described in a separate paper, in many patients the nitinol stents have been gradually integrated into the bronchial wall and in some, have eventually been reepithelialized (11).

As with other metallic meshworks, reocclusion by ingrowth of benign or malignant tissue has been a considerable problem in some patients. Removal of the stent after mechanical debridement by shaving off the

tissue with the edge of the bronchoscope has been possible by grasping a loop at the proximal end of the stent and unraveling the knit work (this is not possible in a different type of nitinol stent where the strings of wire are separately knotted together). For the prevention of occlusion by excessive ingrowth of tissue, we developed prototypes of the nitinol stent that were coated with a biocompatible membrane. By the end of 1993 we implanted 50 of these devices, some of which have been safely in place and providing good function for almost 1 year. A similarly-coated system should be commercially available in the near future.

In our experience, the nitinol stent, in its different configurations, has the potential of becoming the ideal stent system (Figure 4). We have already been able to manage some of the most complex problems, such as sublaryngeal stenoses, extensive tracheobronchomalacia (Figure 5), esophagotracheal fistulas, and even stenting of an extensive tracheal stenosis in a 2-year-old boy after repeated surgical procedures. Interestingly, one of the most recent developments is reinforcement of the silicone stents by nitinol rings for the sake of reduction of the thickness of the wall (Nova stent).

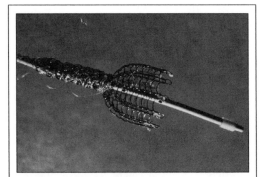

Figure 3. A nitinol stent compressed and fixed onto an introducer by a retaining thread. The device is introduced over a guidewire and the stent is released under endoscopic control by pulling the thread.

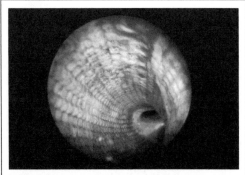

Figure 4. A nitinol stent placed inside the left main bronchus for treatment of stenosis due to tumor compression adapts nicely to the curving contour. At the far end, the opening of the lower and upper lobe bronchi is visible.

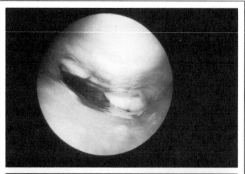

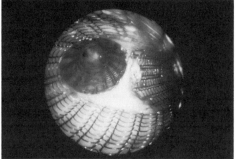

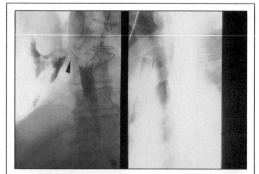

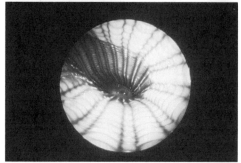

Figure 5. Extensive malacia of the trachea and main bronchi causing severe obstruction of the major airways and retention of purulent secretions *(top)*. After placement of three nitinol stents inside the trachea and main bronchi, the airways were patent, the secretions were cleared, and the patient was breathing easily *(bottom)*.

Figure 6. Contrast medium is dripping from the esophagus into the pleural cavity via a large esophagopleural fistula *(top)* after right pneumonectomy and extensive mediastinal lymph node resection for bronchial carcinoma (arrow on the left). After occlusion by a coated nitinol prosthesis, passage is normal. At the site of the fistula there is a little excavation without any leakage (right). A drainage tube has been placed inside the thoracic cavity for treatment of pleural empyema. The fistula is closed by the coated middle portion of the esophageal stent (clearly marked by its darker color), while the prosthesis is fixed *in situ* by both uncoated ends *(bottom)*.

CONCLUSIONS

In a relatively short time, tremendous progress in stenting of the central airways has been made. "Dedicated" systems (5) that eventually may easily be introduced, even under local anaesthesia by use of the fiberscope, are within reach. By the time of the next International Stent Symposium, stenting of the tracheobronchial tree rather than surgery may have become the treatment of choice in many indications. Furthermore, having solved many of the complex problems of stenting in the central airways, some of the new techniques will surely be applied to other fields of treatment, including esophageal endoprostheses (Figure 6).

REFERENCES

1. Becker HD, van Bodegom PC. Der einsatz des Strecker-stents in der trachea. In: Kollath J and Liermann D, eds. *Stents II.* Konstanz: Schnetztor-Verlag; 1992;S216-225.

2. Macklem and Mead — Zit bei Ulmer WT, Barth J, Hoffarth HP, Hötmann B, Schott D, Sieveking CF. Sieveking Husten. Stuttgart: Verlag W. Kohlhammer; 1990;S52.

3. Masaoka A. Tracheobronchomalacia. J Jap Soc Bronchology 1993;15:719-728.

4. Wehrmeyer B, Kuhn FP. Experimentelle untersuchungen zur druckstabilität vaskulärer endoprothesen. Fortschr Röntgenstr 1993;158:242-246.

5. Dumon JF. A dedicated tracheobronchial stent. Chest 1990;97:328-332.

6. Miyazawa T, Doi M, Mineshita M, Kurata T, Suei T, Yamakido M. The placement of the Dumon stent for airway stenosis. J Jap Soc Bronchology 1993;15:749-756.

7. Becker HD. Derzeitige möglichkeiten und grenzen der bronchoskopischen tracheobronchialen schienung. Pneumologie 1994, in press.

8. Palmaz JC. Intravascular stents. In: Kollath J and Liermann D, eds. *Stents II*. Konstanz: Schnetztor-Verlag; 1992;S162-173.

9. Richter GM. Theoretische grundlagen des ballonexpandierbaren Palmaz-Stents. In: Kollath J and Liermann D, eds. *Stents*. Konstanz: Schnetztor-Verlag; 1990;S50-57.

10. Strecker EP, Liermann D, Barth KH, et al. Expandable tubular stents for treatment of arterial occlusive diseases: experimental and clinical results. Radiology 1990;175:87-102.

11. Grewe P, Krampe K, Müller KM, Becker HD. Macroscopic and histomorphologic alterations of the bronchial wall after implantation of nitinol stents. See related manuscript in this Volume.

12. Do YS, Song HY, Lee HL, et al. Esophagorespiratory fistula associated with esophageal cancer: treatment with a Gianturco stent tube. Radiology 1993; 187:673-677.

13. Bohndorf K, Kurzeja A, Schlöndorff G, Vorwerk D, Günther RW. Implantation selbstexpandierender endoprothesen (Wallstent) bei benignen trachealobstruktionen. In: Kollath J and Liermann D, eds. *Stents II*. Konstanz: Schnetztor-Verlag; 1992;S234-242.

14. Kauffmann GB, Mayo I. The metal with a memory. Invent Technol 1993;18-23.

Macroscopic and Histomorphologic Alterations of the Bronchial Wall After Implantation of Nitinol Stents

P. Grewe[1], K. Krampe[1], K.M. Müller[1], H.D. Becker[2]

[1]Institut für Pathologie, Berufsgenossenschaftliche Krankenanstalten Bergmannsheil,
Bochum, Germany
[2]Departments of Internal Medicine/Oncology and Endoscopy,
Thoraxklinik der LVA Baden, Heidelberg, Germany

INTRODUCTION

Due to the comparatively short time of their application, there have been no extensive investigations on the implantation of metallic stents, especially nitinol stents, in the central airways (1,2). Integration into the bronchial wall is never observed following implantation of silicone prostheses. Fibrinoid depositions, resembling icing, may be seen around the silicone tubes after a period of time which may be later transformed into solid scars. After extraction, the Dumon stent leaves small indentations in the mucosa due to its protrusions; these persist for a short time without further damage into the deeper layers of the bronchial wall. Beneath the silicone stents there is always a metaplastic alteration of the mucosa with impediment of mucus clearance. Sometimes due to excessive pressure onto the bronchial wall, hemorrhagic infarctions and ulcerophlegmonous destruction may be caused.

In contrast to these quasi-inert prostheses, we macroscopically observe a regular but individually different process of integration into the bronchial wall with metallic stents. Depending on the pressure on the bronchial wall (which is related to the diameter of the stent versus the bronchus), the stent initially lays adjacent to the bronchial wall. Due to its expanding force, the stent is pressed to the mucosa a few hours later resulting in a cushion-like edema by which the pale mucosa protrudes through the wire loops. At this time, the stent may be seen only by the cobblestone appearance of the mucosa. If neighboring mucosal cushions come into contact, the stent may become completely embedded and internal epithelialization may begin. In addition, endoluminal occlusion of the stent may also become a problem at this time due to excessive granuloma formation or exophytic tumor growth. Ideally, the stent should eventually be covered by a mucosa-like continuous epithelial layer which provides an almost regular transport of the mucus (3) (Figure 1).

The aim of our study was to investigate these processes by histomorphology and

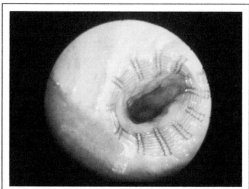

Figure 1. Implantation of a nitinol stent for compression of the left main bronchus after right pneumonectomy for bronchial carcinoma. The suture after pneumonectomy is seen at right. On the nitinol stent all phases of the integration process can be noted: simple indwelling without any mucosal reaction proximally, the cobblestone appearance of the protruding mucosa at the dorsal wall, and complete integration by a mucosal layer at the ventral wall on the left side.

electron microscopy (4). Biopsy specimens were examined from 17 patients at regular intervals during bronchoscopic control. We examined the integration process up to several years after stent implantation in four deceased patients (Figure 2). The alterations were compared to the normal mucosa of children's tracheas. We were also interested as to whether nickel or titanium could be found in the adjacent tissues due to corrosion; this had not been observed macroscopically (5). To this purpose, the bed of the stents and the regional lymphatic tissue were examined by energy dispersive radiomicroanalysis. In some patients with a known allergy to nickel, no reactions could be found after fixation of the alloys to the skin. Adverse reactions may be provoked after some time due to corrosion in the tissue environment. These reactions may also be due to electromagnetic fields. We were unable to further investigate this question, however.

RESULTS

In general, the macroscopic reactions were confirmed by the pathomorphological investigations. Directly after stent implantation, rhythmic indentions by the wires were observed (Figure 3), while polypoid protrusions invaded the gaps (Figure 4). If we had to perform desobliteration mechanically or by laser prior to the insertion of stents, an acellular coating by cellular detritus, fibrinoid membranes, and mucus was observed. In the intact mucosa the stent wires caused superficial lesions. It is from the edges of these tiny lesions that formation of reactive reparative granulation tissue appeared. After a few weeks, the prosthesis may be totally covered by tissue. At that stage, occlusion due to excessive granuloma or exophytic tumor growth may occur. According to our observations, tumor growth at the site of the stent seemed to be much slower than in the adjacent bronchus in many cases. It remains unclear, however, whether this was caused by direct pressure onto the tissue or by impairment of blood flow. After several weeks, the

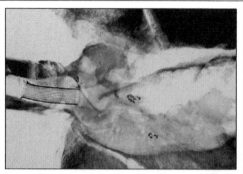

Figure 2. X-ray of a post-mortem anatomical specimen. A nitinol stent had been implanted for treatment of a compression stenosis of the lower trachea. This was due to lymph node metastasis after esophageal resection for carcinoma with adaptation of the stomach to the cervical portion of the esophagus. The calcified lymph nodes in the center are the late residuals of a tuberculous primary complex.

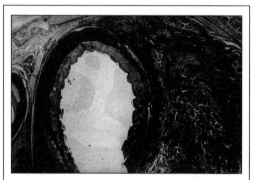

Figure 3. Overview of a tracheal cross section. Rhythmic indentions of the mucosa after removal of the nitinol stent postmortem are apparent. At right, extensive paratracheal tumor spread is seen as the cause for external tracheal obstruction (Magnification: x25).

granuloma tissue resolved and it became replaced by reactive metaplastic epithelial cells of squamous differentiation (Figure 5). As compared to the epithelium proximally and distally to the stent by electron microscopy, these cells are much larger, more flat, and polymorphic, and their ciliation is only rudimentary (Figure 6). Finally, the whole stent may become covered by a continuous layer of tissue.

The reactions described are restricted to the stented area and extended into the submucosal region only. We did not observe any invasive damage such as hemorrhagic infarction or ulcerophlegmonous lesions after implantation of nitinol stents. Fragments

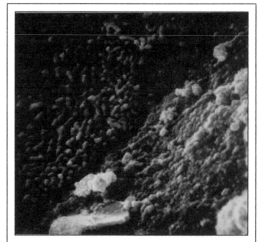

Figure 6.   Boundary running diagonally between two reactive metaplastic epithelial cells inside the prosthesis. Note the rudimentary ciliation. (Electron microscopy; Magnification x1000).

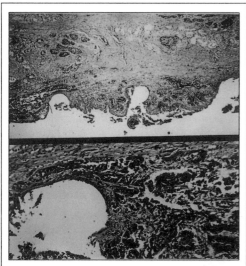

Figure 4.   Detail of diverticulus indentions. Spreading of vital tumor tissue involving all layers of the bronchial wall (Magnification: x140).

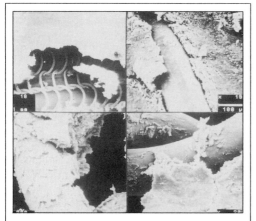

Figure 5.   Cellular coating of a nitinol stent (Electron microscopy; Magnification x10-1300).

of nickel and titanium were also not detected in the bronchial wall, the adjacent lymphatic tissue, or in the regional lymph nodes.

CONCLUSION

In conclusion, we were able to histologically confirm the macroscopic stages of integration after implantation of the nitinol stent. After an early mechanical reaction during which the mucosa was pressed through the wire loops, mucosal islands merged and the stent finally became totally embedded by metaplastic squamous epithelium with rudimentary ciliation. In some cases of excessive granuloma tissue, the stent may become completely occluded, which is a frequent observation after prior mechanical and laser desobliteration or in patients with keloids. The same is true for exophytic tumor growth. Since we have only inserted coated nitinol stents for the prevention of these complications for a relatively short period of time, resulting histomorphologic changes are not available as of yet.

REFERENCES

1. Bohndorf K, Kurzeja A, Schlöndorff G, Vorwerk D, Günther RW. Implantation selbstexpandierender Endoprothesen (Wallstent) bei benignen Tracheal-obstruktionen. In: Kollath J and Liermann D, eds. *Stents II*. Konstanz: Schnetztor-Verlag; 1992;S234-S242.
2. Rauber K, Franke Ch, Syed Ali S, Bensmann G. Experimentelle Erfahrungen mit Nitinol-Prothesen. In: Kollath J and Liermann D, eds. *Stents*. Konstanz: Schnetztor-Verlag; 1990;S65-S70.
3. Becker HD, van Bodegom PC. Der einsatz des Strecker-stents in der trachea. In: Kollath J and Liermann D, eds. *Stents II*. Konstanz: Schnetztor-Verlag; 1992;S216-S225.
4. Grewe P, Schmitz I, Theile A, Becker HD, Müller K.M. Rasterelektronenmikroskopische unter-suchungen der frühen inkorporationsphase von tracheobronchialen endoprothesen (stents). Beitr Elektronenmikroskop Direktabb Oberfl 1992;25:S399-S401.
5. Edie JW, Andreasen GF, Zaytoun MP. Surface corrosion of nitinol and stainless steel under clinical conditions. Angle Ordontodist 1981;51:319-324.

First Experiences with a New Memory Metallic Endoprosthesis in the Tracheobronchial System

D. Liermann[1] and M. Rust[2]

Departments of [1]Radiology and [2]Pulmonology, J.W. Goethe University Hospital,
Frankfurt am Main, Germany

INTRODUCTION

Diseases with a stenotic effect on the lumen are no rarity in the tracheobronchial system. From an etiological point of view, there are differences between acquired and congenital stenoses and occlusions in the tracheobronchial system. In addition to definitive agenesis and atresia of the trachea and anomalies of isolated segmental bronchial branches, stenosis of the respiratory tract results from other deformities or their resulting conditions. The double aorta, which encloses the trachea-like pincers, deserves special mention here as it causes progressive stenosis with tracheomalacia (1-6). Such changes, which can already be relevant during infancy, are only recognized through secondary phenomena such as stridor or recurrent pneumonia caused by ventilation deficiency. This also applies to deformed constricted segment bronchi which must be treated as soon as possible (2,7-11).

It is a peculiarity of the respiratory tract that, in the event of acute blockage, there are only a few minutes available to remove the obstruction, to lay a tracheal tube, or to perform a tracheotomy if the patient is to be kept alive. Less dramatic but equally critical are all measures in the area of the trachea or main bronchus which contribute to the removal of severe stenoses. During these manipulations, the remaining lumen is further constricted with a reduction of respiratory volume.

As far as acquired stenoses and occlusions are concerned, it is important to differentiate between conditions affecting the system from the outside and conditions caused by the system. Cystic fibrosis, a systematic disease of the exocrine glands, results in a thickening of the mucus which leads to blockage of peripheral and segment bronchi (12), particularly among older individuals and those not receiving adequate care and therapy. Cystic fibrosis cannot be treated by recanalizing or dilatative therapies. Similarly, in other conditions characterized by increased mucus production and an inability to repeatedly expectorate, it is usually possible to remove the blockage adequately by medication or aspiration (12). In the case of benign compressive conditions accompanied by respiratory insufficiency such as retrosternal struma in the mediastinum, tracheomalacia, localized strictures, or constriction resulting from iatrogenic injuries between the esophagus and trachea, the high life expectancy favors the selection of primarily surgical methods (13-21).

The situation is completely different in the case of malignant endoluminal tumors or tumors infiltrating and penetrating the lumen from the outside (22-25). Here, palliative therapy is required to maintain adequate respiratory sufficiency for the longest possible period. In these cases, the emphasis is frequently placed on a combined application of alternative methods such as laser, percutaneous transluminal angioplasty, endoluminal splinting, endoluminal afterloading therapy, percutaneous irradiation, and chemotherapy (14,16,20,26-28). A further addition to the range of alternative therapies consists of the use of self-expanding and balloon-expanding stents for the treatment of tracheobronchial stenosis. Compared to surgical treatment of stenoses in the trachea, stent application is a simple method resulting in immediate improvement in the quality of life for the patient. This takes priority, particularly in the case of malignant stenoses with limited life expectancy. The purpose of this paper is to report our initial experiences with a memory metal stent manufactured in one piece.

MATERIALS AND METHODS

The prototype stent consists of a metal lattice braid made of a nickel-titanium alloy (nitinol). The endoprosthesis is inserted in the tracheobronchial system under sedation or anaesthesia, following previous dilatation or laser therapy of the stenotic segment via the positioned guidewire under x-ray and endoscopic control. Dilatation and stent implantation are preceded by precise CT measurement of the tracheal or bronchial segment requiring the stent and by antibiotic prophylaxis. The stent is then positioned at the identified stenosis with the aid of easily identified markers and released by drawing back on a protective membrane covering the stent. This releases the nitinol stent. The stent is completely released once the two markings are congruent. The stent now begins to expand and establishes contact with the surface of the tracheobronchial wall. The memory metal effect, which has been set to body temperature, means that the stent now starts to assume its designated, preprogrammed size and shape. As a rule, it needs 5 minutes to do so. Any manipulation during this expansion process, particularly pulling or pushing forces on the stent, should be avoided at all costs as it could result in compression with deformation of the design or in an extension in the longitudinal axis resulting in a smaller lumen diameter in the stent segment which has not yet expanded. Defects of this nature can no longer be corrected. After 5 minutes the implant set can be easily removed. This is followed by x-ray and bronchoscopic control. Any bleeding caused by expansion of the stent in the tumor tissue should be identified and treated immediately.

The surface of the stent is designed not to hinder adequate transport by the mucus membrane. Although the stent's properties make it relatively rigid, it still retains a certain residual flexibility. The prototype stent we used measured up to 16 mm in diameter with a length of 4 to 10 cm. Use in tracheoesophageal fistulas is ruled out until the stent is designed with a membrane. Further therapy with this uncoated stent type is possible in the form of combined irradiation or laser treatment with recurrent tumors or protruding granulation. In the subsequent follow-up period, endoscopic examinations were performed initially after one week and then at monthly intervals. Additional examinations were required in the case of respiratory insufficiency. Lung function tests were also conducted in order to detect initial signs of a possible constriction before the symptoms became clinically manifested.

INDICATIONS

The indication for implantation of this tracheal stent includes all benign and malignant stenoses of the tracheobronchial system which are accompanied by severe respiratory insufficiency. It is initially irrelevant whether the condition is caused by a primary bronchial tumor gradually constricting the lumen, a tumor penetrating the tracheobronchial system with an ingrowth blocking the lumen, or tumor development with impression of the trachea or bronchus resulting in respiratory insufficiency. Also irrelevant is the genesis of a tracheomalacia in the case of benign stenosis. Benign stenoses in the tracheobronchial system should be discussed individually, but should be treated with reservations because of the initially provisional nature of the results. In addition to the patient's age, it is important to consider disease prognosis along with stenosis type.

Use of an endoprosthesis is usually only considered following unsatisfactory laser therapy. The particular stent type used in this series is accessible for laser therapy in the event of tissue growth through the stent as the remaining lumen allows for use of a laser.

PATIENT DATA

Since 1993, we have implanted 11 Memotherm® (Angiomed, Karlsruhe, Germany) stents in human tracheobronchial systems. The diameter of the stents ranged between 9 and 14 mm in the primary bronchus and between 10 and 14 mm in the trachea. Eight stents with a diameter of 14 mm and three with a diameter of 9 mm were inserted either in the trachea or in one of the two primary bronchi.

Altogether, we have treated four female and seven male patients aged between 51 and 76 years (mean, 65 years). All patients suffered from considerable respiratory insufficiency resulting from constriction of the respiratory tract by malignant tumors. Five patients were initially treated by laser therapy because of lumen-stenosing bronchial neoplasms, without showing any notable or only temporary improvement of the respiratory insufficiency. In the other six patients, the condition was caused by tumorous lumen compression from the outside, in some cases with penetration in the tracheobronchial system. In three cases this consisted of esophageal neoplasia with mediastinal manifestation from ingrowth and lymphomas together with compression of the lumen by mediastinal lymphomas from other primary tumors. There was no fistula growth between the esophagus and tracheobronchial system. All patients were subjected to dilatation treatment before the stent implantation.

RESULTS

All stents were successfully released following prior dilatation. In bent sections, particularly in the area of the two primary bronchi, attention was paid to protracted removal of the implant system in order to give the released stent sufficient time for full expansion. Particular attention was required here to avoid any snaring with the implant system. From a technical point of view there were no problems in any of the cases during implantation. In one case the treatment was followed by a mediastinal emphysema and the patient died within 24 hours. It was not possible to clarify whether the death was a result of overexpansion with a tear in the tumor tissue following stent implantation or a perforation caused by the directly preceding laser treatment. In all other cases there were no peri-interventional complications. No infections were observed following stent implantation.

The average survival period following stent implantation was 6 months, varying from 24 hours in one case to up to 9 months in the longest case followed to date. No further complications developed in stent implantation in the tracheobronchial system (Figures 1 and 2). With one exception, a clinically relevant improvement of the respiratory situation was achieved and all patients felt that their improved respiratory situation after stent implantation enhanced their quality of life. In one of the stented patients, the tumor invaded the stent resulting in deterioration of the respiration situation, but the tumor invasion was eliminated by laser therapy.

DISCUSSION

In the treatment of malignant and benign obstructions with pronounced respiratory insufficiency, only the use of a laser (26) or balloon dilatation (14,27) produces an immediate improvement in the poor respiratory situation. Unfortunately, rapidly occurring reobstruction caused by tumor progression or, in the case of tracheomalacia, by collapse or granulation tissue caused by disease or tumor destruction of the tracheal cartilages, proves detrimental to any immediate treatment success. An improvement in the situation with an extension of the intervals of respiratory sufficiency is frequently possible with a combination of therapies. In 1965, Montgomery was one of the first to insert a

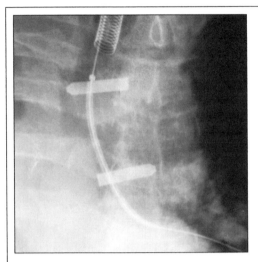
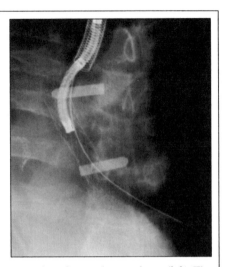

Figure 1. Memotherm nitinol stent placed in the left primary bronchus. Stent prior to release *(left)*. The stenosis is indicated by markings on the skin. Stent after implantation *(right)*. Endoscopic inspection follows to rule out the risk of bleeding.

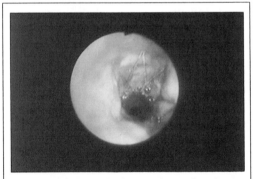

Figure 2. Endoscopic pictures of stenosis and stent.

T-tube tracheal stent to keep the tracheobronchial system open (19). Since then there have been many reports of other internal and external prostheses (18,20,28-32) before Wallace et al published their results using a self-expanding stent in the tracheobronchial system (33). Following reports in 1987 of successful implantation of the Gianturco™ Z-stent (Cook, Bloomington IN), this stent was then implanted in the tracheobronchial system at our clinic as well. In one case of a benign stenosis, the tracheal segment has been kept open for 5 years. Numerous reports have been published by others regarding the use of the Gianturco Z-stent with differing results (34-37). Because of the perforation risk (38) with the Gianturco Z-stent, we began the implantation series described above using a modified Strecker™ stent (Boston Scientific Corp., Denmark) in the tracheobronchial system.

To summarize, the results we obtained from using the Strecker stent in the trachea illustrated an endoprosthesis which was exceedingly simple to position and release, but which was far too rigid in resisting external pressure in comparison to other stents (36,39-41). This relative structural weakness of the stent wall resulted in deformation of the stent with consecutive constriction of the inner lumen. This effect was more pronounced with wider diameters. Even if we had not had evidence of renewed respiratory distress caused by constriction after implantation of this stent type, the risk of deformation or contortion imposes considerable limitations on use. Replacement of the tantalum stent with a nitinol stent (34) has made it possible to obtain positive results (42). We have also obtained good results using the Wallstent™ (Medinvent, Lausanne, Switzerland). The idea of using an even more rigid endoprosthesis comparable to the Palmaz stent (whose characteristics make it unsuitable for use in the tracheobronchial system) was introduced with the development of the nitinol Memotherm stent. This stent combines extreme rigidity with a certain flexibility which seems to be indispensable in the tracheobronchial system. Up to now, the results have satisfied our expectations. One essential disadvantage is the practical impossibility of removing the stent by interventional methods following its release, necessitating strict indication requirements.

Compared to surgery or repeated laser therapy of the tracheobronchial obstruction, stent implantation provides a relatively economical process which places less strain on the patient and results in an immediate improvement in respiratory status. This immediate clinical improvement transforms the patient from being bedridden with respiratory insufficiency to a walking outpatient. This result justifies use of the stent in the human tracheobronchial system. Where malignant stenoses are concerned, the additional combination of endoluminal and percutaneous irradiation provides a palliative improvement of the survival rate. It is also possible to use laser therapy in the event that the tumor penetrates the stent or progresses into other sections of the trachea.

Stent implantation in benign obstructions remains the subject of controversial discussion at the moment because of the impossibility of removing the nitinol Memotherm stent. In spite of the easy-to-handle method, we do not have sufficient long-term results to justify the regular use of this stent for benign stenoses. This treatment should remain second choice for benign stenoses, with surgery taking priority. This applies particularly to young patients with good life expectancy. In older patients, the risk of a full operation must be weighed against the simpler stent implantation. In this case, stent implantation appears to be justified as a first choice even for benign stenoses. Our own previous experimental results seem to indicate that nitinol stents will dominate the future for tracheal stents.

REFERENCES

1. Hagel KJ, Rautenberg HW. Ballondilatation bei angeborenen Pulmonalstenosen im Kindesalter. Herz/Kreislauf 1987;19:343-347.
2. Hartung W. Pathologie der Lungenfehlbildung. Thoraxchirurgie 1975;23:194.
3. Ivemark B. *Kinder-Pathologie*. Berlin: Springer; 1974.
4. Sandritter W, Thomas C, eds. *Histopathologie*. Stuttgart: Schattauer; 1977.
5. Sandritter W, Thomas C, eds. *Makropathologie*. Stuttgart: Schattauer; 1977.
6. Vollmar J. Konnatale Mißbildungen der Arterien: Coarctatio aortae. In: Vollmar J, ed. *Kompendium der Gefäßchirugie*. Stuttgart: Thieme Verlag; 1986;76-88.
7. Hecker W. *Elementare Kinderchirurgie*. München: Urban & Schwarzenberg; 1975.
8. Helbig D. *Chirurgische Pädiatrie*. Stuttgart: Schattauer; 1974.
9. Kloos K, Vogel M. *Pathologie der Perinatalperiode*. Stuttgart: Thieme; 1974.
10. Kunz H. *Operationen im Kindesalter*. Stuttgart: Thieme; 1973.
11. Rehbein F. *Kinderchirugische Operationen*. Stuttgart: Hippokrates; 1976.
12. Windorfer A, Stephan U. *Mucoviscidose — Cystische Fibrose*. Stuttgart: Thieme Verlag; 1968.
13. Becker HC, van Bodegom K. Der einsatz des Strecker-stents in der trachea. In: Kollath J and Liermann D, eds. Konstanz: Schnetztor Verlag; 1992;216-225.
14. Cohen MD, Weber TR, Rao CC. Balloon dilatation of tracheal and bronchial stenosis. Am J Radiol 1984;142:477-478.
15. Grillo HC. Tracheal surgery. Scand J Cardiovasc Surg 1983;17:67-77.
16. Hajek M. Rekonstruktive Operationen bei Trachealstenosen und erworbenen Tracheo-Oesophagealfisteln. Z Erkr Atmungsorgane 1986;166:116-118.
17. Ilberg CV. 7 Jahre erfahrung mit der Tracheaquerresektion. Laryng Rhino Otol 1985;64:40-42.
18. Johnston MR, Loeber N, Hilleyer P, Stephenson LW, Edmunds LH. External

stent for repair of secondary tracheomalacia. Ann Thorac Surg 1980;30:291-296.

19. Montgomery WW. T-tube tracheal stent. Arch Otolaryngol 1965;82:320-321.

20. Neville WE, Bolanowski PJP, Soltanzadeh H. Prosthetic reconstruction of the trachea and the Carina. J Thorac Cardiovasc Surg 1982;83:414-417.

21. Weerda H, Zöllner C, Schlenter W. Die Behandlung der Stenosen des laryngo-trachealen Übergangs und der cervikalen Trachea. HNO 1986;34:156-161.

22. Hartmann, CA, Mollinedo J. Pathologisch-anatomische Gesichtspunkte seltener Bronchustumoren. Prax Pneumol 1981; 35:735-736.

23. Maaßen W. Thorakoskopie: chirugische technik. Pneumologie 1989;43:53-54.

24. Martini N, Goodner TJ, Di Angielo GJ, Beatti EJ. Tracheooesophageal fistula due to cancer. J Thorac Cardiovasc Surg 1970;59:319.

25. Morr H. Tumoren. In: Fabel H, ed. *Pneumologie.* München: Urban & Schwarzenberg; 1989;391-426.

26. Hetzel MR, Nixon C, Edmonstone WM. Laser therapy in 100 tracheobronchial tumors. J Thorax 1985;40:341-345.

27. Rauber K, Kronenberger H. Perorale transluminale Dilatation maligner Bronchusverschlüsse. Fortschr Röntgenstr 1987; 147:261-265.

28. Westaby S, Jackson JW. A bifurcated silicone rubber stent for relief of tracheo-bronchial obstructions. J Thorac Cardiovasc Surg 1982;83:414-417.

29. Andersen HC, Egknud P. Intratracheal tube treatment of stenosis of the trachea. Acta Otolaryngol 1967;224:29-30.

30. Cohen RC, Filler RM, Konuma K, Bahoric A, Knet G, Smith C. A new model of tracheal stenosis and its repair with free periosteal grafts. J Thorac Cardiovasc Surg 1986;92:296-304.

31. Dumon JF. A dedicated tracheobronchial stent. Chest 1990;97:328-332.

32. Nissen R. Tracheaplastik zur Beseitigung der Erschlaffung der Pars membranacea. Schweiz Med Wochenschr 1954;84:219.

33. Wallace MJ, Charnsangavej C, Ogawa K, et al. Tracheobronchial tree: expandable metallic stents used in experimental and clinical applications. Radiology 1986;158:309-312.

34. Rauber K, Franke CH, Syed Ali S, Bensmann G. Experimentelle Erfahrungen mit Nitinol-prothesen. In: Kollath J and Liermann D, eds. *Stents ein aktueller Überblick.* Konstanz: Schnetztor Verlag; 1990;65-70.

35. Rauber K, Weimar B, Hofmann M, Rau, WS. Clinical experiences with endotracheal Gianturco Z-stents. Eur Radiol 1991;1:56.

36. Sawada S, Fujiwara Y, Koyama T, et al. Clinical experience with expandable metallic stent placement for treatment of tracheal and bronchial stenosis. Radiology 1990;177:297.

37. Simonds AK, Irving JD, Clarke SW, Dick R. Use of expandable metal stents in the treatment of bronchial obstruction. J Thorax 1989;44:680-681.

38. Rauber K, Franke C, Rau WS, Syed Ali A. Venendurchwanderung bei Gianturco-Wallace-Stents. Radiology 1990;141:293.

39. Bohndorf K, Günther RW, Huerter T, Kurzewa D, Vorwerk D. Use of metallic self-expandable stent in the tracheobronchial system: first clinical experiences. Radiology 1990;177:297.

40. Fallone BG, Wallace DS, Gianturco C. Elastic characteristics of the self-expanding metallic stents. Invest Radiol 1988;23:370-376.

41. Richter GM. Theoretische Grundlagen des ballonexpandierbaren Palmaz Stents. In: Kollath J and Liermann D, eds. *Stents ein aktueller Überblick.* Konstanz: Schnetztor Verlag; 1990;1:50-57.

42. Liermann D, Lörcher U, Rauber K, et al. Stents in the tracheobronchial system — first results. Eur Radiol 1991:55.

Self-Expandable Stents as an Alternative to Surgical Intervention in the Treatment of Recurrent Stenosis of the Male Urethra

D. Liermann[1] and W.W. Meyer[2]

Departments of [1]Radiology and [2]Urology,
J.W. Goethe University Hospital, Frankfurt am Main, Germany

INTRODUCTION

In addition to other interesting causes of stenoses and occlusions in the urogenital tract, the recurrent stricture of the male urethra poses an unsolved problem. It can occur at increasingly shorter intervals regardless of cause and therapy, and becomes a bane for both patient and doctor (1). In such cases, the endoscopic method of urethrotomy has just as little long-term success as dilatation, bougienage, or open urethroplasty, particularly in the case of strictures having an infectious or iatrogenic genesis. Daughtry et al (2) reported in 1988 about their first successful use of balloon dilatation of urethra strictures. Again in 1988, Milroy was the first to report about the successful use of stents in the urethra (3). In the subsequent period, a series of other publications have appeared regarding the use of stents in the urethra (1, 4-7). The purpose of our study was to provide evidence on whether stent implantation can offer an alternative to surgical methods, and report on the prognosis for a recurrence-free interval in comparison to operative methods.

MATERIALS AND METHODS

Altogether three different stent types were implanted in the urethra. The first stent used was the Wallstent™ (Medinvent, Lausanne, Switzerland) which can be implanted by uroscopic means using a special implant set, or by radiological means using x-ray control. The stent is a self-expanding lattice mesh of stainless steel with notable rigidity. It is available in 2- and 3-cm lengths with a final diameter of 14 mm. Application is relatively simple without requiring the roll membrane application system used in the vascular system. The second type of stent used was the Memotherm® nitinol stent (Angiomed, Karlsruhe, Germany). It consists of a nickel-titanium alloy which expands at body temperature on account of its memory metal properties to a final diameter of 12 mm and lengths between 2 and 4 cm. It also can be implanted by urological and radiological methods. The rigidity of these two stent systems implies that they are only suitable for sub-sphincter sites and not in the bulbar urethra, whereas a third type of stent can be implanted both in the sub-sphincter regions and also in the moving part of the urethra. This is the tubular, woven nitinol stent (Elastalloy™, Boston Scientific Corp., Denmark) whose flexibility is more important than its rigidity. The restoring forces required here can be described as adequate. After deployment, the memory metal properties of the stent make it expand to its designated size of approximately 10 to 12 mm in diameter and 2 to 5 cm in length. Application is preceded by a urethrotomy or dilatation and bougienage. For locations near the sphincter, exceedingly precise positioning is required with x-ray and uroscopic control. As the expansion of all stents is always accompanied by a shortening of the stent length, localizations near the sphincter are exceedingly difficult. Malpositioning makes removal of the stent necessary. Before being used on patients, numerous experimental tests were carried out *in situ* on human cadavers, and the results are reported herein.

PRELIMINARY EXPERIMENTAL INVESTIGATIONS

Application of the nitinol stent system in the urethra without using a guidewire presented no problems for the relatively rigid implant system (Figure 1). The only critical but solvable point was a snaring of the stent filaments in two of ten cases with the sharp-edged back of the applicator system during withdrawal of the system following stent deployment on releasing the back of the guide rod (Figure 2). As this problem also occurred in a straight segment, causing caudal dislocation of the stent, it was essential for the system to be modified before clinical use. In order to counter any possible tearing of the stent filaments during such manipulations, it was better to fix the loop ends to the particular stent ends. Another critical aspect was the ease with which the stent could be displaced in the urethra at a diameter of 8 mm. Although any increase to the stent diameter is tantamount to over-stretching of the corresponding section of the urethra, it would seem sensible to extend the stent diameter to at least 10 mm. Our results tend to indicate that a stent length of 2 cm is suitable to allow for better calculation of stent shortening so that it can also be placed closer to the sphincter. The excellent flexibility, rigidity, and good restoring forces provided by this stent also make it suitable for use in the non-bulbar part of the urethra. It is worth mentioning that, in contrast to the indispensable uroscopic controls under experimental conditions, it is possible to apply this stent under pure radiologic control. Although the poor visibility of the stent does create problems, corresponding urethrographic controls and radiologic control of nitinol stent implantation is still possible even close to the sphincter thanks to the metal markings on the implant set.

Experiments on explantation of the nitinol stent from the urethra showed that it can be removed without any problems, either with a relatively weak polypus forceps (5 Fr) or using stronger forceps which had to be introduced directly through the working canal of the uroscope. The fact that no damage to the urethral wall was caused when removing the stent suggests that it will be possible to remove the stent without any problems in the event of malpositioning. The memory metal effects of the nitinol stent and known restoring forces also allow the stent to be pulled back into the correct position by forceps and deployed again by careful maneuvering, without having completely removed the stent. This was tested in five cases. In four of the five cases, it was possible to move the stent in the event of malpositioning. In these cases, too, no damage to the urethral wall was detected by subsequent uroscopic controls.

The advantage of the Wallstent and the Memotherm nitinol stent is their extreme rigidity once positioned in the urethra. Another advantage is that the stent can be easily positioned under radiologic and uroscopic control, together with the ease with which the implant set can be removed. The differing shortening properties of the self-expanding stents after deployment for a diameter increase of up to 14 mm make the possibility of an implantation near the sphincter without revision a clear risk. However, it emerged that the Memotherm nitinol stent could be removed with relative ease without leaving any macroscopically-visible signs of urethra damage. Consideration of the extraction test results for the Wallstent led to the conclusion that stent revision for malpositioning was only a last resort. The damage is without doubt caused by the outer stent filaments at the top of each particular stent end being positioned like barbs in the expanded stent. Consideration should be given here to modifying the stent design to prevent any damage in the event of extraction.

INDICATIONS

A necessary condition for the implantation of self-expanding stents in the urethra

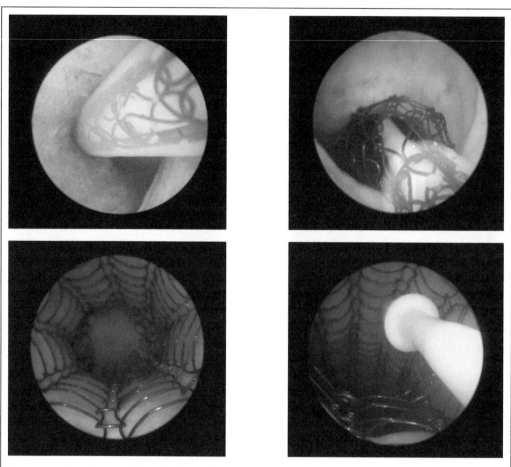

Figure 1. Introduction of the nitinol stent fixed to the implant set into the urethra *(top left)*. The protective sheath is withdrawn to release the stent *(top right)*. The stent has expanded following complete withdrawal of the protective sheath *(bottom left)*. The sharp edged back of the guide rod which tends to interact with the stent filament can be seen. Nitinol stent expanded in the urethra *(bottom right)*.

must be the second or more case of recurrence within a relatively short period of time. The patient should be at least 30 years of age. Clinical symptoms such as stranguria, miction at night, burning during urination, and recurrent urinary tract infections should also be present. The location for the stent is the recurrent stricture of the bulbar urethra underneath the sphincter and above the distal urethra (pendular part). In addition, depending on the case history and with the knowledge of sexual abstinence particularly, flexible nitinol stents were implanted in the bulbar urethra. The patients must be informed in detail about the character of the stent implantation and about possible alternatives, particularly those of a surgical nature.

Contraindications for stent implantation are infected strictures, traumatic strictures following a rupture of the urethra, strictures affecting the external sphincter, strictures which cannot be expanded to 26 Chariere, urethral lesions in the pendular part, the presence of an internal-external fistula in the area to be treated with the stent, and strong bleeding from the urethra following the urethrotomy.

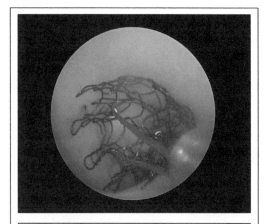

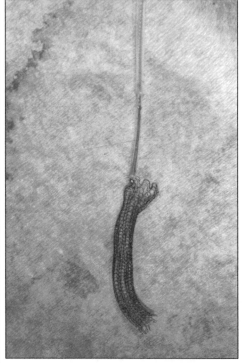

Figure 2. The forceps arms have snared with the stent filaments of the nitinol stent *(top)*. The picture shows the expanded nitinol stent removed from the urethra *(bottom)*.

PATIENT POPULATION

From a final total of 150 patients with recurrent strictures, 60 patients fulfilled the above conditions for participation in the study. Most of the patients were under observation for a period of at least 2 years. The patients

were referred as outpatients by practicing urologists or clinics. The recurrent strictures were severe and all were located under the sphincter in the area of the proximal urethra between the sphincter and pendular part. The patients were aged between 41 and 83 years (mean, 61 years). The number of prior surgical procedures for recurrent strictures ranged from two to ten (mean, 3.9). Urethrotomies had been performed on the 60 patients between two and eight times (mean, four times) with additional urethroplasty performed between once and twice (mean, 1.7 times) before stent implantation. The interval between the initial diagnosis and stricture treatment and the first stent implantation ranged from 1 to 6 years (mean, 2.8 years). The recurrence-free interval following operations ranged from 3 to 8 months (mean, 6.2 months) and the length of the strictures ranged from 0.1 to 3 cm (mean, 1.6 cm). The cause of the stricture was post-infection complications for 75% of the patients, post-traumatic complications for 20%, and iatrogenic complications for 5%. The flow measured in the uroflowmetry before the treatment and stent implantation varied from 1 to 11 mL/s (mean, 5.1 mL/s).

Follow-up examinations were carried out 1, 3, 6, and 12 months after the stent implantation and included uroflowmetry, urethrography, and after 6 and 12 months, urethroscopy. All urethrograms included measurement of the diameter of the urethra at different sections to provide evidence first of growth of the urothel over the stent, and second of premature restenosis, particularly in the sections treated by the stents.

RESULTS

All 60 patients were successfully treated with stents (Figures 3, 4, 5). The first follow-up after stent implantation showed average flow rates of 15 to 45 mL/s (mean, 25 mL/s) with three exceptions (4 to 6 mL/s). The flow rates in the follow-up examination after 3 months resulted in values between 9 and 50 mL/s (mean, 30 mL/s). At the 6-month follow-up, rates ranged from 22 to 49 mL/s (mean, 32.5 mL/s), while after 12 months they ranged from 22 to 50 mL/s (mean, 35 mL/s) and after 2 years between 15 and 49 mL/s (mean, 27.5 mL/s). There was no significant change between the follow-up evaluations at 3 and 12 months. The results after 2 years showed a reduction in the average flow rate, which was caused by the first recurrence.

In the case of the patient with a poor flow value of only 4 mL/s, evidence was found endoscopically of a persistent stricture formation which was not covered by the stent. Unsatisfactory uroflowmetry results from two patients after 3 months resulted in a urethrography being performed. In both cases, this urethrogram indicated a constriction of up to 80% of the stent lumen. The subsequent uroscopy with biopsy revealed an easily-passed hyperplastic urothel. The 6-month follow-up in both cases resulted in a clear flattening of the urothel layer covering the stent with a smooth surface and practically no constriction of the lumen. These results were identical to the 6-month examinations in the other patients treated with the stent.

With the exception of the one patient described above with malpositioning of the stent and correspondingly poor flow, there was no case of irreversible malpositioning. Two malpositionings occurred at a later date, both of which only became evident after complete release of the stent, and could be reversed by removing the stent with bone-holding forceps. In spite of the very sharp edges of the stent, extraction of the stent did not cause any perforation but there were considerable injuries to the urethra on the distal side of the stent, with bleeding and flap growth similar to a condition following urethrotomy of severe stenosis. Follow-up examinations in these

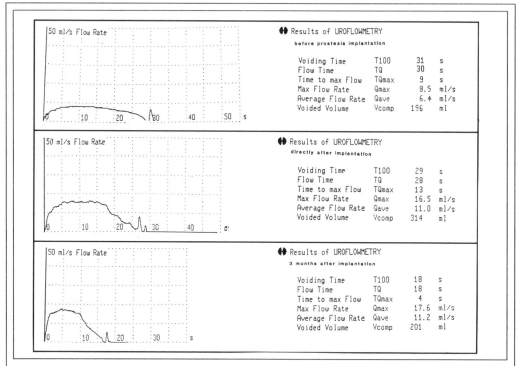

Figure 3. Uroflowmetry for a 75-year-old patient. Uroflow in mL/s before expansion and stent implantation (*top*), after expansion and stent implantation (*middle*), and 3 months after stent implantation (*bottom*).

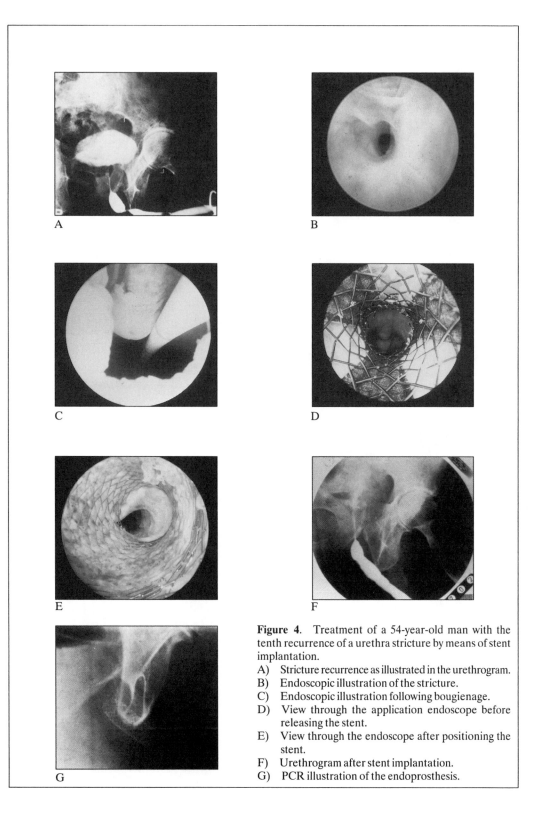

Figure 4. Treatment of a 54-year-old man with the tenth recurrence of a urethra stricture by means of stent implantation.

A) Stricture recurrence as illustrated in the urethrogram.
B) Endoscopic illustration of the stricture.
C) Endoscopic illustration following bougienage.
D) View through the application endoscope before releasing the stent.
E) View through the endoscope after positioning the stent.
F) Urethrogram after stent implantation.
G) PCR illustration of the endoprosthesis.

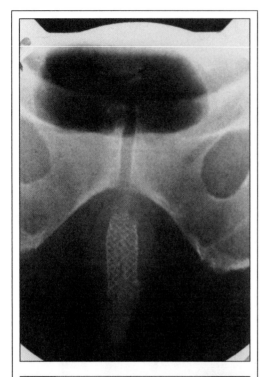

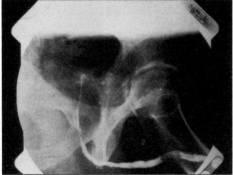

Figure 5. Stent in the urethra of a 79-year-old man after his second stricture recurrence. Illustration of his second stricture recurrence with stenosis in the urethra *(top)*. PCR illustration of the stent *(bottom)*.

two cases revealed identical developments to the other patients treated with stents. At the 12-month follow-up, there was no recurrent stricture either in the section treated with the stent nor in another section of the urethra. In the case where it was necessary to remove the deployed nitinol Memotherm stent, no damage was caused to the urethra. The same

applied to the other nitinol stent which we had implanted in the distal urethra.

Undesirable side effects of stent implantation consisted of trickling after micturition because of the reservoir function of the urethra section treated with a stent which had expanded to up to 14 mm. Discomfort when sitting and during erections over the first few weeks following stent implantation were also noted. This phenomenon was less marked in the case of an implanted Memotherm nitinol stent, and also in the case of the other nitinol stent implanted in the distal urethra. However, it should be noted that the diameter of the latter stent was smaller. After 2 years, the recurrence rate with restenosis was greatest for the Wallstent (approximately 27%), followed by the nitinol stent (22%), and the Memotherm nitinol stent (approximately 21%) (Figure 6).

No long-term results are available for implantation in the distal urethra. Up to now, there has been no recurrences in the five stents which have been implanted at this site.

DISCUSSION

Stents provide an interesting alternative to pure endoscopic urethrotomy or urethroplasty in the treatment of recurrent strictures. Results obtained to date indicate an apparently longer recurrence-free period compared to pure urethrotomy, urethroplasty, or balloon dilatation (2,5,8-11). No recurrence was indicated at the 12-month follow-up and a recurrence rate of up to 27% was seen at the 2-year follow-up. A larger number of cases and longer results over a 5-year period are required before final conclusions regarding the value of stents in the urethra in comparison to other established methods can be made.

The good success rate for our patients treated with stents is due in part to adherence to strict indications for stent use. Donald et al (1) reported on 14 cases of post-intervention recurrences in a 12-month follow-up period for 33 patients treated with stents. Four of these recurrences were in the section

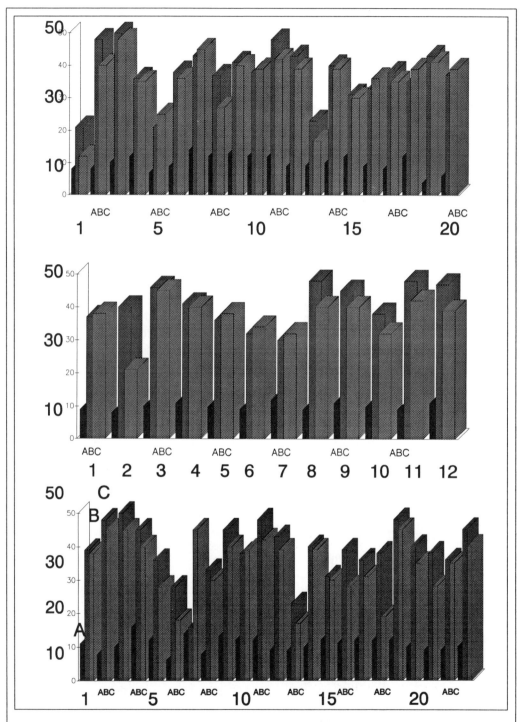

Figure 6. Uroflow (mL) follow-up after implantation of the Memotherm nitinol stent (N=20;*top*), nitinol stent (N=12; *middle*), or Wallstent (N=23; *bottom*) for the treatment of recurrent stenoses in the urethra. (A = before stent implantation; B = 6 or 12 months after implantation; C = 24 months after implantation.)

of the urethra treated with the stent, and were treated by the successful use of additional stents. An interesting phenomenon is the development of further stenoses above or below the section already provided with a stent, e.g. in the vascular system, at the same time that there is clear passage through the stented section. This phenomenon is probably best interpreted as a systemic disease of the entire vascular system, particularly of the vascular walls. Although the hyperplastic urothel reaction in the two cases we described above appears to be clearly different to such processes in the vascular system, it still showed a similar development period and had a similar effect of reducing the lumen by 80% in the section of the urethra treated with a stent. The flattening of the urothel growing over the stent, evident as a strong hyperplastic reaction at the 6-month follow-up with a corresponding development of the uroflow rates, is analogous to results obtained in the vascular system during animal experiments by Barth (12) and Richter (13). Similar phenomena following stent implantation in the bile duct system and in the trachea give rise to presumptions of a similar reaction of the endothel or the myofibroblastic wall structures of various organs to the same type of irritation. Further comparative studies will be necessary before it is possible to predict a typical individual reaction to this irritation in all endothelialized or myoproliferative strictures.

A study of the uroflowmetric curves for each patient treated with a stent indicates a continuous rise in the flow rates up to 6 months, after which the rates remain relatively constant. Only the two cases with hyperplasia of the urothel revealed an expectedly clear jump from the first month to the third month after stent implantation.

Our results indicate that implantation of self-expanding stents is justified with strict indications and results in a prolonged recurrence-free interval compared to urethrotomy or urethroplasty. The self-expanding stent is ideally suitable with its high resistance to compression from the outside; however there

is room for improvement with respect to the sharp edges at the end of the Wallstent. Although this allows for recovery of already released stents, it also conceals an avoidable risk of injury. The relative rigidity of this stent also makes it unsuitable for possible use in the distal urethra. In comparison, the Memotherm nitinol stent performs better, with a moderately lower recurrence rate of around 21% at 2 years. One advantage of this stent is the greater ease with which it can be removed compared to the Wallstent.

The development of the flexible nitinol stent whose material properties combine the advantages of the pronounced rigidity of the Wallstent with the elasticity of the Strecker stent, also allows for implantation of this stent type in the distal urethra. This was only taken into consideration following a detailed series of experiments and for older patients with *de facto* sexual abstinence. The results to date have been most encouraging.

REFERENCES

1. Donald JJ, Rickards D, Milroy EJG. Stricture disease: Radiology of urethral stents. Radiology 1991;180:447-450.
2. Daughtry JD, Rodan BA, Bean WJ. Balloon dilatation of urethral strictures. Urol Radiol 1988;31:231-233.
3. Milroy EJG, Chapple CR, Cooper JE. A new treatment for urethral strictures. Lancet 1988;1:1424-1427.
4. McInerney PD, Vanner TF, Haris SAB, Stephenson TP. Permanent urethral stents for detrusor sphincter dyssynergia. Br J Urol 1991;67:291-294.
5. McLouglon J, Keane PF, Jager R, Gill KP, Machann L, Wiliams G. Dilatation of the prostatic urethra with 35 mm balloon. Urology 1991;67:177-181.
6. Milroy EJG, Chapple CR, Eldin A, Wallsten H. A new stent for the treatment of urethral strictures. Br J Urol 1989;63:392-396.
7. Milroy EJG, Chapple CR, Eldin A, Wallsten H. A new treatment for urethral strictures: a permanently implanted urethral stent. J Urol 1989;141:1120-1122.

8. Castaneda F, Reddy P, Wassermann N, et al. Benign prostatic hypertrophy: retrograde transurethral dilation of the prostatic urethra in humans — works in progress. Radiology 1987;163:649-654.

9. Coleman CC, Kimura Y, Castaneda-Zuniga WR. Interventional techniques in the ureter. Semin Interv Radiol 1984;1:24-37.

10. Johnson CD, Oke EJ, Dunnik NR, et al. Percutaneous balloon dilatation of ureteral strictures. AJR 1987;148-1:181.

11. Smith AD, Lange PH, Miller RP. Percutaneous dilation of ureteral strictures and insertion of Gibbons ureteral stents. Urology 1979;13:24.

12. Barth KH, Virmani R, Strecker EP, et al. Flexible tantalum stents implanted in aortas and iliac arteries: effects in normal canines. Radiology 1990;175:91-96.

13. Richter GM. Theoretische Grundlagen des ballonexpandierbaren Palmaz Stents. In: Kollath J and Liermann D, eds. *Stents ein Aktueller Überblick*. Konstanz: Schnetztor Verlag; 1990;50-57.

PART III

STENTS: BASIC RESEARCH ON MYOINTIMAL HYPERPLASIA AND FUTURE DEVELOPMENTS

Stents: Basic Research and Future Developments

Myointimal Hyperplasia: Research, Therapy, and Future Developments

Stents: New Techniques, Developments, and Future Aspects

Accelerated Stent Ageing: Study by Electrocorrosion

L. Domas, A. Laurent, M. Sapoval, J.J. Merland

Laboratory of Neuroradiology and Therapeutic Angiography, Paris, France

INTRODUCTION

Metallic stents are aged mainly by corrosion (1), particularly in blood (2). Blood is an aggressive medium (temperature, pH, chemical composition, biological effects), while metals are unstable materials that tend to corrode because of thermodynamic equilibria. This instability is increased by mechanical stress and can lead to local toxicity due to the modification of the physico-chemical state of the surface (3), systemic toxicity due to metallic ions released from corrosion phenomena (4,5), misworking of the implant, and mechanical fragility of the implant that can result in its rupture.

A method of accelerated ageing of metallic implants by electrocorrosion has been designed by the Laboratory of Interfacial Electrochemistry (Centre National de la Recherche Scientifique). The method is applied to metallic materials used in dental implantology and has resulted in a French standard (6,7). The method, called chronoamperometry with linear variation of potentials, is based on the premise that the primary way in which metallic materials are aged is by electrocorrosion (8). It consists of applying different electrical potentials, E, to an electrode set in an electrolytic solution (saliva) and measuring the intensity of the current, I. Results are given as voltamograms $[I = f(E)]$.

The aim of our study was to test the feasibility of using this method on ready-to-use devices, i.e., stents, in artificial plasma (9). This test was performed on manufactured products to provide information on their electrochemical behavior as a function of several parameters: the nature of the raw material, the manufacturing steps (cutting, shaping, modalities of soldering, thermic treatment), the nature and quality of the surface treatment, and the sterilization procedure (10).

MATERIAL

Metallic Implants

Four types of stents were studied: Gianturco™ (Cook, Bloomington IN), Wallstent™ (Medinvent, Lausanne, Switzerland), Palmaz™ (Johnson & Johnson Interventional Systems Co., Warren NJ), and Strecker™ (Boston Scientific Corp., Denmark). Each of these implants is different with regards to the raw materials (stainless steel, pure tantalum) and manufacturing processes (cutting, shaping, soldering, setting, etc.) used.

Material for Potentiostatic Technique

The potentiostatic technique consisted of enforcing a potential to an electrode regardless of its behavior. For this technique a potentiostate, a battery that delivers triangular signals so that potentials can be scanned at a pre-chosen speed, was used. In addition, an electrochemical cell was used which consisted of:

- The sample electrode, i.e., the implant we studied. This is the anode of the electrochemical system, the place where the oxidation reaction happens.
- The contra-electrode which is made of a noble material (high equilibrium potential) so that it will not corrode. In our study we used platinum. This is the cathode, the place where the reduction reaction occurs.
- A constant potential reference electrode used for measuring potentials; this was

sulfate electrode (E=650 mV/Normal Hydrogene Electrode) in our study.

Measuring electrical potentials intensities required a differential amplificator and a recording system.

Electrolytic Solution

Blood was modelized by an artificial plasma (7) whose electrolytic composition is given for a liter of distilled water in Table 1.

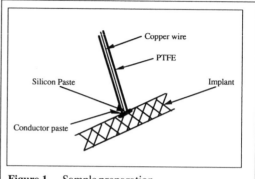

Figure 1.   Sample preparation.

Table 1.   Composition of Standardized Artificial Plasma

Electrolytes	Concentration
NaCl	6.8 g/L
$CaCl_2$	0.2 g/L
KCl	0.4 g/L
$MgSO_4$	0.1 g/L
$NaHCO_3$	2.2 g/L
Na_2HPO_4	0.126 g/L
NaH_2PO_4	0.026 g/L

METHOD

The implant was linked to the circuit with a copper conductor wire (Figure 1). The implant and the electrical wire were soldered with a conductive silver paste (EPO-TEK H21 D, Rhone-Poulenc SA, Courbevoie Cedex, France). This assembling gives a perfect electrical contact between the implant and the rest of the circuit. The copper wire and the silver paste must be insulated from the electrolytic solution so that they do not corrode. The insulation was made with a polytetrafluoroethylene (PTFE) sheath which had been made hermetic by a silicon joint (CAF-4, Rhone-Poulenc SA) around the silver paste soldering. This joint was polymerized for 24 hours at room temperature. The hermicity of the insulation is important because it ensures that the conductor wire and the soldering paste do not participate in the corrosion phenomena.

The vat was filled with artificial plasma. The sample and contra-electrode were immersed in this solution, which was continuously stirred with a magnetic stirring machine during the experiment. The reference electrode was linked to the electrolytic solution by an electrolytic gate. The reference and sample electrodes were linked to the potentiostate by an ohmic contact.

A linear variation of potentials was applied between the sample electrode and the contra-electrode and the intensity of the current through the circuit was measured. This current is the quantification of the electronic exchange between the solution and the metal and thus is representative of the matter loss (ionic exchange) from the sample to the artificial plasma (11). The current density (intensity per surface unit) is a good indicator of corrosion speed (12,13). The test was stopped when the electrical current was high enough to ensure that the corrosion zone had been reached.

Results are given as voltamograms which show the resulting current density as a function of the electrical potential. Voltamograms are characteristic of the resistance to corrosion of material. The following three parameters were measured: the aspect of the samples and the solutions, the polarization potential, and the length of the passivation zone.

RESULTS

Macroscopic Corrosion

Macroscopic manifestations of corrosion such as degradation of the surface, coloring, or gas emission in the electrolytic solution were not observed for the Strecker, Wallstent, and Palmaz stents. With the Gianturco stents the solution became whitish. The aspect of the surface changed macroscopically with morphological heterogeneity around the soldering points.

Microscopic State of the Surface

For the Strecker, Wallstent, and Palmaz stents, microscopic changes in the aspect of the surface were not observed. The soldering points of the Gianturco stent, however, were covered with small pits which were probably due to local pitting corrosion. Table 2 summarizes the results with all four stent types.

The Strecker, Wallstent, and Palmaz stents have a large passivation zone and a high polarization potential, whereas the Gianturco stent does not exhibit any passivation and the polarization potential is quite low.

DISCUSSION

The three parameters examined (length of the passivation zone, polarization potential, aspect of the surface) were intrarelated. The Strecker, Wallstent, and Palmaz stents

did not exhibit any macroscopic or microscopic corrosion and did not change the electrolytic solution; their passivation zones were rather long and their polarization potentials high. Conversely, the Gianturco stent showed macroscopic morphological surface changes and no passivation zone; its polarization potential was low.

A voltamogram typically shows three domains (Figure 2):

* Cathodic reactivity (A), corresponding to the reduction reaction around the contraelectrode.
* Passivation zone (B), where the current is close to 0; this implies that there is no electronic exchange and thus no oxidoreduction reactions. This zone should be as long as possible.
* Anodic reactivity (C), which corresponds to the oxidation of the sample electrode; it is typical of sample corrosion.

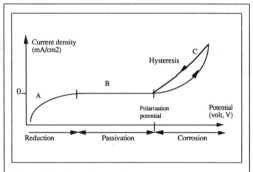

Figure 2.   A typical voltamogram.

Table 2.	Summary of Results			
	Strecker Stent (Tantalum)	Gianturco Stent (Stainless Steel)	Palmaz Stent (Stainless Steel)	Wallstent (Stainless Steel)
Passivation Zone Length	950 mV	0 mV	850 mV	850 mV
Polarization Potential	250 mV	–700 mV	150 mV	150 mV
Remarks	No macroscopic corrosion	Macroscopic corrosion	No macroscopic corrosion	No macroscopic corrosion

The point between the passivation and the corrosion zone is called the polarization potential and is characteristic of a material corrosion behavior because it represents the limit between the corrosion and no corrosion domains. The repetition of the test on the same sample can induce an accumulation of released corrosion products and/or a degradation of the surface state of the material. These modifications of the material and the solution modify the corrosion kinetic of the sample. They are visualized on voltamograms by hysteresis in the anodic reactivity domain (Figure 2, C). The domain of electrical potentials that we used was large enough to recover the domain of biologic potentials (electrical cellular activity).

In the case of the Strecker, Wallstent, and Palmaz stents, the voltamograms were similar to a typical voltamogram, with three domains. With the Gianturco stent, however, the voltamogram was quite different with no passivation domain; this indicates that the implant was never protected against corrosion (Figure 3). The Gianturco, Wallstent, and Palmaz stents are made of stainless steel. The Wallstent and Palmaz stents were resistant to corrosion but the Gianturco stent corroded (Table 2). This indicates that the choice of a good raw material is not enough to obtain a biocompatible, non-bioabsorbable implant. The industrial process (i.e., cutting, shaping, welding, sterilization) confers important properties to the ready-to-use implant (14).

The base material is typically chosen for its mechanical properties, biocompatibility, and eventually, its magnetic properties. The ready-to-use product will not have the same properties as the raw material because the manufacturing steps modify these properties. The choice of the raw material and the manufacturing processes are important for the implant properties but the chronology of these steps is also important. For example, it is important that the shaping step precede the thermic treatment in order to avoid an accumulation of stress in the material.

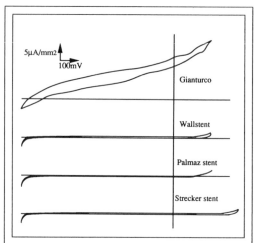

Figure 3. Voltamograms of the Gianturco, Wallstent, Palmaz, and Strecker stents.

The technique we developed discloses the implant's fragility due to the different manufacturing steps. In this regard, this technique can be used to optimize a manufacturing or quality control process because it yields information concerning easy-to-corrode zones, the influence of the manufacturing process on corrosion resistance, and the quality of the coating.

REFERENCES

1. Pourbaix M. Electrochemical corrosion of metallic biomaterials. Biomaterials 1984;5:122-134.
2. DePalma VA, Baier RE, Ford JW, et al. Investigation of three surface properties of several metals and their relation to blood compatibility. J Biomed Mater Res 1972;3:37-75.
3. McFadden JT. Tissue reactions to standard neurosurgical metallic implants. J Neurosurg 1972;36:598-603.
4. Bundy KJ, Luedemann R. Factors which influence the accuracy of corrosion rate determination of implant materials. Ann Biomed Engineer 1989;17:159-175.
5. Merritt K, Brown SA, Sharkey NA. Blood distribution of nickel, cobalt, and chromium

following intramuscular injection into hamsters. J Biomed Mater Res 1984;18:991-1004.

6. AFNOR. NFS 91-141, Biodégradabilité des alliages métalliques utilisés en art dentaire — Normlisation d'essais électrochimiques. 1990.

7. Sella C, Martin JC, Lecoeur J, et al. Biocompatibility and corrosion resistance in biological media of hard ceramic coatings sputter deposited on metal implants. Mater Sci Eng 1991;A139:49-57.

8. Zitter H, Plenk H Jr. The electrochemical behavior of metallic implant materials as an indicator of their biocompatibility. J Biomed Mater Res 1987;21:881-896.

9. Domas L, Laurent A, Sapoval M, et al. Implantable metallic materials: biocompatibility study by electrocorrosion. CIRSE 1992 (30/08/92 3/09/92).

10. Angelini E. Influence of sterilization on the corrosion resistance of high-speed dental handpieces. Quint Ess 1992;23:215-222.

11. Viegas MF, Abrantes LM, Lecoeur J. Metal materials biodegradation: a chronoamperometric study. J Mater Sci 1990;1:105-109.

12. Holland RI. Corrosion testing by potentiodynamic polarization in various electrolytes. Dent Mater 1992;8:241-245.

13. Holland RI. Use of potentiodynamic polarization technique for corrosion testing of dental alloys. Scand J Dent Res 1991;99:75-85.

14. McFadden JT. Metallurgical principles in neurosurgery. J Neurosurg 1969;31:373-385.

Angioplasty Induces Arterial Wall Expression and Release of Smooth Muscle Cell Mitogens

P. Macke Consigny[1] and Glenda E. Bilder[2]

[1]Department of Radiology, Thomas Jefferson University Hospital, Philadelphia, PA USA
[2]Department of Cardiovascular Biology, Rhône-Poulenc Rorer, Collegeville, PA USA

The purpose of this study was to determine if balloon angioplasty induces cells within the arterial wall to produce vascular smooth muscle cell (VSMC) mitogens. Balloon angioplasty was performed on one iliac artery in each of 13 rabbits. In one series of experiments (N=3), the dilated and contralateral control arteries were removed 4 days after angioplasty. Each artery was placed in co-culture with quiescent rabbit VSMC, and 4 days later the change in VSMC number was measured. Co-culture with dilated arteries stimulated a greater increase in VSMC number (+92%) than co-culture with undilated arteries (-10%). In additional experiments (N=10), control and dilated arteries were removed, the intima was denuded of endothelium, and the RNA was extracted. $PDGF_A$ and $PDGF_B$ mRNA concentrations, identified by Northern hybridization, were unchanged 4 hours after angioplasty but were increased 8.7- and 1.7-fold, respectively, 4 days after angioplasty. These results demonstrate that angioplasty induces the release of factor(s) from the arterial wall that stimulate VSMC proliferation; two possible factors are $PDGF_A$ and $PDGF_B$.

INTRODUCTION

Although balloon angioplasty, atherectomy, and stenting of stenotic lesions produce an initial increase in lumen diameter, there is often a gradual reduction in diameter over the ensuing 3 to 12 months (1,2). Histologic studies have demonstrated that this restenosis involves vascular smooth muscle cell (VSMC) migration and proliferation, extracellular matrix deposition, and perhaps macrophage infiltration (2-4). One factor thought to be responsible for restenosis is platelet-derived growth factor (PDGF), since PDGF is a potent VSMC chemoattractant and mitogen which is released from platelets that adhere to the injured artery (5). Smooth muscle cell proliferation continues well beyond the brief interval of platelet deposition, however, suggesting that other mitogens or PDGF from other sources may be involved (6). Recent studies have documented that many cell types, including VSMC, endothelial cells, and monocyte-derived macrophages express the mRNA for one or both chains of PDGF and

secrete factors with PDGF-like activity (2,5,7-9). Based upon these findings, it is possible that cells within the dilated arterial wall are a source of PDGF and other mitogens that stimulate the VSMC proliferation responsible for restenosis.

The purpose of these studies was to test the hypothesis that balloon angioplasty induces cells within the arterial wall to release VSMC mitogens. This test was performed by comparing normal arteries and balloon-dilated arteries for their release of PDGF-like VSMC mitogens and for their expression of the mRNA of the A and B chains of PDGF.

MATERIALS AND METHODS

Bioassay for the Release of Smooth Muscle Cell Mitogens from Rabbit Iliac Arteries

Bioassay experiments were performed to determine if normal and/or dilated rabbit iliac arteries, when placed in co-culture with rabbit VSMC, could stimulate VSMC proliferation.

Balloon Angioplasty

Rabbits weighing approximately 3 kg each were anaesthetized and, using sterile methods, a femoral artery was isolated. An angioplasty catheter with a 2.5-cm diameter balloon was positioned in the external iliac artery and the artery was dilated twice, 60 seconds per inflation. Following angioplasty, the catheter was removed, the femoral artery was ligated, and the skin incision sutured. The contralateral external iliac artery served as an undilated control artery. Heparin was not used during this procedure because it may have antiproliferative properties.

Arterial Removal

Four days after balloon angioplasty, the rabbits were again anaesthetized, and the control and dilated iliac arteries were removed. This 4-day interval was selected because Grunwald and Haudenschild (10) previously demonstrated that balloon injury accelerated the outgrowth of VSMC from explants, particularly if the interval between injury and arterial removal was 4 to 7 days.

Bioassay of Mitogenicity

After removal, the control and dilated arteries were each cut transversely into rings approximately 2 mm in width. The arterial rings were placed in co-culture wells (Millicell-HA, Millipore, Bedford MA), two rings per well, and the wells transferred to the 35-mm dishes containing quiescent rabbit aortic VSMC, two wells per dish. After transfer, the wells were filled with 3 mL of Eagle's minimal essential medium (MEM) supplemented with 5% rabbit platelet-deficient plasma-derived serum (PDS) which lacks platelet-derived mitogens (11). The purpose of the co-culture well was to permit the passage of mitogens through the well's 0.45 µM membranous bottom without permitting cell-artery contact. As a control for the above experiments, additional dishes were filled with MEM supplemented with 5 or 10% rabbit whole blood serum (WBS) to demonstrate that the VSMC

therein were capable of proliferation in media enriched with growth factors. Additional dishes were filled with MEM supplemented with 5% PDS to determine if there was a change in cell number over the course of the experiment in the absence of platelet-derived mitogens. Four days after the arterial rings had been placed in co-culture, the smooth muscle cells in each dish were counted. Cell numbers were then expressed as a percentage of the number of VSMC present in the dishes on the day co-culture was started. A total of three bioassay experiments were performed and the results averaged.

Northern Analysis for $PDGF_A$ and $PDGF_B$ mRNA

Experiments were performed to determine if balloon angioplasty induces the expression of the mRNA for either the A or B chains of PDGF.

Balloon Dilation and Arterial Removal

For these experiments, balloon angioplasty and arterial removal were performed as described above. After removal, however, the arteries were placed in sterile saline, the loose adventitia was removed, the arteries were cut lengthwise, and the luminal surfaces were scraped with a scalpel to remove the endothelium. Finally, the arteries were wrapped in pre-weighed pieces of aluminum foil and frozen (–70°C).

Northern Analysis

After extraction, total RNA (1 to 3 µg) was electrophoretically separated on agarose (0.75%) denaturing formaldehyde (1.3%) gel and transferred to nitrocellulose membranes by capillarity (12). The membranes were baked at 80°C in a vacuum for 90 minutes. cDNA probes, v-sis (Oncor) and A-chain PDGF, a 1.3 kb D1 clone cDNA, were nick translated with ^{32}P-CTP to a specificity of 10^8 CPM/µg and hybridized to membranes at 42°C, 17 hours. Membranes were washed (twice, 2 x SSC/0.1% SDS, room temperature; twice,

0.1 x SSC/0.1%, 50°C) and exposed to Kodak XAR-2 films (-70°C, 2 to 7 days). Autoradiographs were quantitated by densitometry. Laser densitometer measurements of photographic negatives of nitrocellulose membranes (ethidium bromide-RNA) were used to quantitate the total RNA in each lane. Probed mRNA densities were normalized to these values.

RESULTS

Bioassay for the Release of Smooth Muscle Cell Mitogens from Rabbit Iliac Arteries

After 4 days in culture, the number of VSMC in dishes containing MEM supplemented with 5% PDS increased by an average of 1% (Figure 1), indicating that PDS lacked mitogenic activity. This absence of cell proliferation was not due to the inability of the SMC to respond to a mitogen, since when VSMC were cultured in MEM containing 5 or 10% WBS, the cell number increased 38 and 46%, respectively. Most importantly, when VSMC were co-cultured with rings of balloon-dilated artery in MEM containing 5% PDS, the cell number increased to 92%. This increase in cell number was likely due to factors released by the artery in response to balloon dilation, since we observed a 10% decrease in cell number when the VSMC were co-cultured with rings of normal iliac artery.

Northern Analysis for $PDGF_A$ and $PDGF_B$ mRNA

A single 4.3 kb PDGF B-chain mRNA similar to that observed in human umbilical vein endothelial cells was detected in rabbit iliac arteries. Balloon dilation induced a 1.7-fold increase in PDGF B-chain mRNA concentration (relative density, Table 1) and a

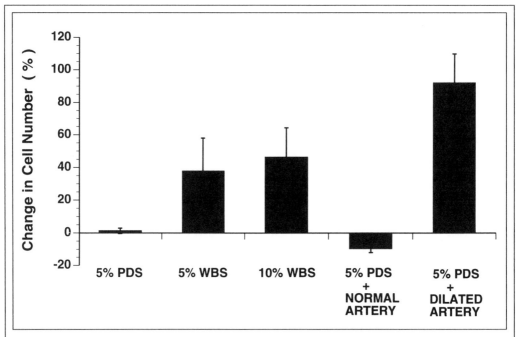

Figure 1.   Effects of different culture conditions on vascular smooth muscle cell proliferation. Changes in cell number are the mean ± SEM for the three experiments.

PDS = plasma-derived serum
WBS = whole blood serum

Table 1. PDGF A- and B-Chain mRNA Expression 4 Hours and 4 Days After Angioplasty[a]

Arterial Treatment	Time After Angioplasty	mRNA Relative Density[b]		Total RNA[c] (μg/mm length)
		PDGF$_B$	PDGF$_A$	
Normal	4 hours	82 ± 16	0	0.16 ± 0.03
Dilated	4 hours	31 ± 30	0	0.16 ± 0.06
Normal	4 days	181 ± 68	78 ± 76	0.23 ± 0.15
Dilated	4 days	305 ± 2	676 ± 8	0.67 ± 0.16

[a] For each measurement, 3 μg total RNA were obtained by pooling two similarly-treated arteries. Results are expressed as the mean ± SEM for arteries removed 4 days (N=8) or 4 hours (N=4) after balloon angioplasty.

[b] Expression of PDGF$_B$ and PDGF$_A$ mRNA are given in relative density which is the ratio of the specific mRNA to total RNA. Specific mRNA was measured by densitometry of autoradiographs; total RNA was measured by densitometry of Polaroid negatives of nitrocellulose membranes stained with ethidium bromide.

[c] Total RNA is expressed as μg RNA per mm of arterial length; arterial length ranged from 19 to 22 mm.

4.9-fold increase in total amount of PDGF B-chain mRNA (relative density x total RNA). These increases were observed in arteries removed 4 days after angioplasty but not in those removed 4 hours after angioplasty.

Two PDGF A-chain mRNAs of approximately 1.7 and 2.4 kb were detected in rabbit iliac arteries. Balloon dilation increased only the 2.4 kb species; the concentration of PDGF A-chain mRNA was increased 8.7-fold and the total content per segment of vessel was increased 26-fold in arteries removed 4 days after balloon dilation (Table 1). PDGF A-chain mRNA was not detected in arteries removed 4 hours after balloon dilation.

DISCUSSION

The results of this study demonstrate that balloon dilation of the rabbit iliac artery induces a measurable increase in mRNA for both the A- and B-chains of PDGF in 4 days. There is a concomitant increase in the release of factor(s) from the arterial wall that stimulate smooth muscle cell proliferation. These two findings suggest that PDGF secretion from cells within the dilated artery are re-

sponsible, at least in part, for the smooth muscle cell proliferation that is responsible for restenosis after angioplasty.

The identity of the mitogen(s) that were released from the dilated arteries and stimulated VSMC proliferation in the bioassay experiments is currently unknown. The fact that these mitogens were able to stimulate proliferation in MEM containing PDS which is deficient in factors released by platelets, however, suggests that one or more of these platelet-derived factors may be involved. Based upon the observation that the expression of the mRNA for PDGF$_A$ and PDGF$_B$ is observed at the same time after balloon injury as the release of mitogens suggests that the mitogenic factor may be PDGF.

Although the identity of the cells producing the PDGF$_A$ and PDGF$_B$ mRNA is unknown, the most likely source is the VSMC in the wall, since PDGF transcripts have been found in cultured VSMC of human, baboon, and rat origin; in human atheroma; and in the neointima of balloon-injured arteries (2,4,7). Endothelial cells are a second possible source of PDGF$_B$ (8). This is probably not the case in our experiments, however, since these cells were removed prior to RNA isolation. Finally, macrophages are a possible source of PDGF$_A$ and PDGF$_B$ (9). It is doubtful, however, that the number of macrophages present in the dilated arteries was sufficient to produce a measurable signal on Northern blots.

The mechanisms by which angioplasty induces mitogen release from the artery remains speculative. We suggest, however, that a feedback system may exist within the arterial wall in which the autocrine or paracrine release of mitogenic factors is under the control of circumferential wall stress. This speculation is based upon our previous observation that circumferential wall stress is increased after angioplasty, secondary to an increase in lumen diameter and a decrease in arterial wall thickness. After arterial repair, however, circumferential wall stress is less than normal, secondary to intimal thickening which decreases lumen diameter and increases arterial wall thickness (13).

In summary, these studies demonstrate that angioplasty induces the release of factor(s) from the arterial wall that stimulate VSMC proliferation. The identity of this factor or factors is currently unknown, but experiments which quantitated the concentration of mRNA for the A- and B-chains of PDGF suggest that these factors may be involved.

REFERENCES

1. Serruys PW, Luijten HE, Beatt KJ, et al. Incidence of restenosis after successful coronary angioplasty: a time-related phenomenon. Circulation 1988;77:361-371.
2. Consigny PM, Cragg AH, Waller BF. Pathophysiology of vascular intervention. In: Strandness Jr ED and van Breda A, eds. *Vascular Diseases: Surgical and Interventional Therapy*. New York: Churchill Livingstone, Inc.; 1993;31-53.
3. Waller BF, Pinkerton CA, Orr CM, Slack JD, Van Tassel JW, Peters T. Restenosis 1 to 24 months after clinically successful coronary balloon angioplasty: a necropsy study of 20 patients. J Am Coll Cardiol 1991;17:58B-70B.
4. Johnson DE, Hinohara T, Selmon MR, Braden LT, Simpson JB. Primary peripheral arterial stenoses and restenoses excised by transluminal atherectomy: a histopathologic study. J Am Coll Cardiol 1990;15:419-425.
5. Consigny PM. Platelet-derived growth factor release after angioplasty. In: Cummins P, ed. *Growth Factors and the Cardiovascular System*. Boston: Kluwer Academic Publishers; 1993;261-274.
6. Wilentz IR, Sanborn TA, Haudenschild CC, Valeri CR, Ryan TJ, Faxon DP. Platelet accumulation in experimental angioplasty: time course and relation to vascular injury. Circulation 1987;75:636-642.
7. Majesky MW, Benditt EP, Schwartz SM. Expression and developmental control of platelet-derived growth factor A-chain and B-chain/Sis genes in rat aortic smooth muscle cells. Proc Natl Acad Sci USA 1988;85:1524-1528.
8. Sitaras NM, Sariban E, Pantazis P, Zetter B, Antoniades HN. Human iliac artery endothelial cells express both genes encoding the chains of platelet-derived growth factor (PDGF) and synthesize PDGF-like mitogen. J Cell Physiol 1987;132:376-380.
9. Shimokado K, Raines EW, Madtes KD, Barrett TB, Benditt EP, Ross R. A significant part of macrophage-derived growth factor consists of at least two forms of PDGF. Cell 1985;43:277-286.
10. Grunwald J, Haudenschild CC. Intimal injury *in vivo* activates vascular smooth muscle cell migration and explant outgrowth *in vitro*. Arteriosclerosis 1984;4:183-188.
11. Rutherford RB, Ross R. Platelet factors stimulate fibroblasts and smooth muscle cells quiescent in plasma serum to proliferate. J Cell Biol 1976;69:196-203.
12. Maniatis T, Fritsch EF, Sambrook J. *Molecular Cloning: A Laboratory Manual*. New York: Cold Spring Harbor Laboratory; 1982.
13. Consigny PM, Tulenko TN, Nicosia RF. Immediate and long-term effects of angioplasty on normal rabbit iliac artery. Arteriosclerosis 1986;6:265-276.

Basic Interactions at the Prosthetic-Blood Interface

Julio C. Palmaz and Eugene A. Sprague

The University of Texas Health Science Center, San Antonio, TX USA

During the past 25 years, increased knowledge of the pathophysiology of the atherosclerotic process has led to significant improvement in the prevention of this disease and its complications. Despite a tremendous investment in research resources, however, progress in non-surgical treatment of atherosclerosis has not been as fruitful as expected. With regard to transluminal balloon angioplasty and related therapeutic modalities, a fair understanding of the mechanism of action and healing modes that may help to decrease the frequency of their failure has been achieved. Furthermore, some of that experience has been extrapolated and expanded upon to interpret the changes that occur after placement of intravascular stents. Our goals, in terms of what we want to further accomplish with implantable vascular prosthetic research, are less clear because of our lack of complete understanding of the intimate relationships between biomaterials and host tissues. In other words, little is known about interfacial bioreactions, particularly critical ones which occur immediately after device implantation.

During the past 10 years, knowledge has been gained about the basic healing modes of arterial stents at the cellular level. We know that the reactive surface of the stent is a thin layer of chromium oxide, which immediately after exposure with circulating blood, is covered with plasma proteins, predominantly fibrinogen (1). Fibrin has the reactive groups to bind platelets which in turn promote further protein deposition. Layer over layer of platelets and plasma proteins deposit in rapid succession in a matter of minutes. Depending on the flow shear, large blood cells attach to this surface which increases the thickness of the material deposited over the prosthetic surface several hundred fold in minutes to hours. Fortunately, this is a self-limiting phenomenon as flow characteristics change with decreasing luminal diameter. A predominantly proteinaceous surface is found 24 hours following stent implantation. This surface, mainly composed of fibrin strands oriented in the direction of flow, is less thrombogenic than the bare prosthetic surface and thus, may be considered "passivated." In a matter of weeks, blood cells are replaced by myointimal cells while neovessels, branching off vasa vasora, proliferate throughout the thickness of the newly deposited tissue. At this point, endothelial cells have already covered the luminal surface, thus rendering it non-thrombogenic, even if slow or turbulent flow develops. Specimens examined 6 years after stent placement show a mature endothelial layer as evidenced by the absence of cellular attachment on the surface and by the appearance of the endothelial cells (Figure 1). These uniformly have flat nuclei and a fusiform shape with the long axis oriented in the direction of the blood flow. The rest of the tissue layer covering the stent is largely composed of collagen with few scattered myointimal cells. These long-term specimens also show almost complete absence of neovessels.

At the biomaterial-host interface, the intimate phenomena are less well understood, particularly at the molecular level. Our understanding is that these phenomena depend on the interaction of three elements: the physico-chemical characteristics of the biomaterial surface, the plasma proteins, and the cell membrane reactivity. A review of the knowledge accumulated in the area of mechanisms of cellular attachment reveals that cells

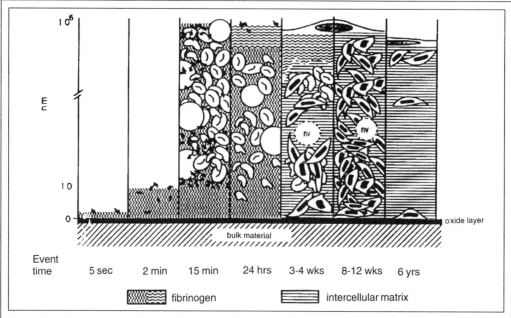

Figure 1. Time sequence of events from immediately after stent placement to 6 years after. (Reproduced from ref. 1).

do not directly attach to prosthetic surfaces but to surface bound proteins known as cellular adhesion molecules or CAMs (2). Activated circulating cells express a group of related membrane receptors called integrins which usually include heterodimers with α and ß subunits (Figure 2).

Integrins react with a high degree of specificity to oligopeptides composed of short amino acid sequences known as adhesive recognition sequences. These oligopeptides are part of usually large and multipotential molecules (CAMs) such as laminin and fibronectin. The structure of laminin and fibronectin is well known (2) and the schematic representation of their components is depicted in Figure 3.

Fibronectin and other CAMs are essential for the attachment, growth, and migration of human aortic endothelial cells (HAEC) on any surface, including the metal stent surface. We have characterized the rate of growth and migration of HAEC over stainless steel 316L (the material used for the construction of balloon-expandable stents) in stationary cul-

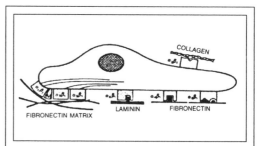

Figure 2. Cell interaction with extracellular proteins by means of cellular adhesion molecules. (Reproduced from ref. 2).

ture conditions to investigate the dynamics of endothelialization over this material. This was performed in an attempt to understand and possibly modify the factors that influence the endothelialization of vascular stents. The rate of endothelialization of the metallic surface was typical for any *in vitro* cell culture, exhibiting a phase of exponential growth followed by a plateau (Figure 4). At present, we are investigating the growth and migration characteristics of endothelial cells over metallic surfaces under variable flow conditions.

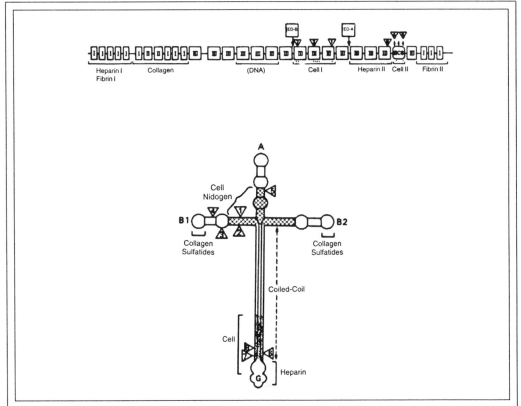

Figure 3. Structure of fibronectin *(top)* and laminin *(bottom)* indicating the adhesive recognition sites and regions. The triangles represent adhesion sites. (Reproduced from ref. 2).

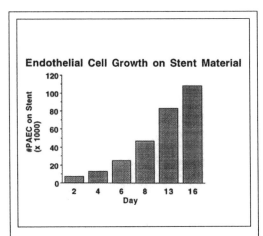

Figure 4. Rate of growth of pig aortic endothelial cells (PAEC) over 10 x 10 mm squares of electropolished 316L stainless steel, the material used for the construction of balloon-expandable stents.

Basic surface chemistry has been shown to affect the growth characteristics of cell cultures. Ratner (3) has shown that hydroxylated surfaces promote little or no cellular growth. Cells initially grow on methyl surfaces but then stop. Methyl-ester surfaces are better than the previous ones but carboxyl surfaces are the best to encourage cell growth.

Unfortunately, prosthetic surfaces of current implantable devices are physically and chemically heterogeneous at the molecular level due to the unavoidable presence of industrial contaminants and the intrinsic heterogeneity of present-day biomaterials. This type of surface causes non-specific, competing reactions with sluggish kinetics when exposed to a biological environment (4). Intrinsic properties of proteins that directly affect their affinity for prosthetic surfaces include size, electrical charge, structure, hydrophobicity, amphipathicity, and solubility (5).

At present, there are new tools available to characterize atomically-smooth substrates that may assist in achieving better biomaterials such as electron spectroscopy for chemical analysis (ESCA), static secondary ion mass spectrometry (SIMS), and scanning tunneling microscopy (STM). These tools may help to engineer surfaces with precise atomic position and range in order to optimize desired biological reactions (6). Ratner (3) indicates that new possibilities to achieve this goal include covering the artificial surface with proteins with specific recognition sites and optimal orientation to facilitate access of cell receptors to those sites. In theory, this can be obtained by several methods such as epitaxial growth and self assembly of protein monolayers. Other ways to achieve defined surface chemistry may be micro- and nanopatterning. These techniques, related to photolithography and etching, may create defined surface patterns that facilitate cell mobility and function. Unlike the present state-of-the-art biomaterials, engineered surfaces on devices may promote orderly, synergistic reactions leading rapidly to a desired outcome.

REFERENCES

1. Palmaz JC. Intravascular stents: tissue-stent interactions and design considerations. AJR 1993;613-618.
2. Yamada KM. Adhesive recognition sequences. J Biol Chem 1991;266:809-812.
3. Ratner BD. New ideas in biomaterials science — a path to engineered biomaterials. J Biomed Mater Res 1993;27:837-850.
4. Cormia R. Engineering polymer surfaces for biological compatibility. R & D Magazine, June 1993.
5. *Proteins at Interfaces: Physicochemical and Biomedical Studies.* Brash JL and Horbett TA, eds. Washington, DC: American Chemical Society; 1987.
6. Ratner BD. Contemporary methods for characterizing complex biomaterials surfaces. Clin Mater 1992;11:25-36.

Microcirculatory Changes Following Stenting

J. Martins Pisco, Miguel Correia, J. A. Esperança Pina, L. Aires de Sousa

Department of Radiology, St. Marta Hospital, Lisbon and
Anatomy and Radiology, Faculty of Medical Sciences, New University of Lisbon, Portugal

INTRODUCTION

Vasa vasorum serve as the vascular support to the wall of the large vessels. They first arise as tributaries of the branches of the main vessels and lay mainly in the groove between the artery and vein, and are oriented longitudinally in perivascular tissue. They ramify in this loose areolar tissue and form a rectangular network around the vessels. The adventitia contains a rich vascular network which supplies the outer third of the media (1,2).

In the normal (non-stenotic) abdominal aorta of the dog, using both scanning electron microscopy and the Spalteholz technique, we saw that the vasa vasorum arise from the collaterals, particularly from the lumbar arteries, and have a caliber of 0.35 mm. The initial trunk has an extension of 4 mm and is situated in the connective tissue of the adventitia of the aorta; it courses laterally to the lateral margins of the aorta. The trunk divides itself dichotomously into two secondary branches that course superiorly and inferiorly parallel to the axis of the aorta. These secondary vessels have a mean length of 0.15 ± 0.06 mm, and they establish anastomosis with the opposite side, as well as upper and lower ones. Thus, a true plexus, whose branches have a mean diameter of 0.15 ± 0.04 mm, is formed in the adventitia. From the inner surface of that plexus arise arterioles with a mean caliber of 0.06 ± 0.03 mm. These arterioles are located in the transition of the adventitia and media and as they form an incomplete arch of 90 to 120°, they are called "arterioles in arch". From the inner surface of those arterioles arise pre-capillary arterioles (mean caliber of $0.02 \pm$ 0.01 mm) which are situated in the outer third of the media.

As stent placement produces neo-intima formation and atrophy of the media, it is possible that it may also damage the vasa vasorum, particularly the above mentioned pre-capillary arterioles.

To evaluate the effects of two different balloon-expandable stents on the vasa vasorum of stenotic arteries, artificial stenoses were created in the abdominal aorta of dogs. Subsequently, a Strecker™ stent (Boston Scientific Corp., Denmark) and a Palmaz™ stent (Johnson & Johnson Interventional Systems Co., Warren NJ) were placed at this level and the results were analyzed.

MATERIALS AND METHODS

Sixteen mongrel dogs of both sexes, weighing 14 to 22 kg, were used. Under general intravenous anaesthesia with sodium pentobarbital, a midline laparotomy was performed to create two focal stenoses in the abdominal aorta, 5 and 10 cm above the aortic bifurcation. The stenoses were created by placing a 3/0 resorbable chromic cat-gut suture which was passed twice around the aorta. To achieve uniform slack in the suture, a piece of 10 Fr Teflon tubing was placed alongside the aorta before applying the suture.

Reabsorption of chromic cat-gut sutures takes about 6 weeks. Therefore, 6 weeks after creation of the focal stenosis, an angiogram was performed to define the stenotic lesions. The diameter of the normal aorta, as measured below the renal arteries, was between 8 and 12 mm. At the stenosis, the diameter was 3.5 mm.

Immediately after angiography, a stent was placed in the most cephalad position. In eight dogs, a Strecker stent was placed while in the other dogs a Palmaz stent was placed. The caudal stenosis was dilated using a polyethylene balloon catheter. The diameter of the balloon used for stent placement was equal to the diameter of the balloon used for the simple angioplasty (PTA) and had the same diameter as the aorta proximal to the stenosis. The balloons were inflated at a pressure of 6 atm. An equal diameter of the stented site and angioplasty site was achieved and was the same as the adjacent proximal portion of the aorta.

The dogs were sacrificed in groups of two animals each at 4, 8, 12, and 18 months after the procedure. Before sacrifice, the animals were intravenously heparinized with 10,000 IU and an abdominal aortography was obtained through a 8 Fr pig-tail catheter. At this time, the aorta caliber at the levels of the stent and of the dilated segment was the same as the normal aorta. After heparinization and complete exsanguination, the aorta was flushed with a normal saline solution at 37°C under 100 mm Hg pressure until clear saline was obtained. The aorta was then ligated above the renals and was filled with a mixture of micropaque and gelatine at 100 mm Hg. The aorta specimen was fixed with 10% formalin for 48 hours.

The specimens were initially processed in a mixture of equal parts of hydrochloric acid and 5% sodium hypochlorite, renewed every 24 hours for 72 hours. The specimens were then dehydrated with increasing concentrations of 60%, 80%, and 100% ethanol, each for 24 hours. The specimens were placed in acetone in a vacuum for 48 hours, followed by placement in a mixture of benzyl benzoate and methyl salicylate in equal parts according to the Spalteholz technique in order to obtain good transparency (3).

MICROCIRCULATORY CHANGES

In the zone where the Strecker stent was placed, the vasa vasorum did not show any

changes in number, distribution, or morphology at 4, 8, 12 or 18 months (Figure 1).

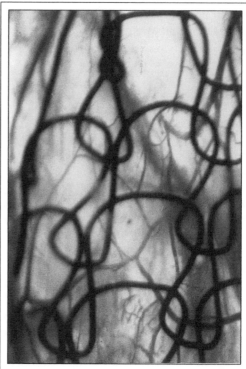

Figure 1. Sagittal section of the aorta 8 months after Strecker stent placement. Spalteholz technique — the distribution of the vasa vasorum is normal and their number is not increased. Magnification x50.

Four months after Palmaz stent placement, early proliferation of the pre-capillary arterioles in the involved segment was seen. These vessels extend medially from the outer-middle junction of the media but do not reach the stent (Figure 2). At 8 months, additional new vessels were noted which were closer to the stent struts. The extension of the pre-capillary arterioles increased up to 12 months (Figure 3). At 18 months the vasa vasora distribution returned to normal patterns (4).

The zone of stenosis of the aorta dilated with a balloon showed proliferation of the pre-capillary arterioles, located in the outer third of the media, which increased up to 8

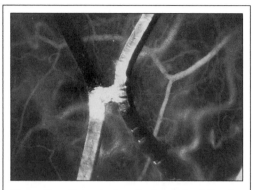

Figure 2. Abdominal aorta 4 months following placement of a Palmaz stent. Spalteholz technique — some new vasa vasorum around the stent.

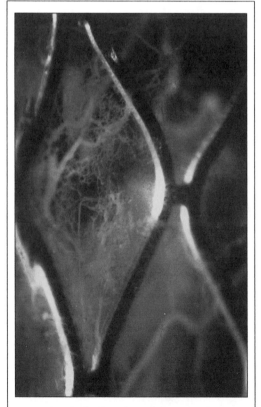

Figure 3. Sagittal section of the aorta 12 months following Palmaz stent placement. Spalteholz technique — increased number of pre-capillary arterioles around the stent struck.

months (5). After 8 months the amount of vasa vasorum began to decrease and at 18 months, the number of vasa vasorum was normal. The proliferation of vasa vasorum following angioplasty was less prominent than following Palmaz stent placement.

At the site of the chromic suture which caused the stenosis, there was interruption of the vasa vasorum and rupture of the elastic and muscle fibers.

Zollikofer et al (6) overdilated the canine aortic segments to more than 100% of the normal size to investigate the acute and long-term effects on the vasa vasorum. In the acute study they found rupture and stretching of the vasa vasorum whereas proliferation of the vasa vasorum was found in the chronic study. All of these changes occurred in the vasa vasorum of the adventitia. In our model all changes following angioplasty occurred in the outer media because we did not overdilate the artery as much.

The vasa vasorum proliferation observed after balloon angioplasty and Palmaz stent placement may be the result of hypoxia of the arterial wall caused by impairment of the blood flow in the vasa vasorum. This may have been caused by temporary compression from the inside towards the outside due to balloon inflation or by permanent compression after the Palmaz stent placement. The intimal hyperplasia observed after these intervention modalities and the thickness of the stent strut may also cause increased oxygen demand and thus further induce proliferation of the vasa vasorum. In normal arteries the intima plus the inner third of the media are avascular and their nourishment comes directly from the main lumen. Beyond the thickness of 0.5 mm, the arterial wall is vascularized and a correlation between intimal hyperplasia and vasa vasorum formation exists. The decreased diffusion of luminal nutrients subsequent to mural thrombus organization after Palmaz stent placement may also induce neovascular proliferation.

The lack of proliferation of vasa vasorum following Strecker stent placement may be due to increased flexibility and reduced rigidity of the stent structure resulting in less outwards compression.

The plexus of the new vessels in the media was more prominent after Palmaz stent placement than after PTA alone. This was probably due to long-term hypoxia as a result of prolonged compression of the vasa vasorum.

The vascular changes of improved arterial vascularization caused by the mechanical effects of stents, although temporary, may have an important role in determining long-term patency due to the support of the metabolic changes in the arterial wall.

CONCLUSIONS

In an experimental dog model, the microvascular changes related to increased vasa vasorum circulation in the aortic wall, caused by the mechanical effects of Palmaz stent placement, are temporary but more prominent than following angioplasty alone. The Strecker stent caused no significant changes in the microcirculation of the aortic wall in this experimental model.

REFERENCES

1. Robertson HF. Vascularization of the thoracic aorta. Arch Path 1929;8:881-893.
2. de Sousa A, Alves L. Microangiographic study of the vasa vasorum of the thoracic aorta. Radiology 1960;75:91-96.
3. Spalteholz W. Das Durchsichtigmachen als biologische. *Arbeistsmethode Handbuch der Biologischen.* Arbeistsmethoden 1927;8:409-432.
4. Pisco JM, Correia M, Esperança Pina JA, de Sousa LA. Vasa vasorum changes following stent placement in experimental arterial stenoses. JVIR 1993;4:269-273.
5. Pisco JM, Correia M, Pina JAE, de Sousa LA. Vasa vasorum changes following angioplasty and stenting. In: Castaneda-Zuniga WR, ed. *Percutaneous Revascularization Techniques.* New York: Thieme; 1993; 64-69.
6. Zollikofer CL, Redha FH, Bruhlman WF, et al. Acute and long-term effects of massive balloon dilation of the aortic wall and vasa vasorum. Radiology 1987;164:145-149.

New Therapeutic Options for Intimal Hyperplasia

Thomas Roeren

Department of Radiodiagnostics, University Hospital Heidelberg, Heidelberg, Germany

INTRODUCTION

As intimal hyperplasia develops following percutaneous transluminal angioplasty (PTA), research for therapies directed toward intimal hyperplasia did not begin prior to the first clinical series of percutaneous transluminal coronary angioplasty (PTCA) which showed recurrence rates of approximately 30%. Over the last 15 years, hundreds of experimental and clinical studies have been undertaken to understand intimal hyperplasia. New pharmacological regimens, as well as new mechanical devices for treatment of vascular stenosis have, however, not reduced the rate of restenosis. Although the underlying mechanisms of percutaneous balloon angioplasty are well understood, induced biochemical reactions are not.

While inflating a balloon in a stenosed, atherosclerotic artery, the plaque material as well as the unaffected arterial wall are often dissected (Figure 1). By this mechanism, the vascular lumen of the endothelium is denuded and the collagen and smooth muscle cells (SMC) exposed to flowing blood. The reactions that follow have been covered in previous manuscripts. It appears at this point that research in angioplasty has provided us with more profound knowledge of the process surrounding intimal hyperplasia, but attempts at therapeutic interventions have not as yet been successful. This paper describes new options for the treatment of intimal hyperplasia.

THERAPEUTIC STRATEGIES

Currently, the development of a therapeutic strategy resembles a 4-step stairway. The first developmental step includes mechanical devices such as atherectomy cath-

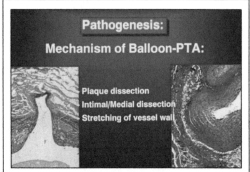

Figure 1. Histologic specimen from a rabbit femoral artery one month after percutaneous angioplasty. On the left, there is an intimal crack through the hyperplastic neointima into the medial tissue. On the right, an old crack of an atheromatous plaque has been filled with extensive intimal hyperplasia (metachromatic stain, original magnification x40).

eters and rotational devices which try to remove at least part of the plaque material from the arterial wall. Johnson and co-workers, however, have shown that the restenosis rate will increase proportional to the percentage of medial tissue removed from an atherectomized artery. This and other studies could not prove that mechanical devices other than simple balloons are able to decrease restenosis rates after PTA. The second step includes pharmacological regimens. Some of these are intended to reduce platelet adherence and induction of coagulation processes. In addition, drugs have been developed that supposedly reduce smooth muscle cell proliferation and migration. The best known substances that are pathophysiological factors for the induction of restenosis are platelet-derived growth factor (PDGF), basic fibro-blast growth factor (b-FGF), and other endothelium- or media-derived growth factors. All pharmacological substances that have been tested thus far in controlled studies after PTCA were not able to unequivocally reduce the incidence of intimal hyperplasia. The most widely used drugs include aspirin, warfarin, steroids, fish oil, and prostacycline, as well as calcium channel blockers.

The third and fourth steps on the stairway toward effective therapy for intimal hyperplasia will include research aimed at the molecular and cellular level, perhaps with the ultimate end result of genetically-engineered endothelial cells or platelets which can suppress or block all of the processes that contribute to the origin of intimal hyperplasia. We know that normal and undamaged endothelial cells are crucial for prevention of unwanted thrombosis. Angioplasty will always destroy the integrity of the endothelial surface, however, and thereby induce platelet adherence and release of various growth factors. It is also known that the integrity and function of the endothelial cells depend on the presence of adequate flow. Low-flow or no-flow situations (Figure 2) lead to deformity of the endothelial cells with a rougher surface and a superficial structure that is more prone to platelet adherence than the smooth endothelial surface in a well-perfused vessel. The methods employed to reconstitute normal endothelial layers, even in the presence of foreign bodies like stents, are either direct cell impregnation of these devices *ex vivo*, i.e., the impregnation of either balloon surfaces or stent surfaces with functional endothelial cells or direct cell impregnation by carrier devices onto the luminal surface of the vessel during the intervention. This "artificial endothelium" will grow as normal endothelium cells do and thereby rapidly cover the injured area. The result should be a reduction in intimal hyperplasia.

A more elegant, but nevertheless more sophisticated and difficult way, is to create specific receptor sites on artificial surfaces that will bind circulating endothelial cells, thereby creating a true endothelial surface within a short period of time. Research in this area is currently ongoing. At present, the time

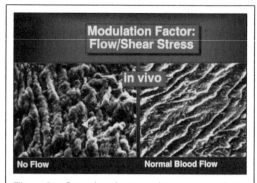

Figure 2.   Scanning electron microscopy specimen of endothelial cells in a non-perfused artery *(left)* and a regularly perfused artery *(right)*.

necessary to induce a new endothelial surface is approximately 4 to 8 hours; while this is impractical for clinical applications, the feasibility of this method seems very promising.

Apart from these molecular biology approaches, genetic engineering is also being used to solve the problem of intimal hyperplasia. The activation of certain proto-oncogens during the mitosis of subintimal myocytes can already be blocked by specific messenger-RNA. Modulation of endothelial cell secretion by gene transfer so that endothelial cells secrete large amounts of fibrinolytic or anti-thrombogenic substances is also being investigated.

CONCLUSIONS

In the past, research has shown that mechanical approaches to the prevention of restenosis left us standing where we started without any significant progress. In addition, pharmacological agents have not been proven to reduce the incidence of restenosis. Future therapies, including custom-made devices or changes at the molecular level that can interact with biologic reactions, as well as the genetic expressions of those cellular and surface components that are responsible for the induction of hyperplastic processes, seem promising. These future new therapeutic options for intimal hyperplasia may one day reduce the levels of restenosis currently seen with percutaneous angioplasty.

Endovascular Afterloading with 192 Iridium HDR in the Treatment of Recurrent Intimal Hyperplasia in Stented Peripheral Arteries

D. Liermann[1], G. Herrmann[3], B. Schopohl[2], K. Gregel[3], K.H. Breddin[4], J. Kollath[1], K. Hübner[3], H.D. Böttcher[2]

Departments of [1]Radiology, [2]Radiotherapy, [3]Pathology, and [4]Internal Medicine J.W. Goethe University Hospital, Frankfurt am Main, Germany

INTRODUCTION

Treatment for the revision of stenoses in stented vascular segments causes injuries to the vascular wall, almost always resulting in intimal hyperplasia (1-16). Some authors presume that because of this, the use of stents alone does not appreciably improve patency rates compared to percutaneous transluminal angioplasty (PTA) (17-22). One possible alternative is to combine the methods available for treating intimal hyperplasia. The good results obtained in treating keloids by means of irradiation therapy (23-34) was the basis for our therapeutic concept for the prophylactic irradiation of hyperproliferative vascular wall reactions. The development of small-caliber probes for afterloading therapy in the biliary tract (35) allowed us to use these for therapy in the vascular system. Together with the initiator of the method, H.D. Böttcher, our considerations were converted into a clinical trial. Before proceeding further, all risks and problems, together with ethical reservations in the context of using afterloading methods for treating arterial occlusive disease in the peripheral vascular system, were discussed in detail and taken into consideration when planning the procedure. In addition to interventional management, significance was also accorded to stipulation of the individual dose, follow-up regimen, and adequate patient information.

MATERIALS AND METHODS

The entire treatment was carried out under heparin therapy (100 IU/kg body weight). On conclusion of recanalization and PTA of the restenosed, stented vascular segment, a 9 Fr recanalization catheter was inserted through the positioned 9 Fr sheath via a guidewire, and positioned so that its tip was just below the affected vascular segment. The inner diameter of this catheter permitted insertion of a special catheter having a diameter of 5 Fr. The pointed tip of the catheter means that the measuring rod and special catheter can only be pushed forwards to just before the tip of the recanalization catheter without being able to pass through the catheter opening. This particular feature allowed for exact measurement and calculation of the length of the stented vascular segment and of the insertion length of the afterloading probe under stable, reproducible conditions.

After stipulation of the distal point of the catheter, the sheath and recanalization catheter were fixed on the skin to avoid any displacement. The measuring rod whose distal segment marks the lower end of the irradiation field and protrudes 1-cm distally beyond the actual irradiation field, was then exchanged with the 5 Fr special catheter. This catheter was inserted through the 9 Fr catheter as far as possible with its independently-sealed tip, and was again firmly fixed (Figure

1). It later accommodated the iridium probe with its 1.1-mm diameter. This was inserted during the afterloading procedure, after the proximal end of the special catheter had been connected to the outlet valve of the iridium 192 HDR source. We used a Nucletron (Micro) Selectron HDR planning system version 10.10 for exact calculation, monitoring, and control of the afterloading procedure. Our source was iridium 192 with a strength of 10 Ci. The reference dose was 1200 cGy. After calculation of the exact irradiation dose for the afterloading method, the program controls and monitors the insertion and removal of the iridium probe from the source into the special catheter through to the tip, and monitors the irradiation duration. The exposure time depends on the condition of the source and was around 200 sec. During this time, a surface dose of 12 Gy was applied to the vascular wall in one session in the affected region.

Subsequently, the catheter material was removed and pressure carefully applied by hand to the puncture point for 10 to 20 minutes. An elastic pressure bandage was then applied for 24 hours and the patient was treated for 72 hours with a dose of heparin 1000 IU/hour via a perfusor. A 6-month course of Marcumar® therapy was then initiated.

Follow-Up

Follow-up examinations were carried out at precisely-defined intervals, and consisted of routine ankle-arm indices (AAI) before and during the intervention, after 3 and 6 months, and later at 6-month intervals, together with a study of the case history and examination of the patient. Additionally, magnetic resonance imaging (MRI) examinations were carried out before and after treatment and at 6-month intervals. The examinations were performed in a FLASH (Fast Low Angle Shoot) gradient, spin echo sequence with a flip angle of 30°, in vertical and coronary sections [1.0 Teslar unit in a cervical coil (300)]. An intravenous digital subtraction angiography (DSA) was also carried out

after 6 months or upon MRI evidence of stenotic lesions. The clinical parameters were stipulated according to the Fontaine classification.

INDICATIONS

Indications for endovascular afterloading therapy were restricted to clinically-relevant stenoses or recurrent occlusions in the stented vascular segment occurring within less than 8 months after preceding, repeated PTA treatment. All patients must have had a long history of arterial occlusive disease, with recurrent vascular occlusions following PTA treatment in a vascular segment of the superficial femoral artery prior to stent implantation. In the event of restenosis or occlusion in the stented vascular segment, at least one successful treatment of the recurrence must have been carried out by conventional PTA or by using the Nd:YAG laser with matted sapphire tip. Prior to repetition of the PTA in the stented segment with subsequent irradiation therapy, an angiogram control must have been performed, together with diagnostic atherectomy by means of the Simpson catheter to obtain histological material.

In order to minimize the somatic tumor risk as a consequence of the radiation therapy, only patients in their seventh decade of life or older were admitted for such treatment. Contraindications to heparin and Marcumar therapy were not to be present following stent implantation and irradiation therapy.

PATIENT POPULATION

To date a total of 20 patients (7 women, 13 men) have been treated with endovascular afterloading. All patients suffered from clinically-relevant reocclusions or restenoses in stented vascular segments of the superficial femoral artery following successful laser or PTA treatment, within 6 to 8 months after the last therapy. The patients were aged from 60 to 84 years (mean, 68.6 years). All patients had generalized arterial occlusive disease.

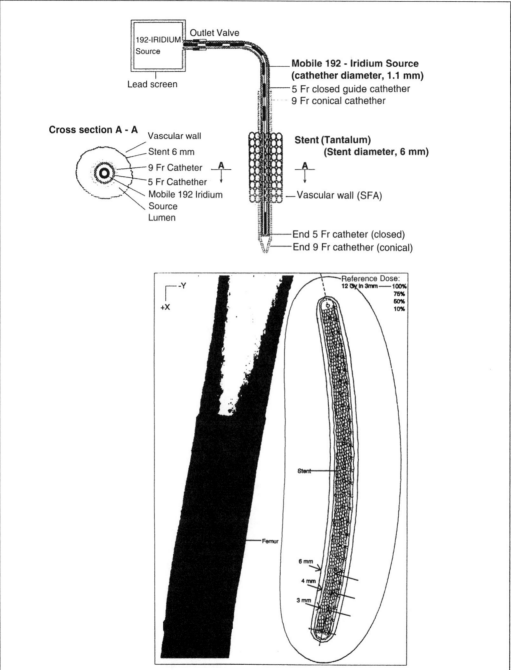

Figure 1. Iridium 192 afterloading irradiation within the stent of the superficial femoral artery. Application of endovascular irradiation. Diagram showing the catheter and loading system for endovascular irradiation *(top)*. Distribution of the isodoses in endovascular irradiation in the region of the stented superficial femoral artery *(bottom)*.

(We would like to thank Professor Dr. H.D. Böttcher and the Radiotherapy Department for letting us have the plans and diagrams for calculating the isodoses).

Eleven patients had concurrent diabetes mellitus, 16 had high blood pressure, and 14 abused nicotine over a period of more than 20 years. According to the Fontaine classification before the repeated PTA treatment (18 cases) or laser therapy (two cases), eight of the patients were in clinical stage IIb and twelve patients were in stage III. The histological analysis indicated intimal hyperplasia as the cause for restenosis in all 20 patients.

The case histories for all patients revealed several PTAs as a treatment for reocclusion in the superficial femoral artery prior to implantation of one or more stents. The length of stented vascular segments ranged from 4.5 to 14 cm (mean, 6.7 cm), with the stent diameter ranging from 6 to 7 mm. Prior to the afterloading radiation therapy, five patients had suffered from recurrent stenosis after PTA and laser treatment within 8 months, after stent implantation within 7 months after the first re-PTA, within 7 months after the

first laser therapy, or within 6 months after the second laser therapy. Fifteen patients had two recurrent stenoses after PTA within 5 to 8 months (mean, 6.6 months) and after stent implantation within 5 to 7 months (mean, 6.1 months) after first re-PTA treatment, or within 5 to 6 months (mean, 5.8 months) after the second re-PTA (Figure 2).

RESULTS

In all 20 patients it was possible to perform re-PTA treatment without remaining residual stenoses in the stented region. Subsequent irradiation therapy with the 192 iridium HDR afterloading method was successfully performed. In all cases, the dose was 12 Gy in the plane of the vascular wall; the exposure time was approximately 200 sec. The additional time required in comparison to a sole PTA procedure was approximately 45 minutes, with most of this time consisting

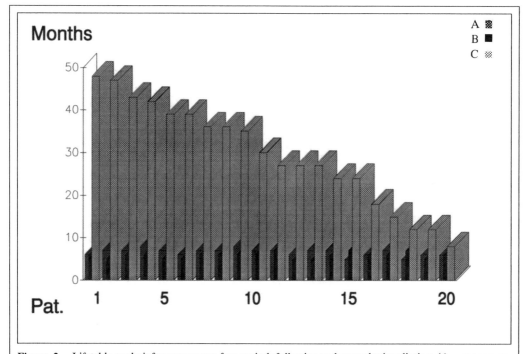

Figure 2. Lifetable analysis for recurrence-free periods following endovascular irradiation. (A = recurrence free time after stent implantation; B = recurrence-free time after re-PTA in stent; C = recurrence-free time after radiation and re-PTA).

of transport between the treatment room and afterloading room. After conclusion of the treatment, there was no bleeding from the puncture sites.

The follow-up period for the 20 patients ranged from 6 to 53 months (mean, 28 months). According to the Fontaine classification, it was possible to improve the clinical stage for seven patients from stage IIb to stage I, and for nine patients from stage III to stage I. It was only possible to improve one patient from stage II to stage IIa, and two patients from stage III to stage IIa. In these three cases, contralateral occlusion was present as a limiting factor. In a fourth case, it had been possible to improve the clinical stage from III to IIa, but after approximately 2 years this patient suffered from an occlusion which became manifest in the exit region of the superior femoral artery, resulting in a bypass.

During the follow-up examinations, there was no deterioration of the clinical stage and no recurrent stenosis for 18 patients. One patient suffered from an acute thrombosis approximately 3 months after stent implantation, without a cause being found. Histological examination using the atherectomy catheter revealed fresh thrombotic material, as expected. Following local lysis therapy, the thrombosis was entirely eliminated. We suspect that the thrombosis was due to an underdose of Marcumar in an otherwise physically active patient. One other patient had a stenosis 3 cm above the stented vascular segment 12 months after irradiation treatment. During treatment to eliminate the severe stenosis, angioscopic and angiogram controls revealed no evidence of constrictions or intimal hyperplasia in the stented and irradiated region. The restenosis above the stent was successfully eliminated. In a third case, approximately 10 months after the combined therapy, restenosis occurred in a vascular segment approximately 8-cm long which had not been included in the irradiation treatment. It occurred between two treated sections in the superficial femoral artery, and was success-

fully removed by PTA treatment. In this case also, there was no intimal restenosis in the vascular segment previously treated by stent implantation, PTA, and irradiation.

Follow-up examinations have revealed no evidence of nerve lesions following irradiation therapy. The tissue surrounding the artery showed no recordable change following irradiation therapy, either in the CT, color-coded Doppler, endovascular ultrasonic scan, or MRI. No complaints of discomfort were reported during or after irradiation. With the exception of the changes described above, and the one acute thrombosis likely caused by an underdose of Marcumar, there was no evidence of any complications (Figures 3-9).

DISCUSSION

In view of the early stage of development, afterloading irradiation is a therapeutic concept for treating recurrent intimal hyperplasia in stented vascular segments which must be applied under extremely strict provisos. From an ethical point of view, the method should be compared with radiation therapy of non-malignant disorders (23,30,31,34) and it is essential to make a strict distinction between this kind of radiation therapy and irradiation of malignant growths where a far higher dose is required and there is a greater risk of induction of malignant secondary disorders. The afterloading technique allows for drastic reductions in the radiation load for the tissue surrounding the affected organ, which in turn reduces somatic risk. The decreased dose for iridium 192 HDR afterloading has a surface dose of 1200 cGy at a depth of 3 mm, a dose of 877 cGy at a depth of 4 mm, 551 cGy at a depth of 6 mm, 396 cGy at a depth of 8 mm, and 303 cGy at a depth of 10 mm (Figure 2). The risk to the nearby nerves can be considered as slight. In the medical literature, the tolerance for a maximum single dose is 15 Gy (36,37).

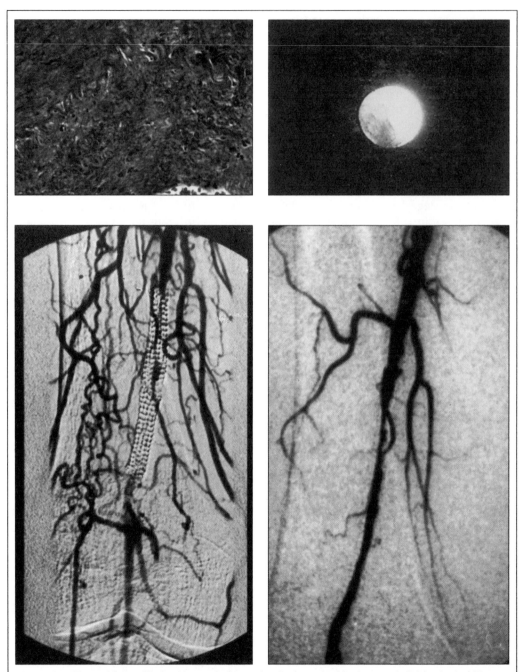

Figure 3. The problems of intimal hyperplasia are clearly shown in this characteristic histological illustration *(top left)*. The histological section with Ladewig coloring shows, from bottom to top, isolated erythrocytes in the vascular lumen, over which there is a clearly thickened hyperplastic intima demarcated from the media by the visible tape-like internal elastic tissues. Endoscopy *(top right)* shows the plaque-shaped hyperplasia as lumen-constricting compression. Wall thickening in the stent is clearly visible with lumen constriction in the stented region of the superficial femoral artery *(bottom left)*. After laser recanalization and endovascular afterloading with iridium 192, there is once again a patent lumen in the stent *(bottom right)*.

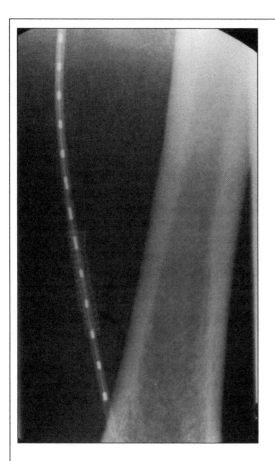

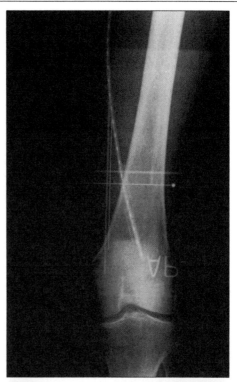

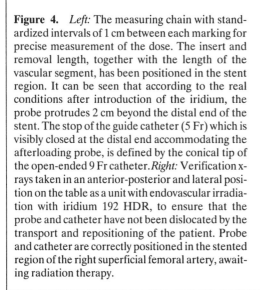

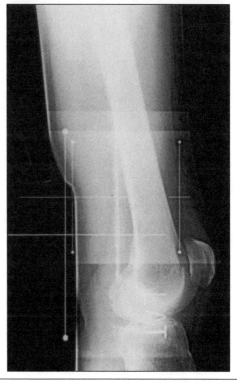

Figure 4. *Left:* The measuring chain with standardized intervals of 1 cm between each marking for precise measurement of the dose. The insert and removal length, together with the length of the vascular segment, has been positioned in the stent region. It can be seen that according to the real conditions after introduction of the iridium, the probe protrudes 2 cm beyond the distal end of the stent. The stop of the guide catheter (5 Fr) which is visibly closed at the distal end accommodating the afterloading probe, is defined by the conical tip of the open-ended 9 Fr catheter. *Right:* Verification x-rays taken in an anterior-posterior and lateral position on the table as a unit with endovascular irradiation with iridium 192 HDR, to ensure that the probe and catheter have not been dislocated by the transport and repositioning of the patient. Probe and catheter are correctly positioned in the stented region of the right superficial femoral artery, awaiting radiation therapy.

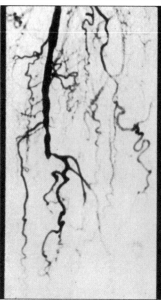
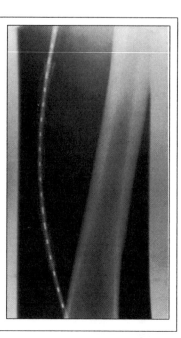

Figure 5. The angiogram shows a complete occlusion in the stented left superficial femoral artery *(left)*. Following the third recurrence at short intervals, after revision in the form of re-PTA treatment, in the same session the measuring probe has been positioned prior to irradiation and can be clearly seen in this plain film *(right)*.

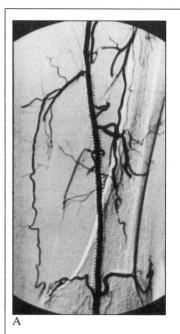
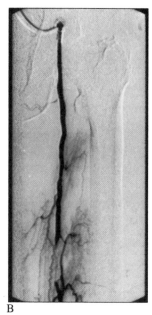
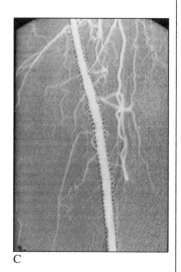

A　　　　　　　　　　　　　　B　　　　　　　　　　　　　　C

Figure 6. The case shown in this set of pictures is an example of the use of endovascular irradiation, histological monitoring, and interpretation in the case of occlusion of the left superficial artery in an 80-year-old female patient.

A) The angiogram shows free passage following re-PTA and irradiation treatment.
B) The control examination 1 year after revision and irradiation therapy shows occlusion of a segment of the superficial femoral artery above the radiated, stented region.
C) Under the occlusion, the 12-month control examination shows free passage without any indication of intimal hyperplasia in the stented area.

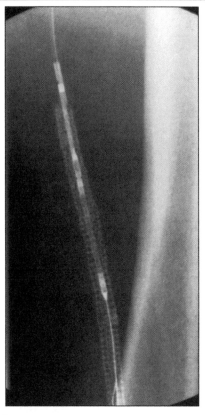

D

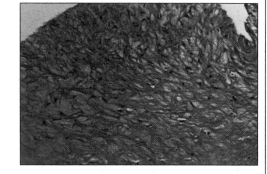

E

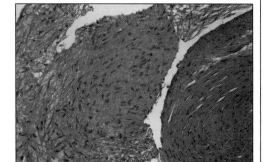

F

Figure 6 continued.

D) Tissue material is sampled from various sectors of the vascular wall in the stented region and the vascular lumen is not exposed to irradiation by means of the Simpson atherectomy catheter in order to proceed with histological analysis.

E) This Anti Actin Monoclonal (Mouse) Clone HHP 35 coloring in histological analysis shows smooth muscle cells and myofibroblasts in irregular distribution, as in florid atherosclerosis.

F) HE coloring of a section with material from the vascular segment not exposed to irradiation, showing expansive, myoxide degeneration of the basic substance, with irregular distribution of the smooth muscle cells and myofibroblasts, as in highly active, florid atherosclerosis.

G) HE coloring of a section with material from the stented region shows a more compact arrangement of the smooth muscle cells and myofibroblasts, indicating lesser florid intimal lesion possibly the result of the mitosis inhibiting effects of irradiation.

G

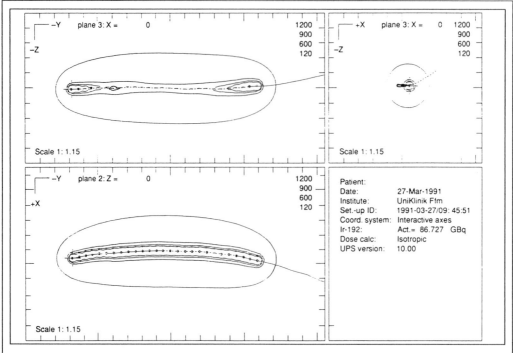

Figure 7. Printout of an original calculation plan for dose penetration depth during vascular therapy.

For ethical reasons, this pilot study was restricted to older patients. In addition, the case histories of prospective patients had to reveal multiple restenosis with short recurrence intervals for the vascular segment concerned, together with a clinical stage of IIb to IV. Our therapeutic approach was discussed in detail with the patients, together with other possible alternatives.

Interarterial afterloading therapy became possible because the diameter of the afterloading probes had been considerably reduced during further development of this treatment for malignant growths in the biliary tract (35). In contrast to percutaneous irradiation which has to be applied in a fractionated form to avoid severe side effects to the surrounding tissue, the endovascular afterloading method reaches the same effect in the vascular wall with only a single application lasting 200 seconds with a strong dose decrease for the surrounding tissue.

Based upon experience with antihyperproliferative treatment of keloids (23-34), we thought it possible that irradiation would have a suppressive effect on hyperproliferative reactions following stent implantation. The initial small number of patients, however, does not allow us to make any definitive statements. Our follow-up results, however, are sufficiently encouraging to prompt us to proceed with further development of afterloading irradiation as an antihyperproliferative therapy following stent implantation. With the exception of the somatic risk during irradiation therapy described above, we saw no other relevant short- or long-term complications. Potential short-term effects possibly include an increased thrombosis risk following an edema or inflammatory reaction to irradiation, although such effects were not detected (38,39). Cicatrization with corresponding lumen constriction of the iliac artery is a feared long-

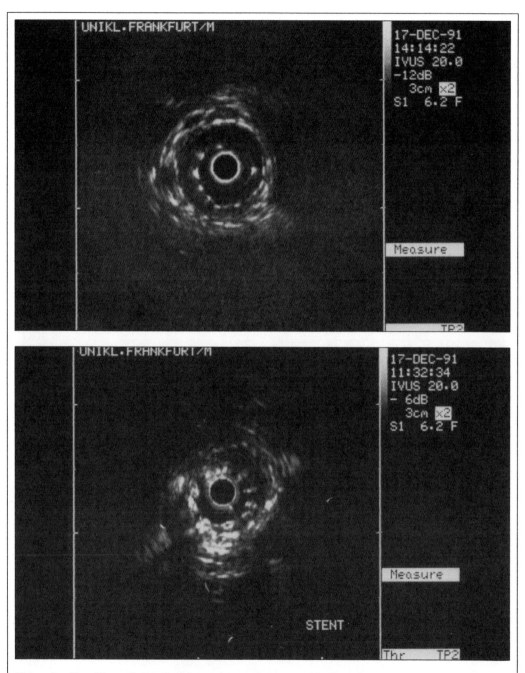

Figure 8. *Top:* The endovascular ultrasonic scan shows centrally from the inside outwards the ultrasonic probe, then the dark ring showing the patent lumen, with the outer border formed by the stent (outward triangles in circular arrangement representing the stent filaments of the tantalum stent). *Bottom:* The condition 12 months following re-PTA and endoluminal irradiation with a 12 Gy surface dose without evidence of intimal hyperplasia occluding the lumen. Behind the circular stent filaments grouped around the probe, there is a highly reflexogenic zone to be interpreted as calcium deposits in the formerly recanalized, occluded vascular segment.

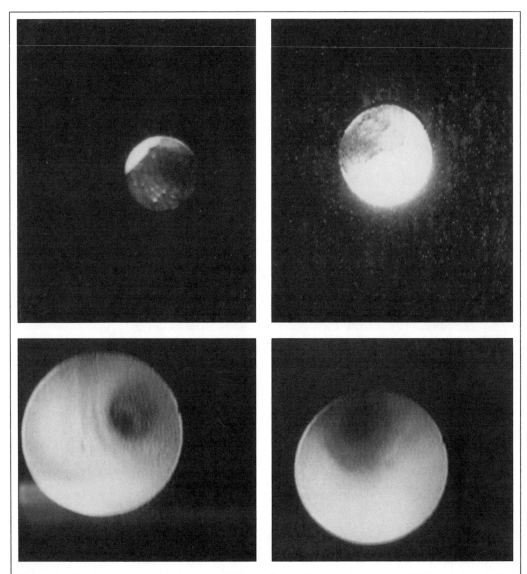

Figure 9. Angioscope immediately after positioning of a tantalum stent in the superficial femoral artery *(top left)*. Six months after stent implantation, the lumen is severely constricted by material resulting from intimal hyperplasia *(top right)*. Angioscopic findings 12 months after re-PTA and endovascular irradiation therapy in the afterloading method with a 12 Gy surface dose. Shows a freely patent lumen with a smooth surface in the stented vascular region *(bottom left and right)*.

term effect of high-dose radiation therapy (40-44). Various analyses about the effect of irradiation show that cicatrization in the vascular system only occurs following high doses with complete tissue necrosis. Cicatrization is not anticipated following endovascular application of low doses of 12 Gy. The dose we have used in our therapy only causes a significant reduction of mitosis in the most exposed cells with only isolated cell necrosis (39,43,45-53). This effect, combined with reduction in myofibroblast migration velocity, is possibly responsible for the lack of restenoses in our patient population (54).

It should be noted that recurrences have also been observed in our patients. Zeitler and colleagues, who also use our procedure, have indicated a higher recurrence rate than our group using a single dose of 10 Gy applied to the vascular wall. Our application of 12 Gy also gives rise to doubts whether the dose is always homogeneously distributed in the vascular wall, achieving the same antiproliferative effect all over, or whether certain adjacent areas may be differentially exposed resulting from the decentral position of the probe. In order to minimize this effect, I have developed a catheter which can accommodate the probe system with an inner lumen of just 6 Fr, but which has an outer diameter of approximately 8 Fr with balloons for centering the catheter in the lumen during dose application. Preliminary experimental tests have already been successfully completed.

In comparison to alternative methods for the treatment of intimal hyperplasia, endovascular afterloading irradiation is the only method which is used locally in the stented region with success under clinical conditions. Some models use heparin, Marcumar, aspirin, low-molecular weight heparin, corticoids, or other substances to influence intimal hyperplasia, but therapeutically effective doses all have systemic side effects (55-70). Knowledge about the mediators responsible for prolific growth after any kind of damage to the vascular wall led to the development of substances aimed at interrupting or reducing this process. Unfortunately, such processes are always only aimed at one or two growth factors, while leaving others largely unaffected (19,56,59,69,71,72). Another model favors the genetic influence on the vascular wall (73-76). A few animal experiments have been carried out with rather discouraging results following implantation of so-called "coated stents". Hyperproliferation has been observed at the transition zones between stent end and vascular wall (77,78). Finally there are a few initial models in which the stent is prepared with heparin or other chemotherapeutic substances to reduce intimal hyperproliferation following implantation (58,78). Finally it is worth mentioning the development of so-called biocompatible stents which have been tested in animal experiments (79,80). Most of these models are still only in the experimental stage, so that it is necessary to wait for further developments. When all is said and done, it is only the use of a functioning antihyperproliferative therapy, of whatever type, which makes it possible to proceed with routine use of stents for the treatment of arterial occlusive disease in the peripheral vascular system.

REFERENCES

1. Clowes AW, Karnovsky MJ. Suppression by heparin of smooth muscle cell proliferation in injured arteries. Nature 1977;265:625-626.
2. Clowes AW, Reidy MA, Clowes MM. Kinetics of cellular proliferation after arterial injury. Lab Invest 1983;49:327-334.
3. Cox JL, Gottlieb AL. Restenosis following percutaneous transluminal angioplasty: clinical, physiological and pathological features. Can Med Assoc J 1986;136:1129-1132.
4. Essed CE, Van den Brand M, Becker AE. Transluminal coronary angioplasty and early restenosis: fibrocellular occlusion after wall laceration. Br Heart J 1983;49:393-396.
5. Faxon DP, Sanborn TA, Weber VJ. Restenosis following transluminal angioplasty in experimental atherosclerosis. Arteriosclerosis 1984;4:189-195.
6. Faxon DP, Sanborn TA, Haudenschild CC. Mechanism of angioplasty and its relation to restenosis. Am J Cardiol 1987;60:5B-9B.
7. Friedman JR, Burns R. Role of platelets in the proliferative response of the injured artery. Prog Hemost Thromb 1978;4:249-278.
8. Garth EA, Ratliff NB, Hollman J, Tabei S, Phillips FD. Intimal proliferation of smooth muscle cells as an explanation for recurrent coronary artery stenosis after percutaneous transluminal coronary angioplasty. J Am Coll Cardiol 1985;6,2:369-372.
9. Hashizume M, Yang Y, Galt S. Intimal response of saphenous vein to intraluminal trauma by simulated angioscopic insertion. J Vasc Surg 1987;5:862-868.

10. Imparato AM, Bracco A, Kim GE, Zeff R. Intimal and neointimal fibrous proliferation causing failure of arterial reconstructions. Surgery 1972;172:1007-1017.

11. Ip JH, Fuster V, Badimon L, Badimon J, Taubman MB, Chesebro JH. Syndromes of acceleration atherosclerosis: role of vascular injury and smooth muscle cell proliferation. J Am Coll Cardiol 1990;15:1667-1687.

12. Laerum BF, Vlodaver Z, Castaneda-Zuniga WR, Edwards E, Amplatz K. The mechanism of angioplasty. Fortschr Röntgenstr 1982;136:573-576.

13. Nobuyoshi M, Kimura T, Ohishi H, Horiuchi H. Restenosis after percutaneous transluminal coronary angioplasty: pathologic observations in 20 patients. J Am Coll Cardiol 1991;17:433-439.

14. Spaet TH, Stemermann MB, Veith FJ, Lejnieks I. Intimal injury and regrowth in the rabbit aorta. Medial smooth muscles cells as a source of neointima. Circ Res 1975;36: 58-70.

15. Ueda M, Becker AE, Fujimoto T. Pathological changes induced by repeated percutaneous transluminal coronary angioplasty. Br Heart J 1987;58:635-643.

16. Zollikofer CL, Cragg AH, Hunter DW, Yedlicka JW, Castaneda-Zuniga WR, Amplatz K. Mechanism of transluminal angioplasty. In: Castaneda-Zuniga WR and Tadavarthy SM, eds. *Interventional Radiology*. Baltimore: Williams and Wilkins; 1992;249-298.

17. Leung DYM, Glagov S, Matthews MB. Cyclic stretching stimulates synthesis of matrix components by arterial smooth muscle cells *in vitro*. Science 1976; 191:475-477.

18. Liermann D, Böttcher HD, Kollath J, et al. Prophylactic endovascular radiotherapy to prevent intimal hyperplasia after stent implantation in femoropopliteal arteries. Cardiovasc Intervent Radiol 1994;17:12-16.

19. Liu MW, Roubin GS, King SB. Restenosis after coronary angioplasty: potential biologic determinants and rose of intimal hyperplasia. Circulation 1989;79:1374-1387.

20. Palmaz JC, Windeler SA, Garcia F. Atherosclerotic rabbit aortas: expandable intraluminal grafting. Radiology 1986; 160:723-726.

21. Rollins N, Wright KC, Charnsangavej C, Gianturco C. Self-expanding metallic stents:

preliminary evaluation in an atherosclerotic model. Radiology 1987;163:739-742.

22. Rousseau H, Joffre F, Raillat C, et al. Self-expanding endovascular stent in experimental atherosclerosis. Radiology 1989;170: 773-778.

23. Baensch W. Über die Strahlenbehandlung der Keloide. Strahlentherapie 1937;60: 204-209.

24. Craig RDP, Pearson D. Early post-operative irradiation in the treatment of keloid scars. Br J Past Surg 1965;18:369-375.

25. Crocett DJ. Regional keloid susceptibility. Br J Plast Surg 1964;17:245-253.

26. Dalicho W. Zur Therapie der Keloide mit besonderer Berücksichtigung der Radiumbestrahlung. Stahlentherapie 1949:78.

27. Enhamre A, Hammar H. Treatment of keloids with excision and postoperative x-ray irradiation. Dermatologica 1983;167: 90-93.

28. Graul EH. Zur Klinik des Keloids. Strahlentherapie 1955;98:119-132.

29. Kovalic JJ, Perez CA. Radiation therapy following keloidektomie: a 20 year experience. Radiation oncology. Biol Phys 1989;17: 77-80.

30. Krüger A. Über Keloide und ihre Behandlung unter besonderer Berücksinchtigung der Strahlentherapie. Strahlentherapie 1945;93:426-433.

31. Levy DS, Salter MM, Roth RE. Postoperative irradiation in the prevention of keloids. Am J Roentg 1981;127:509-510.

32. Ollstein RN, Siegel HW, Gilloley JF, Barsa JMM. Treatment of keloids by combined surgical excision and immediate postoperative x-ray therapy. Ann Plast Surg 1981;7: 281-284.

33. Scherer E. Kontaktbestrahlung mit radioaktiven Stoffen. In Hdb Med Radiol, Bd XVI/2, Springer 1970:136-146.

34. Wagner W, Schopohl B, Böttcher HD, Scheppner E. Ergebnisse der Narbenkeloidprophylaxe durch Kontaktbestrahlung mit Strontium 90. Röntgenpraxis 1989; 42:248-252.

35. Brambs HJ, Freund U, Bruggmoser G, Wannenmacher M. Kombinierte intraduktale perkutane Radiotherapie bei malignen Gallengangsobstruktinonen mit anschließenderprothetischer Versorgung. Onkologie 1987;10:84-89.

36. Kinsella TJ, Sindelar WF, De Luca AM. Threshold dose for peripheral nerve injury following intraoperative radiotherapy (IORT) in a large animal model. Int J Radiat Oncol Biol Phys 1988;I:205.

37. Le Couteur RA, Gilette EL, Powers BE, Child G, McChesney SL, Ingram JT. Peripheral neuropathies following experimental intraoperative radiation therapy (IORT). Int J Radiat Oncol Biol Phys 1989;17:583-590.

38. Rosen EM, Vinter DW, Goldberg ID. Hypertrophy of cultured bovine aortic endothelium following irradiation. Radiat Res 1989;117:395-408.

39. Schwartz RS, Koval TM, Edwards WD, et al. Effect of external beam irradiation on neointimal hyperplasia after experimental coronary artery injury. J Am Coll Cardiol 1992;19:1106-1113.

40. Drescher W, Basche St, Schumann E. Arterielle Spätkomplikationen nach Strahlentherapie. Strahlentherapie 1984; 160:505-507.

41. Johnson AG. Large artery damage after X-radiation. Br J Radiol 1969;42:937-938.

42. Kolar J. Strahlenfolgen am Herz und großen Gefäßen. Med Klin 1971;66:661-668.

43. Scherer E, Streffer C, Trott KR, eds. Radiopathology of Organs and Tissues. Berlin: Springer; 1991.

44. Schwartz RS, Murphy JG, Edwards WD, Camrud AR, Vliestra RE, Holmes DR. Restenosis occurs with internal elastic lamina laceration and its proportional to severity of vessel injury in a porcine coronary artery model. Circulation 1990;82(Suppl III):656.

45. Amronin GG, Gildenhorn HC, Solomon RD, Nadkarni BB, Jacobs, MI. The synergism of X irradiation and cholesterol fat feeding on the development of coronary artery lesions. J Atheroscler Res 1964;4:325-334.

46. Artom C, Lofland HB, Clarkson TB. Ionizing radiation, atherosclerosis, and lipid metabolism in pigeons. Radiat Res 1965;26:165-177.

47. Battegay EJ, Raines EW, Seifert RA, Bowen-Pope DF, Ross R. TGF-B induces bimodal proliferation of connective tissue cells via complex control of an autocrine PDGF loop. Cell 1990;63:515-524.

48. Fischer JJ. Proliferation of rat aortic endothelial cells following X irradiation. Radiat Res 1982;92:405-410.

49. Hirst DG, Denekamp J, Hobson B. Proliferation studies of the endothelial and smooth muscle cells of the mouse mesentery after irradiation. Cell Tissue Kinet 1980;193:91-104.

50. Kirkpatrick JB. Pathogenesis of foam cell lesions in irradiated arteries. Am J Pathol 1967;50:291-309.

51. Liermann D, Schopohl B, Herrmann G, Kollath J, Böttcher HD. Endovaskuläres Afterloading als Therapiekonzept zur Prophylaxe der intimalen Hyperplasie in peripheren Gefäßen nach Stentimplantation. In: Kollath J and Liermann D, eds. Stents II. Konstanz: Schnetztor Verlag; 1992;80-92.

52. Narayan K, Cliff WF. Morphology of irradiated microvasculature: a combined in vivo and electron microscopic study. Am J Pathol 1982;106:47-62.

53. Sholley MM, Gimbrone MA, Coltran RS. The effect of leukocyte depletion on corneal neovascularization. Lab Invest 1978;38:32-40.

54. Sholley MM, Gimbrone MA, Cotran RS. Cellular migration and replication in endothelial regeneration: a study using irradiated endothelial cultures. Lab Invest 1977;36:18

55. Betz E, Hämmerle H, Strohschneider T. Vergleich von Wirkungen einzelner Pharmaka auf die Proliferation von Gefäßmuskelzellen in vivo und in vitro. In: Fischer H and Betz E, eds. Gefäßwandelemente In Vivo und In Vitro. Stuttgart: Wiss Verlagsgesellschaft; 1984;43-57.

56. Betz E, Hämmerle H, Strohschneider T. Inhibition of smooth muscle cell proliferation and endothelial permeability with fluranizine in vitro and in experimental atheromas. Res Exp Med 1985;325-340.

57. Courrier JW, Power TK, Haudenschild CC, Miniham AC, Faxon DP. Low molecular weight heparin (enoaparin) reduces restenosis after iliac angioplasty in the hypercholesterolemic rabbit. J Am Coll Cardiol 1991;17:118-125.

58. Cwikiel W, Stridbeck H, Stenram U. Electrolytic stents to inhibit tumor growth: An

experimental study *in vitro* and in rats. Acta Radiologica 1993;34:1-5.

59. Dartsch PC, Betz E, Ischinger T. Wirkung von Dihämatoporphyrin-Derivaten auf kultivierte glatte Muskelzellen des Menschen aus normalen und atherosklerotisch veränderten Gefäßsegmenten.-Übersicht über bisherige Ergebnisse und Impliktationen für eine photodynamische Therapie. Z Kardiol 1991;80:6-14.

60. Ellis SG, Roubin GS, Wilentz J. Results of a randomized trial of heparin and aspirin vs aspirin alone for prevention of acute closure and restenosis after angioplasty (PTCA). Circulation 1987;76:213.

61. Guyton J, Rosenburg R, Clowes A, Karnowsky M. Inhibition of rat arterial smooth muscle cell proliferation by heparin: *in vivo* studies with anticoagulant and non anticoagulant heparin. Circ Res 1980;46: 625-634.

62. Hagen B. Einflüsse der medikamentösen Nachbehandlung auf die mittelfristigen Ergebnisse von Stent-Implantationen der A Femoropolitea: In: Liermann D, ed. *Stents*. New York: Marianne Liebert; 1993; in press.

63. Heras, M, Chesebro JH, Penny WJ, Baily KR, Badimon K, Fuster, V. Effects of thrombin inhibition on the development of acute plateletthrombus deposition during angioplasty in pigs. Heparin versus recombinant hirudin, a specific thrombin inhibitor. Circulation 1989;79:657-665.

64. Hoepp LM, Elbadawi M, Cohn M, Dachelet R, Peterson C, De Weese JA. Steroids and immunosuppression effect on anastomotic intimal hyperplasia femoral arterial dacron bypass grafts. Arch Surg 1979;114:273-276.

65. Hoover R, Rosenburg R, Hearing W, Karnovsky M. Inhibition of rat arterial smooth cell proliferation by heparin: II *in vitro* studies. Circ Res 1980;47:578-583.

66. Kramsch DM, Aspen AJ, Rozler LJ. Suppression of experimental atherosclerosis by the Ca++ antagonist lanthanum. J Clin Invest 1980;65:967-981.

67. Liu MW, Roubin GS, Robinson KA. Trapidil in preventing restenosis after balloon-angioplasty in the atherosclerotic rabbit. Circulation 1990;81:1089-1093.

68. Pepine CJ, Hirschfeld JW, MacDonald RG. A controlled trial of corticosteroids to prevent restenosis after coronary angioplasty. Circulation 1990;81:1753-1761.

69. Powell JS, Clozel JP, Müller KM. Inhibitors angiotensin-converting enzyme prevent myointimal proliferation after vascular injury. Science 1989;245:186-188.

70. Reis GJ, Boucher TM, Sipperly ME. Randomized trial of fish oil for prevention of restenosis after coronary angioplasty. Lancet 1989;2:1753-1761.

71. Castellot Jr JJ, Addonizio ML, Rosenberg R, Karnovsky MJ. Cultured endothelial cells produce a heparin like inhibitor of smooth muscle cell growth. J Cell Biol 1990;373-379.

72. Nilsson J, Sjölund M, Palmberg L, Thyberg J, Heldin CH. Arterial smooth muscle cells in primary culture produce a platelet-derived growth factor like protein. Cell Biol 1985;82:4418-4422.

73. Dichek DA, Neville RF, Zwiebel JA, Freeman SM, Leon MB, Anderson WF. Seeding of intravascular stents with genetically engineered endothelial cells. Circulation 1989;80:1347-1353.

74. Leclerc G, Isner JM, Kearny M, et al. Evidence implicating nonmuscle myosin in restenosis: use of *in situ* hybridization to analyze human vascular lesions obtained by directional atherectomy. Circulation 1992; 85:1-11.

75. Nabel EG, Plautz G, Nabel GJ. Site specific expression *in vivo* by direct gene transfer into the arterial wall. Science 1990;249: 1285-1288.

76. Wilcox JN. Analysis of local gene expression in human atherosclerotic plaques by *in situ* hybridization. Trends Cardiol Med 1991;1: 17-24.

77. Roeren T, Palmaz JC, Garcia O, Rees CR, Tio FO. Percutaneous vascular grafting with a coated stent. Radiology 1990;177-202.

78. Strecker EP, Hagen B, Liermann D, Kuhn FP. Komplikationen bei der Implantation arterieller Tantalstents und deren Behandlung. Zentralblatt der Radiologie, Radiology 1993;147:799.

79. Murphy JG, Schwartz RS, Kennedy K, Edwards RE, Vliestra RE, Holmes DR. A new biocompatible polymeric coronary stent: design and early results in the pig model. J Am Coll Cardiol 1990;1:10.

80. Slepian MJ, Schindler A. Polymeric endoluminal paving/sealing: a biodegradable alternative to intracoronary stenting. Circulation 1988;78:409.

The Potential of a Beta Particle-Emitting Stent to Inhibit Restenosis Following Catheter-Based Revascularization: Work in Progress

Robert E. Fischell[1], David R. Fischell[1], Tim A. Fischell[2]

[1]*IsoStent, Inc., Fair Haven, NJ USA*
[2]*Vanderbilt University Medical Center, Nashville, TN USA*

Catheter-based revascularization techniques, including PTA and PTCA, have been limited by acute complications secondary to intimal dissection and elastic recoil leading to acute or subacute closure and unreliable, long-term patency due to restenosis. This paper presents preliminary data that suggest that a beta particle (electron)-emitting intravascular stent may prove effective in minimizing these acute and long-term limitations of percutaneous revascularization. A series of experiments performed in cell culture examined the ability of external beam and localized beta particle irradiation from a P32-impregnated titanium wire source to inhibit the growth and/or migration of proliferating smooth muscle and endothelial cells. Using the dose-response data from the in vitro studies, the appropriate activity of a P32-coated intravascular stent, and the tissue irradiation levels required to inhibit smooth muscle cell proliferation and possibly neointimal hyperplasia in vivo, were calculated. The results from cell culture studies demonstrated that external irradiation in the range of 400 to 600 cGy, delivered as a single dose, completely inhibited the clonal proliferation of smooth muscle cells. Endothelial cells appeared much more radioresistant with doses of > 800 cGy required to eliminate the proliferative capabilities. A P32-impregnated titanium wire source with wire activity as low as 0.006 μCurie caused maximal inhibition of localized smooth muscle cell growth near the wire. Using these data, the calculated activity of a P32-coated intravascular stent required to inhibit smooth muscle cell proliferation is estimated to be only 0.13 μCurie, yielding a localized tissue radiation dose of only 25 cGy.

INTRODUCTION

The CAVEAT trial which compared directional coronary atherectomy with percutaneous transluminal coronary angioplasty (PTCA) in 1012 patients indicated 6-month restenosis rates of 50% for atherectomy and 57% for PTCA (1). Furthermore, abrupt vessel closure in 7% of the atherectomy cases and 3% of the PTCA patients was reported. Nicolini et al (2) have reported restenosis rates between 35 and 40% subsequent to percutaneous transluminal angioplasty (PTA) and PTCA, and an acute closure rate of 4%. It is widely understood that the principle cause of restenosis is neointimal hyperplasia secondary to smooth muscle cell migration and proliferation; this occurs over a period of

months following the revascularization procedure. Elastic recoil has also been reported by Nicolini et al (2) and others (3, 4) as a contributing factor to restenosis.

Recent publications have indicated that intravascular stents can decrease restenosis. Columbo et al (5) reported a restenosis rate of only 19% after placement of the Palmaz-Schatz stent in restenosed coronary arteries of 97 consecutive patients. This study suggests that stents can have a significantly beneficial effect in decreasing restenosis subsequent to arterial dilatation.

An analysis of acute and long-term complications resulting from revascularization procedures such as PTA, PTCA, and coronary or peripheral atherectomy indicates that a beta particle-emitting stent might provide a therapeutic modality that is capable of decreasing acute post-procedure complications and improving long-term patency. Clinical trials have demonstrated the efficacy of stents in the treatment of acute and threatened vessel closure. The ability of stents to decrease elastic recoil has also been demonstrated. The fact that stents can serve as a platform for a radioisotope which can decrease neointimal hyperplasia over an extended period of time after the interventional procedure has only recently been reported (6). Specifically, Hehrlein et al have shown that low levels of radioactivity can completely inhibit neointimal proliferation in the iliac arteries of New Zealand White rabbits. Hehrlein et al (6) state that: "Radioactive coronary stents completely inhibited neointimal proliferation in non-atherosclerotic rabbits and may be suitable to eliminate restenosis after stent implantation in humans." The fact that radioactivity combined with stenting can reduce or eliminate restenosis in human subjects was recently described by Liermann et al (7). Specifically, they described the successful use of endovascular radiotherapy with a surface dose of 12 Gy using an iridium 192 source on the distal end of an afterloading probe for 200 seconds. This procedure was performed following PTA or laser recanalization in superficial femoral arteries which had restenosed after stenting.

The authors have previously described the use of a radioisotope intraarterial stent for inhibiting intimal hyperplasia subsequent to PTA, PTCA, or atherectomy (8). Specifically, a beta particle-emitting metallic stent is described which contains a radioisotope that has a comparatively short half-life. The rationale for such a stent is that because of its mechanical structure, the stent can minimize acute vessel closure caused by intimal dissection and elastic recoil. The prevention of neointimal proliferation is accomplished by electrons that are spontaneously emitted from a radioisotope that is integral to the stent wire or plated onto its outer surface. The purpose of the electrons emanating from the stent's

surface is to prevent the migration and/or growth of cells through the stent wires. If electron irradiation could prevent proliferating cells from entering the stent's interior lumen, the rate of acute, subacute, and chronic complications subsequent to revascularization procedures could be significantly reduced.

Based on cell culture studies using titanium wires coated with the beta particle (electron)-emitting isotope, phosphorous 32 (P32), we have analyzed the potential advantages of such a beta particle-emitting stent to decrease complications associated with percutaneous revascularization.

MATERIALS AND METHODS

An important consideration in the use of a beta particle-emitting stent to reduce post-angioplasty complications is whether such a stent would prevent endothelial cells from relining the arterial wall. To quantitate the relative effectiveness of radiation in inhibiting smooth muscle cell growth as compared to the growth of endothelial tissues, experiments were performed in cell cultures by one of the authors (TA Fischell) and associates at Stanford University (9).

Bovine aortic and coronary artery smooth muscle and endothelial cells were grown in culture for 2 days and then exposed to a single x-ray radiation dose ranging from 0 to 800 rads in increments of 100 rads. Six days after irradiation the number of cell colonies surviving was measured and compared to new colonies in the control (non-irradiated) cell culture.

Additional experiments were performed with smooth muscle and endothelial cells exposed to beta particle emission from a straight section of stent wire which included a beta particle-emitting radioisotope within the wire structure. For this purpose, the radioisotope P32 was selected because it is a pure beta particle-emitting radioisotope with no gamma radiation. P32 emits electrons with an average energy of 0.695 MeV having an average range in tissue or water of approximately

3.5 mm. The wire material was titanium and the wire diameter was 0.2 mm.

RESULTS

Data from the experiments on x-ray irradiation of smooth muscle and endothelial cells are presented in Figure 1. These experiments indicate that at 600 rads there were no surviving colonies of smooth muscle cells, whereas approximately 40% of the endothelial cell colonies survived.

The results of experiments with P32 in titanium wires showed that an activity of only 0.006 μCurie/cm of wire was sufficient to fully inhibit smooth muscle cell growth to a distance of at least 3.5 mm. In contrast, endothelial cells appeared to be unaffected at wire activity levels as high as 0.019 μCurie/cm; i.e., approximately three times the activity level that completely inhibited the growth of smooth muscle cells. Since P32 has a half-life of 14.3 days, this would mean that the endothelial cells could grow over the stent wires for a period of approximately 24 days (1.7 half-lives of the P32) during which time the smooth muscle cells would still be completely inhibited.

These two *in vitro* studies both demonstrate the potentially favorable finding that endothelial cells appear to be considerably less sensitive to radiation than smooth muscle cells.

It can be shown that the desired radioactivity level for an entire stent using a beta particle-emitting radioisotope to inhibit neointimal proliferation would be given by:

$$A_o = \frac{2^{T/\tau}\pi\, a\, L\, D}{2\, r} \quad (\mu Curie) \qquad (1)$$

where a = minimum activity level per cm of a wire that would fully inhibit smooth muscle cell growth (μCurie/cm)

T = desired shelf life for the stent (days),
τ = half-life of the radioisotope (days),
L = stent length (cm),
D = stent diameter (cm), and
r = average range of electrons emitted by the stent's radioisotope (cm).

Let us assume a P32 (14.3 day half-life), electron-emitting, 0.3 cm diameter stent having a length of 2 cm and a desired and practical shelf life of 43 days (approximately 6 weeks is selected). Based on the P32 in titanium wire studies showing full inhibition of

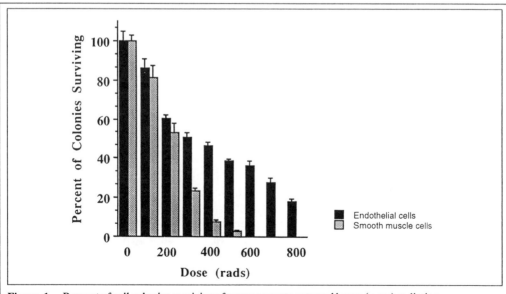

Figure 1. Percent of cell colonies surviving after exposure to external beam (x-ray) radiation. Courtesy of M. Abbas, Stanford University.

smooth muscle cell proliferation at 0.006 μCurie/cm of wire and a range of 0.35 cm, the initial activity in such a stent is given by:

$$A_o = 2^{43/14.3} \frac{\pi(0.006)(2)(0.3)}{2(0.35)} = (0.13 \mu Curie)$$

This represents an extremely low level source of radiation activity.

The dose rate to tissue surrounding the stent would be given by:

$$\dot{D} = \frac{A \Delta \phi}{m} \text{ rad/hr} \qquad (2)$$

where A = stent activity (μCurie), and
$\Delta = 2.13 \bar{E}_\beta$.

where $\bar{E}_\beta$ = mean energy of the electrons (0.695 MeV for P32),

ϕ = the fraction of stent-emitted electrons that enter the surrounding tissue, and

m = mass of the surrounding tissue (gm).

The mass m is given by:

$$m = \pi \rho \, (r^2 + Dr) \, (L + 2r) \qquad (3)$$

where ρ = density of the tissue (~ 1 gm/cm^3).

Assuming that one-half the electrons from the stent are absorbed by the blood and the other half are absorbed in the first 0.35 cm of surrounding tissue, then from equation (3)

$$m = 1.93 \text{ gm}$$

and from equation (2)

$$\dot{D}_o = 0.05 \text{ rad/hr.}$$

The integrated dose rate to the tissue surrounding the stent for the lifetime of the stent is given by:

$$H = \dot{H}_o \int_0^\infty 2^{-1/\tau} dt \text{ (rem)} \qquad (4)$$

where H_o = initial radiation dose rate (in rem/hr) of the tissue surrounding the stent.

As the emitted electrons from P32 are all absorbed by the tissue,

$$\dot{H}_o \text{ (rem/hr)} = \dot{D}_o \text{ (rad/hr)},$$

therefore $H = \dot{H}_o \tau \ln 2$ (rem).   (4)

Using $H_o = 0.05$ rem/hr
and $\tau = 14.3$ days
gives   H = 0.25 Gy.

DISCUSSION

These data and calculations suggest that a P32-impregnated, beta particle-emitting intravascular stent with very low levels of radioactivity (≈ 0.13 μCurie) may prove to be effective in substantially inhibiting neointimal hyperplasia following catheter-based revascularization. It is difficult to conceive that this very low level radiation dose could kill smooth muscle cells, although at even lower doses we have found a zone of complete inhibition around P32-impregnated stent wires placed in cultures of proliferating smooth muscle cells. One possibility is that sublethal levels of comparatively high energy electrons from the P32 isotope can prevent cell proliferation. Another possibility is that the electron irradiation causes the proliferating smooth muscle cells to migrate away from the P32 source. If either of these phenomena occurs *in vivo*, then any neointimal proliferation which might occur would remain exterior to the stent lumen and thus would dramatically reduce restenosis. Therefore, if the proliferative cell growth surrounding a P32 stent *in vivo* behaves like the cells *in vitro*, then neointimal hyperplasia could be reduced with very limited radiation exposure of the surrounding tissue.

Since these stents should have a zone of inhibition that extends for approximately 3.5 mm beyond the end of the stent, endointimal proliferation should also be significantly reduced in that end region. This could be important since stents may promote proliferative growth at their extremities.

Since neointimal proliferation takes place for at least several weeks following a revascularization procedure, an optimum solution for inhibiting such proliferation may be a stent which includes a radioactive component that irradiates the arterial wall over a comparable period of time. Thus, although the endovascular therapy of Liermann et al (7) was effective using only a 200 sec radiation exposure period at the completion of the revascularization procedure, the source strength was extraordinarily high (10 Curie) compared to the less than 1 μCurie source strength suggested herein for the implanted beta particle-emitting stent. The beta particle-emitting stent would therefore provide a less hazardous radioisotope handling situation in the catheterization laboratory. Furthermore, since neointimal proliferation occurs for at least several weeks after a revascularization procedure, radiation applied over a comparable period of time can be accomplished with less total radiation of the blood and the tissue surrounding the stent.

The improved efficacy of radiation therapy initiated at a significant time after the revascularization procedure is borne out by the work of Shefer et al (10). They have reported that the same beta particle radiation exposure performed on the second day after a balloon overstretching injury in rabbits was considerably more effective in decreasing neointimal proliferation compared to this level of radiation exposure accomplished immediately after the injury.

It is also important to note that thrombotic complications associated with intravascular stents might be reduced if the diameter of the implanted stent was deliberately oversized as compared to the normal vessel diameter. Unfortunately, oversizing can result in increased neointimal hyperplasia. For example, if a beta particle-emitting stent is 10% oversized when placed within the vessel, then we are suggesting the possibility of a decreased thrombogenicity without excessive neointimal hyperplasia.

SUMMARY

In summary, it is suggested that an oversized, beta particle-emitting stent could simultaneously minimize the complications of acute or subacute vessel closure caused by intimal dissection vasospasm and elastic recoil as well as long-term failure due to restenosis caused by neointimal hyperplasia. Extensive animal and human trials will be required to determine if in fact such a stent can reduce these complications without causing other adverse effects due to radiation exposure of blood and surrounding tissues. The extremely low doses and localized delivery of radiation as proposed for such a stent provides some encouragement that radiation-related adverse effects will not occur from the use of this beta particle-emitting stent.

Experiments in laboratory pigs are currently underway using a multiplicity of titanium stents which have various levels of pure beta particle radioactivity ranging from 0 to 0.4 μCurie. These experiments will provide additional data addressing the efficacy of a beta particle-emitting stent to reduce neointimal hyperplasia.

REFERENCES

1. Topol EJ, Leya F, Pinkerton CA, et al. A comparison of directional atherectomy with coronary angioplasty in patients with coronary artery disease. N Engl J Med 1993;329:221-227.
2. Nicolini FA, Pepine CJ. Biology of restenosis and therapeutic approach. Endovasc Surg 1992;72:919-940.
3. Hjemdahl-Monsen CE, Ambrose JA, Borrico S, et al. Angiographic patterns of balloon inflation during percutaneous transluminal coronary angioplasty: role of pressure-diameter curves in studying dispensability and elasticity of the stenotic lesion and mechanism of dilation. J Am Coll Cardiol 1990;16:569-575.
4. Waller BF, Pinkerton CA, Orr CM, et al. Two distinct types of restenosis lesions after coronary angioplasty: intimal proliferation and atherosclerotic plaque only: an analysis of 20 necropsy patients. Circulation 1990;82(Suppl III):311-314.
5. Columbo A, Almagor L, Maiello L, et al. Results of coronary stenting for restenosis. J Am Coll Cardiol 1994;22:118A.

6. Hehrlein C, Zimmermann M, Metz J, et al. Radioactive coronary stent implantation inhibits neointimal proliferation in non-atherosclerotic rabbits. Circulation 1993;88:1-65A.

7. Liermann D, Bottcher HD, Kollath J, et al. Prophylactic endovascular radiotherapy to prevent intimal hyperplasia after stent implantation in femoropopliteal arteries. Cardiovasc Intervent Radiol 1994;17:12-16.

8. Fischell RE, Fischell TA. Intra-arterial stent with the capability to inhibit intimal hyperplasia. U.S. Patent No. 5,059,166, 1989.

9. Fischell TA, Abbas MA, Kallman RF. Low-dose radiation inhibits clonal proliferation of smooth muscle cells: a new approach to restenosis. Arteriosclerosis and Thrombosis 1991;11:1435A.

10. Shefer A, Eigler NL, Whiting JS, Litvack FI. Suppression of intimal proliferation after balloon angioplasty with local beta irradiation in rabbits. J Am Coll Cardiol 1993;21:185A.

Research, Development, and Use of a Matted Sapphire Tip for Sole Laser Recanalization of Occluded Stents

D. Liermann

Department of Radiology, J.W. Goethe University Hospital, Frankfurt am Main, Germany

INTRODUCTION

Peri-interventional and post-interventional problems following stent implantation result in the use of percutaneous transluminal angioplasty (PTA), laser, or atherectomy to eliminate restenosis or reocclusions, with good primary success, but with a tendency towards shorter and shorter reocclusion intervals for the individual patient. Because of these unsatisfactory results, an alternative method for vascular recanalization was sought. A large number of experimental and clinical studies have appeared with apparently acceptable results for laser recanalization (1-6). The problem with using laser energy to recanalize occlusions and stenoses consists of the fact that use of the laser probe alone only creates a canal with a relatively narrow lumen. Additional therapy to expand the vascular lumen, usually PTA, is unavoidable. Only one report exists in the recent literature concerning the sole use of a laser probe for recanalization of infrapopliteal vessels (7). Laser therapy was possible here because the diameter of the infrapopliteal vascular system was almost identical to that of the laser probe being used.

Reports in the medical literature and experience with laser use confirm that the maximum vascular canal which can be generated corresponds to that of the laser probe. The sapphire with the largest diameter of 3 mm, which can still just be inserted through a 9 Fr sheath, is consequently only capable of creating a lumen with a diameter of 3 mm. The original lumen of the distal superficial femoral artery normally has a diameter of between 5 and 6 mm. In order to solve this problem, in cooperation with an engineer in Darmstadt, I developed a matted sapphire tip which allowed for energy transmission not only forwards into the vascular lumen but also laterally to the vascular wall. These properties make it possible to achieve recanalization with a maximum lumen diameter between 5.5 and 6 mm, and thus eliminate the need for further expansion methods such as PTA. No experience with this specially developed sapphire tip was available, so experimental examinations on human cadaver preparations were necessary prior to its actual clinical use.

LASER MATERIAL, TECHNIQUE, AND METHODS

The laser equipment used was a Neodymium Yttrium Aluminum Granat (Nd:YAG) laser (Surgical Laser Technologies, Malvern PA) with a wavelength of 1.064 nm. The actual recanalizing effect can be achieved more easily and more reliably with a narrower sapphire contact probe rather than with a large probe, so that as a rule we first use a probe with a diameter of 2.2 mm, then expand the canal with the matted 3-mm sapphire probe. Output varies between 10 and 25 watts in a 1-second pulsed mode or in a continuous mode. Continuous, non-pulsed release of laser energy was particularly effective when using the matted sapphire tip for extending the lumen to a diameter of 5.5 to 6 mm and to smooth the vascular surface.

In contrast to the conventional 3-mm sapphire tip, which concentrates 95% of the laser energy at the top and emits the same in a forward direction, the matted sapphire tip known as the "Frankfurt tip" only concentrates 65 to 70% of the output at the tip.

Thirty percent of the laser energy is emitted radially to the vascular wall (Figure 1). This mode of energy release by the sapphire requires higher laser energy, but at the same time creates a larger canal diameter so that the laser can be used as the sole recanalization method. The laser is used as ipsilateral and percutaneous therapy under x-ray control in a road mapping technique. The patients receive heparin 100 IU/kg body weight as anticoagulation therapy. Following conclusion of the intervention and placement of a pressure dressing on the puncture site for 24 hours, patients receive heparin 1000 IU/hour via a perfusor for 72 hours. Marcumar® therapy is gradually introduced at the same time and is maintained for a period of at least 6 months.

EXPERIMENTAL SERIES

Test Method

In the first part of the examination, muscle preparations were separated out of the psoas group and spread out on a wooden board. Attempts were made to pre-form holes in the muscles, corresponding to a recanalization canal, using different energy levels. In doing so, a conventional 3-mm diameter sapphire was compared in five experiments to our 3-mm diameter matted sapphire tip for recanalization of a 5- to 6-mm canal. In a second test, vascular system segment preparations were selected in which the case history of the patient indicated severe arterial occlusive disease combined with a clinical stage of III to IV according to Fontaine. In cooperation with our pathology center, preparations consisted of either a severely constricted or occluded proximal femoral artery segment including a remnant of the superficial femoral artery measuring approximately 5 cm, or a severely constricted or occluded common femoral artery with a section of the external iliac artery measuring approximately 5 cm in length. The vascular preparation was fixed to a wooden board in the normal man-

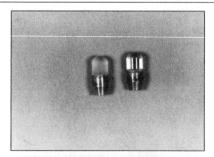
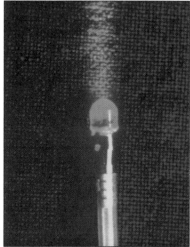
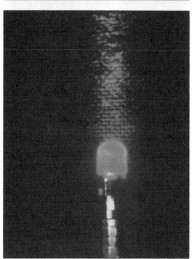

Figure 1. Conventional and new matted sapphire tip *(top)*, each with a diameter of 3 mm. The non-matted sapphire concentrates 95% of the laser energy at its tip *(middle)*. The matted sapphire emits 30 to 35% of its energy radially to the vascular wall, thus making it possible to create a wider vascular lumen of up to 6 mm in diameter *(bottom)*.

ner, spread out, and prepared for the experimental use of the laser. Using the technique described above, five further tests were carried out comparing the normal and the matted 3-mm sapphires. The experiments were conducted under x-ray control, and the vascular section was subsequently cut open and examined.

Results

The results obtained following experimental use of the two laser sapphires in muscle tissue revealed a difference in canal diameter in all five cases. When using the normal 3-mm sapphire and pulsed energy up to 20 watts, there were no problems in obtaining a hole corresponding to the sapphire diameter. The diameter varied from 2.9 mm (caused by the tissue's recoiling forces) to 3.2 mm. When using the matted laser sapphire under the same conditions, the laser catheter moved forwards in the muscle tissue at a far slower speed because the energy current was now not only directed in a forward direction. It was frequently necessary to increase the energy output to above 25 watts and to switch over from pulsed energy output to continuous energy output in order to obtain the desired effect. The diameter of the hole created in the muscle tissue varied from 5.5 to 6.1 mm.

The second series of tests carried out in partly occluded or stenosed vascular segments brought essentially the same results. As in the tests with muscle tissue, a greater energy output was necessary to create a correspondingly large lumen with the matted 3-mm sapphire. It was also necessary to switch from a pulsed to a continuous energy mode in order to achieve a corresponding canal diameter between 5.5 and 6.0 mm. However, in all five cases a larger lumen was obtained compared to the regular unmatted sapphire. Subsequent inspection of the vascular segment revealed no signs of any vascular wall damage or perforation caused by the laser. Following successful conclusion of the experimental series, it was possible to commence the clinical studies.

CLINICAL INVESTIGATIONS

Indications and Patient Population

Before treatment was initiated, a clinical examination was performed together with a detailed case history. The clinical examination included assessments of walking distance, ankle-arm indices (AAI) from Doppler and pressure values, and stipulation of the precise stage according to Fontaine's classification together with intravenous (i.v.) digital subtraction angiography (DSA). In the follow-up phase, the corresponding parameters were performed after 3, 6, and 12 months and at yearly intervals thereafter or whenever complaints occurred so that any recurrent stenosis could be detected and eliminated as soon as possible. Routine i.v. DSA was restricted to 6-month intervals.

The case histories of all patients revealed several recurrent stenoses or occlusions treated by PTA before they received stent implantation. The mean age of the four female and six male patients monitored in this study was 67 years (range, 56 to 83 years). Before endoprosthesis implantation started, the clinical stage according to Fontaine ranged from class IIb to IV, with three patients in stage IIb, five patients in stage III, and two patients in stage IV. Prior to stent implantation, six patients had two recurrences following PTA treatment, three patients had three recurrences, and one patient had four recurrences.

The duration of the first recurrence-free interval following stenting varied from 6 to 10 months. Three patients had a recurrence in the stent after only 6 months, two after 7 months, four after 8 months, and one patient after 10 months. The numbers of re-PTA treatments in the stent varied from none to two. The clinical stage according to Fontaine was improved in six cases to stage I, in three cases to stage IIa, and in one stage to stage IIb. Indication for use of the modified laser was therefore limited to patients with relatively short-term recurrences in the stented vascular segment.

Results

All ten patients were treated successfully with the method described above. In all cases, a vascular lumen of between 5- and 6-mm diameter was obtained using the laser with the matted 3-mm sapphire. The final diameter of the canal, and thus of the vascular lumen, were directly dependent on the duration of laser energy emission. Normally, laser treatment started with an output of 10 watts in pulsed mode, increasing to 25 watts depending on progress made in the vascular segment. Once a diameter of approximately 4 mm had been reached, energy emission was switched from a pulse rate to a continuous mode in order to widen the canal. Here also the energy output was slowly increased from 10 to 25 watts in order to widen the canal. Careful backwards and forwards movement of the laser while in continuous mode created maximal smoothness of the vascular canal surface with the aim of reducing the thrombogenic tendency of the vascular wall surface. The degree of energy output in continuous mode was controlled by x-ray according to the mobility and friction of the probe while carefully pushing and pulling. The actual diameter of the canal was registered by parallel angiograms. Continuous laser energy output was only tolerable when the probe was kept constantly moving in order to avoid any local injuries by overheating the deeper vascular wall layers. Discomfort such as feeling heat in the leg indicated excessive local energy output, which had to be corrected by immediate interruption of the laser energy supply and subsequent reduction of the laser energy level. Pain in the vascular wall indicated a possible change in the adventitia.

There were no cases of perforation, dissection, or any other interaction between the laser probe and implanted stent in this study. Later angioscopic controls also revealed no defects in the tantalum stent from use of the laser. The follow-up results after use of the laser as the sole recanalizing measure are summarized in comparison to previously com-bined methods for eliminating restenosis in Figure 2. The results obtained to date have not achieved any significant extension of the recurrence-free interval for recurrences in the stent compared to PTA (Figures 3 and 4).

Discussion

The combined use of the Nd:YAG laser with the sapphire contact probes revealed acceptable ablation conditions, both in the experimental series and in the first clinical studies (1,2,8-10). Three years after the start of a prospective multicenter study, Lammer et al found no significant differences in the results following PTA in comparison to the results obtained after laser recanalization (3,8,9,11-14). One possible explanation is the fact that, as a rule, each use of the laser for recanalization of the vascular system is supplemented by a PTA in order to create a sufficiently wide vascular lumen to maintain good flow. The advantages of using the laser for recanalization of the vascular system, such as the smooth surface of the created canal with an accompanying lower thrombotic tendency of the vascular wall surface together with a lack of mechanical interference with the vascular wall, are completely negated by the following PTA. Thus, the results obtained when PTA follows laser treatment must be expected to be comparable with results obtained with PTA only. Even following recanalization by means of wire, Rotacs, or other techniques, PTA always remains the last of the vascular extension measures (15). It is always the limiting factor, resulting in mechanical alteration and traumatic effects on the vascular wall and subsequent intimal hyperplasia.

In light of our experience with the sensitive situation in the region of the adductor canal, and the extremely hyperproliferative reaction to mechanical irritation or trauma of the vascular wall with prolific repair requirements, I decided to develop the a matted sapphire for the Nd:YAG laser. The objective of the sole use of this sapphire tip was to keep mechanical irritation of the vascular wall as low as possible by eliminating the

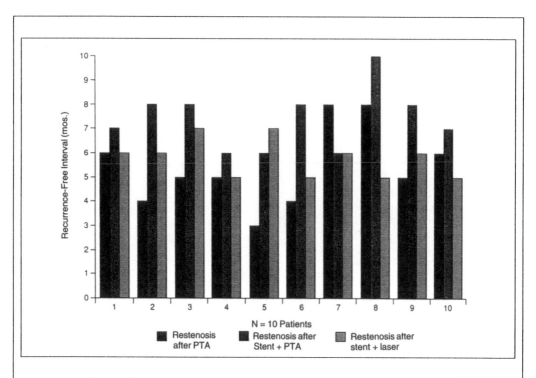

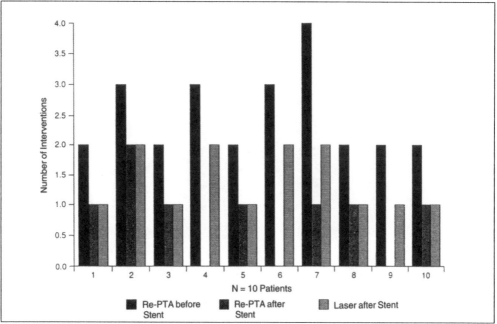

Figure 2. Lifetable analysis after sole laser treatment in the stent *(top)* compared to preceding therapies after reocclusions in the stent *(bottom)*.

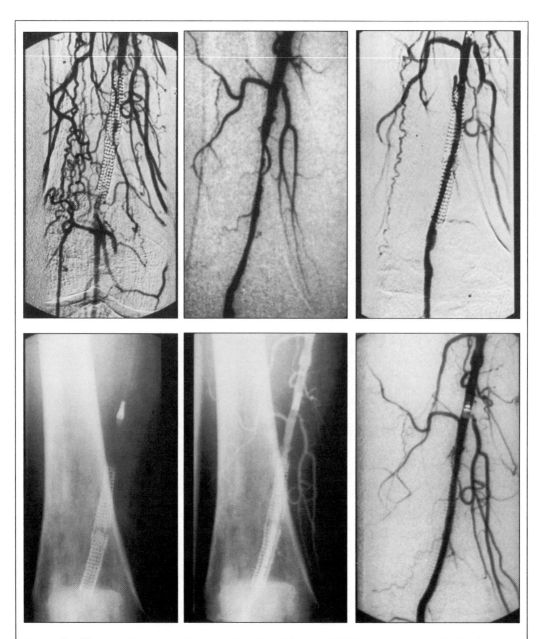

Figure 3. The second recurrence in a stented section of the superficial femoral artery can be clearly seen in this 80-year-old woman. The vascular lumen is nearly completely occluded with good collateralization *(top left)*. A 2-mm sapphire laser has no problems in creating a canal; however, considerable hyperplastic wall thicknesses remain at the edges *(top middle)*. The angiogram shows that after use of the 2-mm laser, there is still considerable hyperplastic wall thickness along the edges of the canal. The 3-mm laser head can be detected above this vascular segment *(top left)*. The 3-mm laser sapphire tip in a plain film image before the stented section of the superficial femoral artery. The disconnection between the two originally overlapping implanted stents can be clearly seen. The stents were pushed apart during redilatation *(bottom left)*. Continuous movement of the laser fitted with 3-mm matted tip backwards and forwards succeeded in ablating the lumen to approximately 6 mm under a 25-watts energy output *(bottom middle)*. Angiogram DSA result following use of the 3-mm laser *(bottom right)*.

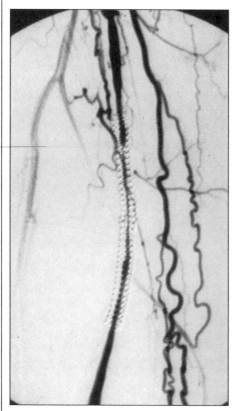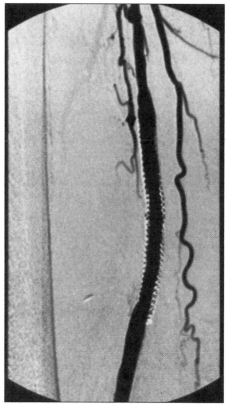

Figure 4. Typical recurrence of intimal hyperplasia of the superficial femoral artery. Pronounced collateralization can also be clearly seen, with increasing constriction of the main vessel *(left)*. Following treatment with the matted laser *(right)*, the lumen can be expanded to the required stent diameter of 6 mm. At the same time, there is a considerable reduction in flow through the collateral blood vessels.

traumatic use of balloon angioplasty. Comparison of the results obtained from the use of the laser alone with consideration of the recurrence-free interval following stent recurrences by PTA indicates that, contrary to our theoretical considerations, no significant extension of the recurrence-free interval has been obtained by avoiding mechanical trauma induced by PTA. There are two possible explanations for these results. One, the thermal strain or irritation of the vascular wall may also have been sufficient to induce regenerative hyperproliferation by myofibroblastic migration, thus causing early reocclusion of the stented vascular segment. Alternatively, it is also possible that the mechanism underlying regenerative hyperproliferative vascular wall reactions involves mediators which are currently unknown. The comparatively small number of patients and their extreme clinical condition, however, precludes any final conclusions regarding the value of sole laser use compared to PTA treatment in the peripheral vascular system.

REFERENCES

1. Lammer J, Pilger E, Kleinert R, Ascher PW. Laserangioplastie peripherer arterieller Verschlüsse: Experimentelle und klinische Ergebnisse. Fortschr Röntgenstr 1987;147: 1-5.

2. Lammer J, Karnel F. Percutaneous transluminal laser angioplasty with contact probes. Radiology 1988;168;733-737.

3. Lammer J, Kleinert R, Pilger E. Contact probes for intravascular recanalization: experimental evaluation. Invest Radiol 1989;24:190-195.

4. Lammer J, Pilger E, Karnel F, et al. Laser angioplasty: results of a prospective, multicenter study. A 3-year follow up. Radiology 1991;178:335-337.

5. Lee G, Lkeda RM, Kozina J, Mason DT. Laser dissolution of coronary atherosclerotic obstruction. Am Heart J 1981;102:1074-1075.

6. Lee G, Ikeda RM, Chan LM. Dissolution of human atherosclerotic disease by fiberoptic laser-heated metal cautery cap. Am Heart J 1984;107:777-778.

7. Sanborn TA, Mitty HA, Train JS, Dan SJ. Infrapopliteal and below knee popliteal lesions: treatment with sole laser thermal angioplasty. Radiology 1989;172:89-93.

8. Cumberland DC, Taylor DI, Proctor AE. Laser assisted percutaneous angioplasty: initial clinical experiences in peripheral arteries. Clin Radiol 1986;37:423-428.

9. Lammer J, Pilger E, Kleinert, R. Laser angioplasty by sapphire contact probe: experimental and clinical results. J Interv Radiol 1988;3:53-58.

10. Vollmar J. Rezidiveingriffe an der Aorta abdominalis und den Beckenarterien. Langenbecks Arch Chir Suppl, Kongressbericht 1991:514-518.

11. Abela GS, Normann S, Cohen D, Feldman RL, Geiser EA, Conti CR. Effects of carbon dioxide, ND-YAG and argon laser radiation on coronary atheromatous plaques. Am J Cardiol 1982;50:1199-1205.

12. Daikuzono N, Joffre SN. An artificial sapphire probe for contact photocoagulation and tissue vaporization. Med Instrum 1985;19:173-178.

13. Geschwind H, Boussignac G, Teisseire B. Percutaneous transluminal laser angioplasty in man (letter). Lancet 1984;1:844.

14. Geschwind H, Dubois-Randé J, Bonner F, Boussignac G, Prevosti L, Leon M. Percutaneous pulsed laser angioplasty with atheroma detection in humans. J Am Coll Cardiol 1988;11:2-107A.

15. Vallbracht C, Kollath J, Roth FJ, et al. Grundlagen, Technik und Ergebnisse der Rotanionsangioplastie. In: *Gefäßchirurgie im Fortschritt*. Stuttgart: Thieme Verlag; 1991;249-254.

Temporary Stenting

D. Liermann

Department of Radiology, J.W. Goethe University Hospital, Frankfurt am Main, Germany

INTRODUCTION

The introduction of interventional measures in the treatment of arterial occlusive disease (AOD) has seen the development of new recanalization techniques (1) which are capable of successfully recanalizing old, long occlusions, without being able to keep these vascular segments open in all cases by means of percutaneous transluminal angioplasty (2-9). This resulted in a marked reduction in the PTA success rate for our patients and prompted us to look for a more promising method of keeping the vascular lumen open. Following our own experimental studies, we initially decided to use the tantalum endoprosthesis and later other prostheses for the clinical treatment of the vascular system. The preferred location was always the distal superficial femoral artery with recurring stenoses or occlusions. Following considerable initial success, there was a particularly high restenosis rate of up to 60% in peripheral vessels treated with stents. Revision of these occlusions and stenoses was inevitable. Measures for revision of stenoses in vessels treated with stents cause damage to the vascular wall, and thus almost always lead to intimal hyperplasia (2,3,5-7,9-19). Some authors presume that use of the stent itself also causes vascular wall damage and thus would not necessarily lead to any notable improvement in patency rates compared to simple PTA (17,20-25). One alternative could possibly be a combination of methods for treating intimal hyperplasia. The good results obtained in treating keloids by radiation therapy (26-37) formed the basis for our therapeutic concept involving prophylactic irradiation of the hyperproliferative vascular wall reaction. The development of small-caliber probes for afterloading treatment of the biliary tract (38) allowed us to use the same in vascular therapy. This method, however, is initially reserved for only a small group of patients, and routine use is not yet in sight.

The experimental studies I conducted with the implantation and explantation of various prostheses gave me the idea that an endoprosthesis which can be easily removed after a certain period of time could possibly help avoid the myointimal hyperplasia caused by permanent implantation. The most suitable target for the temporary use of these stents in stenoses and occlusions seemed to be dissections of iatrogenic genesis during recanalization.

MATERIALS AND METHODS

After experimental studies, the only stent remaining suitable for no-risk implantation and explantation in the peripheral arterial vascular system without causing damage to the vascular walls was the tantalum Strecker™ stent (Boston Scientific Corp., Denmark). The Wallstent™ (Medinvent, Lausanne, Switzerland) and Palmaz™ stent (Johnson & Johnson Interventional Systems Co., Warren NJ) failed completely during explantation, and the nitinol stent could not be recovered without damaging the vascular walls. Consequently, the tantalum stent was used for the treatment of dissections with observation to a strict anticoagulation protocol, when other means of treating the dissection failed. The temporary use of tantalum endoprostheses for 24 hours was preceded by several long-term PTA tests. Repeated dilatation for at least 5 minutes made it possible to affix the dissection in more than 70% of the cases, and thus treatment could be successfully concluded.

Temporary stent implantation was only relevant for the remaining 30% of cases.

For this purpose, each particular tantalum stent was implanted using normal techniques. The sheath remained in position for 24 hours and the patient was infused with heparin 1000 IU/hour through the sheath. A control angiogram was performed after 24 hours. The stent was then removed from its position. A commercially available polypus forceps (Boston Scientific Corp., Watertown MA) (7 Fr) or (Cook, Europe) (9 Fr) was carefully inserted as recovery forceps, and gradually pushed the forceps through to the stented area. The three forceps arms were opened by pulling on a handle at the back of the forceps. The arms are rounded on the outside and at the tip to avoid vascular damage, but have a sharp hook on the inside so that when the forceps is carefully pushed forward in an open condition, it can snare in the mesh of the stent. After ensnaring the stent, the forceps arms are closed again by moving the handle forwards and the stent is carefully pulled into the sheath. It does not matter in which section of the stent the forceps are applied. When using the relatively stable Terumo sheath, we always managed to pull the stent-forceps combination completely into the sheath, without damaging the sheath in doing so. When using a soft or thin-walled sheath, it is possible for an undesirable concertina effect to occur which can only be removed by surgery under anaesthesia. The seal valve of the sheath was destroyed when the stent-forceps combination was pulled through. It is advisable to apply a new sheath via wire in routine cases to avoid blood loss. A subsequent angiogram on several levels provides a control.

EXPERIMENTAL STUDIES

For the experimental studies, we were provided with commercially available tantalum stents fixed on a 5 Fr Meditech balloon catheter with diameters ranging from 8 to 11 mm and lengths from 3 to 8 cm. They were positioned according to the vascular anatomy and degree of stenosis. The stents were positioned through an 8 or 9 Fr Terumo sheath through which the stents were also recovered. Stent implantation was preceded by vascular x-ray with contrast medium and, on evidence of corresponding stenoses, probing by means of a guidewire and dilatation with a commercially available balloon catheter. The stent was then deployed using normal techniques by balloon insufflation with pressure injection. Following this procedure, four different experiments were performed. In the first series, 10 stents were deployed in human cadaver arteries and removed using special recovery forceps. The human cadaver arteries were made available by the Pathological Institute of our clinic after review of the case histories and autopsy findings. For our experiments, we used only stenosed pelvic arteries of patients with a known history of AOD.

The following procedure was performed for all series of experiments under x-ray control. After deployment of the stent, it was carefully recovered from its position using forceps as described above, and pulled through the sheath. In addition to the described tantalum stent, extraction tests were also carried out with Palmaz, Wallstent, and nitinol stents. As indicated, the results with these tests indicated that only the tantalum stent could be recovered without causing injuries (Table 1-4, Figures 1-3). Experimental stent extraction of the tantalum stent from human cadaver arteries using the recovery forceps and Terumo sheath was successful in all attempts. Apart from damage to the valve of the Terumo sheath and notches to the tip of the sheath, no other damage was seen. All tantalum stents were completely recovered and no damage to the vascular walls was caused in any extraction attempt. The stents were localized seven times in the common iliac artery and three times in the external iliac artery. All patients had suffered from AOD, although the degree of atherosclerosis in the pelvic artery did not always coincide with the clinical stage

Table 1. Experimental Implantation of Tantalum Endoprostheses in the Iliac Arteries of Human Cadavers: Endoprosthesis Removal with Special Forceps

Sex	Age	Localization	Atherosclerosis Severity	Fontaine Stage	Complete Extraction?	Damage to Vascular Wall?
Male	72	I. com.	Severe	III	Yes	No
Male	78	I. com.	Minor	II	Yes	No
Female	65	I. com.	Severe	II	Yes	No
Male	78	I. ext.	Minor	II	Yes	No
Male	75	I. com.	Severe	IV	Yes	No
Female	70	I. com	Severe	II	Yes	No
Female	68	I. ext.	Minor	II	Yes	No
Female	82	I. ext.	Severe	II	Yes	No
Female	70	I. com.	Minor	II	Yes	No
Male	89	I. com.	Severe	III	Yes	No

KEY: I. com. = common iliac artery; I. ext. = external iliac artery

Table 2. Experimental Implantation of Palmaz Endoprostheses in Iliac Arteries of Human Cadavers: Endoprosthesis Removal with Special Forceps

Sex	Age	Localization	Atherosclerosis Severity	Fontaine Stage	Complete Extraction?	Vascular Wall Damage?
Female	67	I. com.	Minor	II	No *	(No) *
Male	79	I. com.	Minor	II	No *	(No) *
Male	59	I. ext.	Severe	II	No *	(No) *

KEY: I. com. = common iliac artery; I. ext. = external iliac artery

* It was not possible to remove the stent correctly from its position or to mobilize the stent from its position. Vascular wall damage was not caused because we dispensed without stent extraction with the use of force on account of the preliminary tests.

Table 3. Experimental Implantation of Nitinol Endoprostheses in the Iliac Arteries of Human Cadavers: Endoprosthesis Removal with Special Forceps

Sex	Age	Localization	Atherosclerosis Severity	Fontaine Stage	Complete Extraction?	Damage to Vascular Wall?
Male	78	I. ext.	Minor	II	Yes	No
Male	81	I. com.	Minor	II	Yes	No
Female	62	I. ext.	Severe	III	Yes	No
Female	56	I. com.	Minor	II	(Yes) *	No
Male	78	I. com.	Severe	III	(Yes) *	No
Male	63	I. ext.	Severe	II	(Yes) *	No

KEY: I. com. = common iliac artery; I. ext. = external iliac artery

* The stent was completely recovered but caused material damage to the sheath.

Table 4. Experimental Implantation of Wallstent Endoprostheses in Iliac Arteries of Human Cadavers: Endoprosthesis Removal with Special Forceps

Sex	Age	Localization	Atherosclerosis Severity	Fontaine Stage	Complete Extraction?	Damage to Vascular Wall?
Male	64	I. ext.	Minor	II	No *	Yes *
Male	69	I. com.	Minor	II	No *	Yes *
Female	71	I. com.	Severe	III	No *	Yes *

KEY: I. com. = common iliac artery; I. ext. = external iliac artery

* It was not possible to remove the stent correctly. The result was concertina deformation of the sheath, ring-shaped change to the stent, and following additional force, tearing of the vessel at the puncture site.

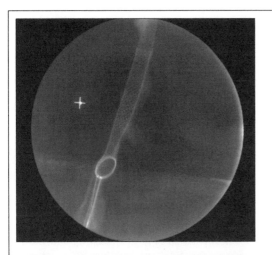
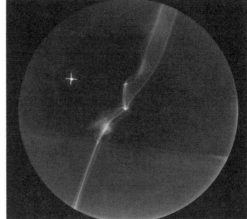
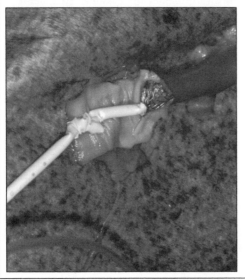

Figure 1. During an attempt to remove the implanted Wallstent from the iliac artery using forceps, the lower end changed to a ring shape without the stent moving *(top left and right)*. During the attempt to remove the stent from the vascular system through the sheath, the sheath was pushed together like a concertina without it being possible to extract the stent *(bottom)*.

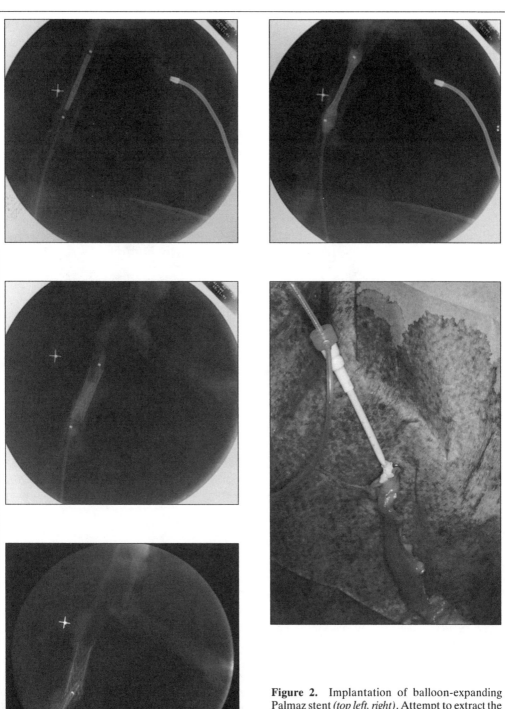

Figure 2. Implantation of balloon-expanding Palmaz stent *(top left, right)*. Attempt to extract the Palmaz stent using forceps. During extraction, the stent was merely deformed in the caudal area *(middle, bottom left)*. The extraction attempt resulted in deformation of the sheath *(bottom right)*.

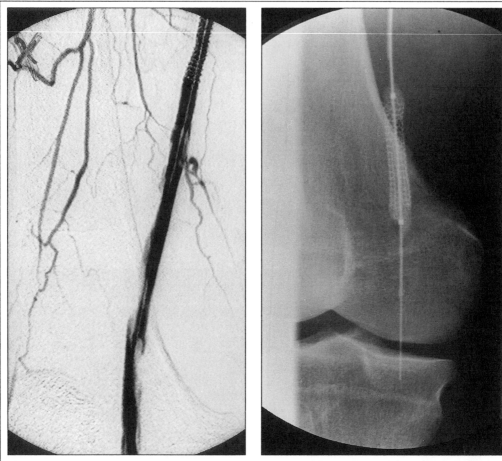

Figure 3. Recanalization of an occlusion of the superficial femoral artery in the adductor channel resulted in extended dissection, which could only be mastered following repeated PTA attempts by implanting a stent.

according to Fontaine. Altogether, we had six slight and four severe changes. Clinical analysis of the case histories of the patients using Fontaine's classification revealed seven cases of stage II, two cases of stage III, and one case of stage IV.

INDICATIONS

All cases with iatrogenic dissections were accepted as indicated, without any specific age or sex restrictions. Pre-condition for use of the temporary stent was merely the futile attempt to affix the dissection by prolonged PTA balloon time exceeding 5 or more minutes. The patients were informed in detail about the risks of the 24-hour stent implantation and particularly about the risk of bleeding with the positioned sheath, together with possible surgical alternatives. This study did not include cases with unsatisfactory PTA results but no dissection. This group of patients was to be included in a second study following successful completion of this first study. In contrast to permanent stent implantation, Marcumar® therapy of the patients was not necessary.

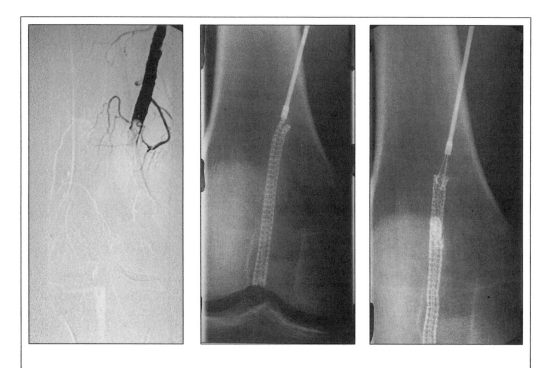

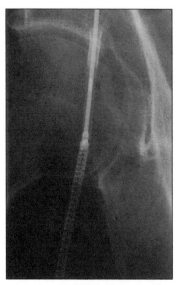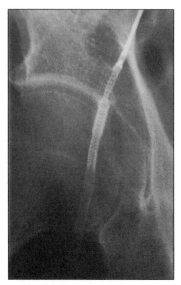

Figure 4. Treatment of a dissection following PTA of an occlusion in the right femoral artery following reocclusion with implantation of a temporary stent. Reoccurred, thrombotic occlusion in a previously recanalized occlusion *(top left)*. The forceps was positioned in front of the stent so that it could be used for recovery 24 hours later *(top middle)*. Interaction between the open, ensnared arms of the forceps and the expanded stent in the superficial femoral artery resulted in the stent initially being squashed together and then extracted *(top right)*. The forceps-stent tandem was pulled into the introduction sheath *(bottom left)*. The stent was removed easily through the sheath valve *(bottom right)*.

PATIENT POPULATION

This study involved 45 patients with pronounced AOD (Fontaine stages III and IV). They were suffering from long-length occlusions of the femoral artery which had been recanalized either by rotation angioplasty or by means of Terumo wire and bent catheter (Beerenstein), resulting in dissection with clear drain blockage through to stasis. This was the case in up to 2% of all recanalizations with the prerequisites described above. A further condition included repeated, prolonged, long-term PTA without success, which was the case in 25% of all therapies.

This resulted in a group of 13 patients satisfying the study conditions defined above. The patients included seven men and six women, aged between 56 to 87 years (mean, 71 years). All had advanced AOD according to Fontaine with ten patients having stage III and three having stage IV. Corresponding ankle-arm indices (AAI) were between 0.23 and 0.4 for the affected side before the treatment. Walking distance was clearly reduced to under 200 m. Other risk factors included nicotine abuse (75%), diabetes mellitus (45%), and long-term dialysis treatment (20%).

The post-treatment protocol for temporary stent implantation covered peri-interventional heparin therapy with heparin 1000 IU/hour by a perfusor, together with corresponding further treatment for 72 hours with the same dose. Aspirin was administered as long-term therapy. Follow-up examinations included assessments of AAI, painless walking distance, and clinical condition, together with intravenous (i.v.) digital subtraction angiography (DSA) at 6-month intervals.

RESULTS

Between 1982 and 1993, we have performed 5,400 dilatations, with 3,125 in the femoral arteries alone. Looking at femoral artery occlusions with iatrogenic dissections during recanalization, we had to expect long-length occlusions with dissections in approximately 2% of all recanalization cases. Forty-five of the dissections in the adductor canal thus registered were treated with this prolonged dilatation for at least 5 minutes. In 32 cases, this therapy was successful on its own. In 13 cases, the failure of this therapy led to temporary stent implantation, of which 11 cases were treated successfully (Figure 5). Only in two cases was it necessary to proceed with permanent stent implantation. We used stents with diameters between 6 and 7 mm and lengths between 4 and 8 cm. Following stent implantation, the patients were returned to the ward for 24 hours with a positioned sheath and under heparin therapy. Extraction of the stent with the forceps described above also succeeded without any difficulties. No evidence was found of damage to the vascular walls. The 11 patients with successful therapy were treated in the usual manner with a pressure dressing and given heparin therapy for a further 72 hours. The two therapy failures were given a permanent stent (Palmaz stent). Surgery was not necessary in any of the cases. The AAI increased to values between 0.65 and 0.95 (mean, 0.78), and the free walking distance improved from at least 300 m in some cases to unlimited in others. The clinical condition according to Fontaine improved from stage II to IV pre-treatment to stage IIb in three cases, stage IIa in eight cases, and stage I in two cases.

DISCUSSION

The results of the experimental series indicate that the tantalum stent is the only stent suitable for extraction. All other currently available stents are either not extractable or can only be extracted with considerable damage to the vascular wall. Therefore, the tantalum stent was considered the only possible stent for temporary use in the vascular system. Although the tantalum stent can be compressed with relative ease, this phenomenon was not observed. In all patients, the 7 Fr recovery forceps was adequate under clinical conditions. Consideration of the success rate for temporary stent implantation allows this method to be called successful. The dissection was successfully treated in 11 of 13 cases.

Initial experiments are already being performed for the development of alternative temporary stents. One development concerns a memory metal stent; it is hoped that by changing the temperature, the stent can be caused to collapse, facilitating extraction. Other models which also aim at avoiding stimulation of myointimal hyperproliferation, involved so-called resorbable stents which are incorporated into the vascular wall after a set period of time, where they are epithelialized and then dissolve. Here again, research is still limited to the animal experiment stage. The exciting aspect of this particular idea is that the use of temporary stents may possibly cause a lower degree of hyperproliferative reaction, thus resulting in a lower restenosis risk compared to permanent stent implantation. The described secondary problems of permanent stent implantation would thus possibly become avoidable.

REFERENCES

1. Vallbracht C, Kollath J, Roth FJ, et al. Grundlagen, Technik und Ergebnisse der Rotationsangioplastie. In: *Gefäßchirurgie im Fortschritt*. Stuttgart: Thieme Verlag; 1991;249-254.
2. Clowes AW, Reidy MA, Clowes MM. Kinetics of cellular proliferation after arterial injury. Lab Invest 1983;49:327-334.
3. Cox JL, Gottlieb AL. Restenosis following percutaneous transluminal angioplasty: Clinical, physiological and pathological features. Can Med Assoc J 1986;134:1129-1132.
4. Faxon DP, Sanborn TA, Haudenschild CC. Mechanism of angioplasty and its relation to restenosis. Am J Cardiol 1987;60:5B-9B.
5. Ip JH, Fuster V, Badimon L, Badimon J, Taubman MB, Chesebro JH. Syndromes of accelerated atherosclerosis. Role of vascular injury and smooth muscle cell proliferation. J Am Coll Cardiol 1990;15:1667-1687.
6. Laerum BF, Vlodaver Z, Castaneda-Zuniga WR, Edwards E, Amplatz K. The mechanism of angioplasty. Fortschr Röntgenst 1982;136:573-576.
7. Spaet TH, Stemermann MB, Veith FJ, Lejnieks I. Intimal injury and regrowth in the rabbit aorta. Medial smooth muscle cells as a source of neointima. Circ Res 1975;36:58-70.
8. Wissler RW. Principles of the pathogenesis of atherosclerosis. in: Braunwald E, ed. *Heart Disease: A Textbook of Cardiovascular Medicine. Vol 2*. Philadelphia: WB Saunders; 1984;1183-1204.
9. Zollikofer CL, Cragg AH, Hunter DW, Yedlicka JW, Castaneda-Zuniga WR, Amplatz K. Mechanism of transluminal angioplasty. In: Castaneda-Zuniga WR and Tadavarthy SM, eds. *Interventional Radiology*. Baltimore: Williams & Wilkins; 1992; 249-298.
10. Clowes AW, Karnovsky MJ. Suppression by heparin of smooth muscle cell proliferation in injured arteries. Nature 1977;265:625-626.
11. Essed CE, Van den Brand M, Becker AE. Transluminal coronary angioplasty and early restenosis: fibrocellular occlusion after wall laceration. Br Heart J 1983;49:393-396.
12. Faxon DP, Sanborn TA, Weber VJ. Restenosis following transluminal angioplasty in experimental atherosclerosis. Arteriosclerosis 1984;4:189-195.
13. Gall FP, Franke F. Chronische Veshlußprozesse der Arteria fesoropoplitea. In: Heberer G and Dongen RJAM, eds. *Gefäßchirurgie*. Berlin: Springer; 1987; 404-414.
14. Friedman JR, Burns R. Role of platelets in the proliferative response of the injured artery. Prog Hemost Thromb 1978;4:249-278.
15. Garth EA, Ratliff NB, Hollman J, Tabei, S, Phillips FD. Intimal proliferation of smooth muscle cells as an explanation for recurrent coronary artery stenosis after percutaneous transluminal coronary angioplasty. J Am Coll Cardiol 1985;6:369-372.
16. Hashizume M, Yang Y, Galt S. Intimal response of saphenous vein to intraluminal trauma by simulated angioscopic insertion. J Vasc Surg 1987;5:862-868.
17. Imparato AM, Bracco A, Kim GE, Zeff R. Intimal and neointimal fibrous proliferation causing failure of arterial reconstructions. Surgery, 1972;172:1007-1017.

18. Nobuyoshi M, Kimura T, Ohishi H, Horiuchi H. Restenosis after percutaneous transluminal coronary angioplasty: pathologic observations in 20 patients. J Am Coll Cardiol 1991;17:433-439.

19. Ueda M, Becker AE, Fujimoto T. Pathological changes induced by repeated persutaneous transluminal coronary angioplasty. Br Heart J 1987;58:635-643.

20. Leung DYM, Glagov S, Matthews MB. Cyclic stretching stimulates synthesis of matrix components by arterial smooth muscle cells *in vitro*. Science 1976;191:475-477.

21. Liermann D, Böttcher HD, Kollath J, et al. Prophylactic endovascular radiotherapy to prevent intimal hyperplasia after stent implantation in femoropopliteal arteries. Cardiovasc Intervent Radiol 1994;17:12-16.

22. Liu MW, Roubin GS, King SB. Restenosis after coronary angioplasty. Potential biologic determinants and rose of intimal hyperplasia. Circulation 1989;79:1374-1387.

23. Palmaz JC, Windeler SA, Garcia F. Atherosclerotic rabbit aortas: expandable intraluminal grafting. Radiology 1986; 160:723-726.

24. Rollins N, Wright KC, Charnsangavej C, Gianturco C. Self-expanding metallic stents: preliminary evaluation in an atherosclerotic model. Radiology 1987;163:739-742.

25. Rousseau H, Joffre F, Raillat C, et al. Self-expanding endovascular stent in experimental atherosclerosis. Radiology 1989;170: 773-778.

26. Baensch W. Über die Strahlenbehandlung der Keloide. Strahlentherapie 1937;60: 204-209.

27. Craig RDP, Pearson D. Early post-operative irradiation in the treatment of keloid scars. Br J Past Surg 1965;18:369-375.

28. Crocett DJ. Regional keloid susceptibility. Br J Past Surg 1964;17:245-253.

29. Dalicho W. Zur Therapie der Keloide mit besonderer Berücksichtigung der Radiumbestrahlung. Strahlentherapie 1949;78.

30. Enhamre A, Hammar H. Treatment of keloids with excision and postoperative x-ray irradiation. Dermatologica 1983;167:90-93.

31. Graul EH. Zur Klinik des Keloids. Strahlentherapie 1955;98:119-132.

32. Kovalic JJ, Perez CA. Radiation therapy following keloidectomy: A 20 year experience. Radiation Oncology. Biol Phys 1989;17:77-80.

33. Krüger A. Über Keloide und ihre Behandlung unter besonderer Berücksichtigung der Strahlentherapie. Strahlentherapie 1945;93:426-433.

34. Levy DS, Salter MM, Roth RE. Postoperative irradiation in the prevention of keloids. Am J Roentg 1981;127:509-510.

35. Ollstein RN, Siegel HW, Gilloley JF, Barsa JMM. Treatment of keloids by combined surgical excision and immediate postoperative X-ray therapy. Ann Plast Surg 1981;7:281-284.

36. Scherer E. Kontaktbestrahlung mit radioaktiven Stoffen in Hdb.Med.Radiol., Bd.XW2. Springer; 1970;136-146.

37. Wagner W, Schophol B, Böttcher HD, Scheppner E. Ergebnisse der Narbenkeloidprophylaxe durch Kontaktbestrahlung mit Strontium 90. Röntgenpraxis 1989;42: 248-252.

38. Brambs HJ, Freund U, Bruggmoser G, Wannenmacher M. Kombinierte intraduktale perkutane Radiotherapie bei malignen Gallengangsobstruktionen mit anschließender prothetischer Versorgung. Onkologie 1987;10:84-89.

Polymeric Endoluminal Paving: Evolving Therapeutic Methods for Extending the Spectrum of Local Endovascular Interventions

Marvin J. Slepian

University Heart Center, University of Arizona, Tucson, AZ USA

INTRODUCTION AND RATIONALE FOR DEVELOPMENT OF AN ENDOLUMINAL PAVING APPROACH

Over the past decade, great strides have been made in the percutaneous treatment of atherosclerotic coronary and peripheral vascular disease. Balloon angioplasty has emerged as the primary therapy for high grade, obstructive, atherosclerotic coronary artery disease. Newer therapies such as atherectomy, lasers, and stents have appeared as alternative or adjunctive therapies for revascularization (1). Acute procedural success rates have improved, and the scope of lesions approachable by these non-surgical technologies has increased. Despite these significant advances in percutaneous revascularization therapy, the overall long-term success of these approaches remains limited by vessel reclosure several months post-procedure (2-5). Beyond this significant and expensive shortcoming, a much broader conceptual limitation exists with regard to the current overall approach to revascularization. From its inception, the central focus of percutaneous revascularization has been on the mechanical process of creating a large, stable vessel lumen. Despite our ability to access arterial stenoses percutaneously and mechanically re-establish a larger lumen, to date we have not attempted to treat or alter the underlying natural history of either the primary atherosclerotic lesion or the secondary post-intervention lesion following initial mechanical revascularization. With recent increased insight into the contributory role of cellular and biochemical factors in atherosclerotic progression and restenosis, a need exists for therapies which go beyond current, predominately mechanical, interventions.

Of the new interventional technologies to emerge over the past few years, the most promising thus far has been endovascular stenting (6-8). Stents have proven effective as arterial wall supports to prevent abrupt reclosure (9-11), and more recently have been demonstrated to partially limit the development of restenosis (12-14). Despite the success of current metal stents, they remain limited as first generation endoluminal implants by a propensity for thrombosis with subsequent subacute closure (15-20), difficult placement (21), stiffness (22), migration (14,23), wall thinning (24), aneurysm formation (25,26), limited flexibility (21), compliance mismatch (27,28), spasm (29), and progressive intra-stent restenosis (30-36).

In an effort to overcome these experimentally-demonstrated limitations of stents, as well as begin development of a broad-based endovascular therapeutic approach to biomanipulate *de novo* and post-interventional atherosclerotic lesions, efforts began in 1987 to examine the potential of applying biodegradable polymers locally as "form in place", therapeutic endoluminal liners. The basic operating tenant of this approach has been that biodegradable polymers, custom-molded in place, provide the potential for a broad-scope means of addressing several mechanisms which contribute to vessel reclosure or other local, endovascular, pathological processes. A custom-molded endoluminal polymeric liner, uniquely conforming to a given lesion topography, would address vessel wall recoil and lumen-protruding dissection flaps which mechanically contribute to vessel reclosure. A polymeric liner might also serve as a local barrier to overflowing thrombogenic and inflammatory blood elements, thereby interfering with their contribution to vessel reclosure mechanisms. Through selection of a particular polymeric substrate for a given lesion or arterial wall pathology, the polymer as a therapeutic biomaterial itself might exert a locally desirable effect by virtue of its individual material or chemical properties. Further, application of a drug-laden polymeric liner would provide a means for altering arterial wall or lesion pathology through focused, localized, controlled release of bioactive pharmacologic agents at the lesion site associated with degradation of the polymer excipient. Use of biodegradable polymers as a local therapeutic platform would provide a specific advantage in that lesion-directed therapy could be temporary, without the necessity for device removal, and multi-targeted, addressing several operative pathophysiologic mechanisms. Thus, incorporation of a drug-laden polymeric liner would go beyond the restricted focus of a mechanical stent and provide the physical targeting unachievable with systemically-administered drugs.

In 1988, we described the initial embodiment of this broad therapeutic approach known generically as polymeric endoluminal paving. In this method, thin tubes or sheets of biodegradable polymers are locally applied percutaneously to vessels as endoluminal liners, resurfacing (paving) the underlying arterial wall and functioning as local wall supports (37,38). In its initial prototype form, a slitted tube of biodegradable polymers was applied to a specific endovascular site via a balloon catheter and locally thermoformed to yield an adherent, conformal, structurally-supportive, thin polymer film. Over the last few years, polymer paving has evolved from this initial point and has been transformed from a generic methodological approach into several actual prototype treatment systems involving different types of polymeric materials. An update on paving is provided in this paper. Specifically, the overall process of polymeric endoluminal paving is described with the generic paving process outlined, and several possible therapeutic embodiments of paving emerging from this generic process discussed. Recent experimental studies with two forms of paving — solid paving and gel paving — are reviewed. Finally, the role of these paving forms in future approaches to vascular therapy are discussed.

THE POLYMER PAVING PROCESS

Generic Description of the Paving Process

Polymeric endoluminal paving in its most generic form is a process in which biocompatible polymers may be applied to the endoluminal surface of an organ or organ component and custom contoured *in situ* via a catheter to yield a polymeric layer or film in intimate contact with the underlying tissue surface. The polymer application process reconfigures the polymer, allowing it to mold and adapt to the underlying tissue topography, while at the same time generating a smooth balloon-molded endoluminal surface. The overall "tissue resurfacing" process has been termed 'paving'.

In a cardiovascular application, the target for paving typically is an artery, vein, or graft. Extending beyond vascular applications, many other tubular organs or organ component structures, e.g., esophagus, trachea, bile or pancreatic duct and others amenable to balloon catheter polymer application, are also potential therapeutic targets for paving (39).

Three Forms of Paving

Polymer paving in its current state of development may be thought of as a family of therapeutic approaches. Depending upon the choice of polymer system utilized as the substrate for paving, a variety of physical forms of endoluminal paving layers may be formed. As such, utilizing materials of differing consistencies raises the possibility for differing types of therapeutic effects and residence times for polymers locally at the site of application. Specifically, three forms of polymer paving have been envisioned and experimentally demonstrated to date: solid paving, gel paving, and liquid paving.

Solid Paving

Solid or structural paving was the initial form of paving to be experimentally demonstrated (40). In this form, thin tubes or sheets of biodegradable polymers are transported intravascularly via catheter, positioned at the lesion site, and locally remolded intraluminally via catheter-based thermoforming of the baseline material. In contrast to stenting which relies on either the inherent expansile tendency of a constrained stent (i.e., self-expanding stents) or active mechanical deformation (i.e., balloon-expanding stents) for deployment and expansion, solid paving relies on catheter-based mechanical deformation combined with controlled phase changes of the polymer material, typically through a local heating and cooling process. The phase changes involved include conversion of the polymer locally from solid to liquid and back to solid at the site of deployment. Advantage is taken of the thermoplastic nature of several biodegradable polymers, co-polymers, or blends in that localized simultaneous polymer heating and balloon molding allows the polymer substrate to flow and conform to the irregularities and interstices frequently encountered in many endoluminal surface pathologies while maintaining a balloon-dictated smooth luminal surface. Further, by pre-modifying the polymer substrate with fenestrations, the flow can be "directed" with predictable shapes and forms resulting. The resultant polymer lining may have partially open walls, thereby presenting a reduced foreign material load to the vessel as well as allow for blood flow through the side branch ostia if desired or dictated by a given therapeutic application. Solid paving offers multiple therapeutic possibilities (see below), including endoluminal wall support, physical

barrier layer imposition, and localized controlled and sustained intraluminal drug delivery.

To more fully appreciate the process of polymer paving, sequential photographs taken during an early polymer deployment experiment in a "mock" blood vessel are presented in Figure 1. A small fenestrated tube of pre-deployed polymer, in this case poly(ε-caprolactone), is seen positioned at the desired location within the vessel on a modified balloon dilatation catheter (Figure 1B). A distal flow occluding catheter is then inserted in the vessel (Figure 1C). In this sequence of photographs, two catheters are utilized for deployment for purposes of illustration, the catheter on the left serving as a distal flow occluding catheter and the one on the right serving as a polymer dilating catheter. In actual *in situ* experiments, a single, dual balloon catheter is utilized. The polymer tube is rapidly heated through infusion of warm saline (60°C) (Figure 1E), facilitating an instantaneous polymer melt with subsequent thermoforming of the polymer through balloon-directed flow (Figure 1F). During this flow, the polymer walls thin and fenestrations expand, creating partial wall openings. This flow also causes the polymer to envaginate into vessel surface irregularities, i.e., with the external polymer surface contour being dictated by the underlying surface of the vessel wall, while the new manufactured surface contoured by the balloon remains smooth and regular. The vessel surface therefore becomes polymer "paved and sealed" (Figure 1G). Immediately following expansion and application of the polymer, the warmed fluid surrounding the polymer is rapidly replaced by "cool" overflowing blood which leads to rapid polymer setting in place. Poly(ε-caprolactone), with a narrow transition temperature range, undergoes a rapid phase change to a semicrystalline solid form, thereby regaining mechanical stability at the "new" balloon-dictated configuration. By virtue of specific paving polymer substrate selection, through use of polymers with varying degrees of

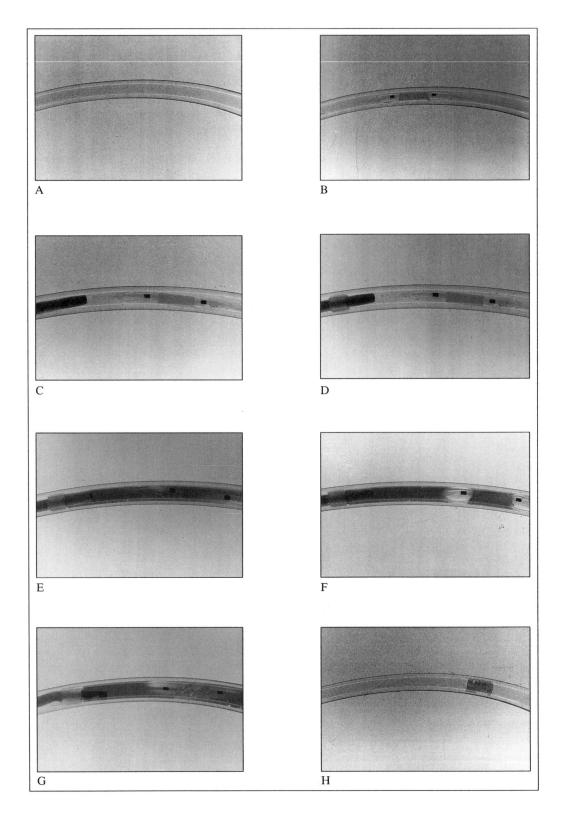

crystallinity, the material properties (rigidity, flexibility, collapse resistance) of a paving layer may be tailored to a specific endoluminal application.

The intravascular melt-flow thermoforming of the polymer substrate which takes place within a vessel may be more clearly appreciated in Figure 2, in which a pre-deployed polymer paving layer may be seen on the left (with this film having minimal fenestrations) and post-deployed polymer removed from an actual acute *in vivo* paving experiment seen on the right. Of note, with pressure-directed flow, the polymer reconfigures the bulk material resulting in the development of macroporous regions in the polymer surface (Figure 2). In addition, while the external configuration of the polymer layer on the right appears somewhat irregular as it has been contoured as a relief of the underlying vessel surface, the internal surface is smooth.

Several different prototype catheter systems for use in applying thin films of structural polymer materials have been designed. Initial catheter systems consisted of a distal compliant occlusion balloon and a proximal non-compliant "paving" balloon. The distal occlusion balloon was used to transiently restrict blood flow allowing for zone isolation and heating, while the paving balloon functioned as a thermoforming balloon. Thermo-

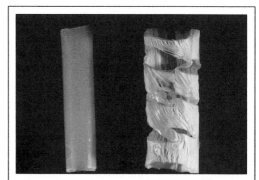

Figure 2. Pre-deployed tube of polymer for structural paving with microscopic fenestrations *(left)*. Expanded, post-deployed tubular polymer paving layer removed from vessel *(right)*. Note development of open regions, engineered to occur in this case.

forming was accomplished via rapidly perfusing the occluded paving zone with warmed saline, both surrounding the polymer via ports in the catheter proximal and distal to the paving balloon, as well as via recirculation of warmed saline within the thermoforming balloon. More recently, several methods of heating have been integrated into paving catheter systems including resistance heating, microwave heating, and fiber optic laser heating.

Recently, a new paving system has been developed which achieves local polymer melting and flow through a thermoselective method (41,42). In this system, described in detail

Figure 1. *In Vitro* solid "structural" paving in transparent mock blood vessel. (See page 342)

A) Mock blood vessel, normal 37°C "blood" flow from right to left.

B) Tubular polymer substrate positioned at desired location within vessel on balloon deployment catheter.

C) Distal, balloon occlusion catheter placed. Balloon deflated.

D) Occlusion catheter balloon inflated to create stagnant column of blood around polymer substrate.

E) Heated saline (60°C) is injected via infusion port to create a column of hot saline surrounding the polymer to facilitate an instant polymer melt.

F) Polymer remains in original form after being surrounded by hot fluid until mild radial dilating force is exerted by deployment balloon with resultant progressive expansion.

G) Further balloon expansion results in pressure-directed polymer flow forming a vessel encasing "polymer paving layer", with the external polymer surface geometry being dictated by the shape of the vessel wall, while the new intraluminal surface is smooth.

H) Following deflation of distal flow occlusion balloon, with return of 37°C blood flow, the polymer paving layer achieves increased mechanical stability. Upon removal of deployment catheter, the applied polymer is left intact with the vessel locally "paved".

below, a photosensitive dye is incorporated within the polymer films to be deployed. Local catheter-based illumination of the polymer at the time of deployment results in selective absorbance of light by the polymer, with local conversion to heat, resulting in polymer melting. Through selection of a dye-illumination wavelength (near infrared) combination, with absorbance characteristics distinctly different form those of tissue, illumination results in transmission of light through tissue with minimal tissue photothermal heating.

Gel Paving

Aside from using solid or structural polymers as substrates for paving, the use of polymeric hydrogel or colloidal systems as the applied polymeric material formed the basis for the second type of paving which has been developed — gel paving (43-45). The rationale for this approach was to develop a modified paving form which would allow creation of *in situ* short-term, non-structural physical barrier layers which are (1) permeable to fluid, gases, and low molecular weight solutes, (2) exclusionary of larger molecular weight compounds, and (3) physically limiting of cell-cell and cell-matrix interactions with the underlying tissue surface. The cardiovascular therapeutic motivation for this type of paving arose in an attempt to develop a physical, non-pharmacologic method of preventing or limiting early interactions between blood (i.e., platelets, white blood cells, and soluble endocrine-functioning mediators) and underlying exposed arterial subintima, which play an essential role in localized thrombosis and the development of intimal hyperplasia (46-48). Specifically, early platelet-wall interactions with the release of platelet-containing growth factors, thrombin deposition, and progressive thrombus formation have all been shown to be contributory mechanisms leading to smooth muscle cell proliferation and extracellular matrix synthesis, ultimately resulting in neointimal hyperplasia and restenosis. By interposing a physical barrier

layer, definitively limiting contact between platelets, white blood cells, and blood-borne growth factors and the arterial wall, a more complete inhibition of these early interactions is likely compared with soluble pharmacologic means which result in a reduction in the activity of platelets, white blood cells, or other factors though with persistent physical contact of these factors with the underlying surface. Through use of polymeric hydrogel or colloidal materials as the substrate for paving, short-term, "bandage-like", semipermeable endoluminal barriers could be created transiently on the vessel wall. The period that these would be in place, days to weeks, is shorter than would be possible with more rigid structural polymer systems which typically take months to biodegrade. These types of materials would also allow creation of either thin or thick polymer barriers, depending upon the particular end use indication and the chemistry and mode of application of the gel system selected. Gel systems also afford advantage in that, depending upon the particular gel chemistry, they may either biodegrade through bond scission or bioerode through solvation or physical thinning. This type of paving may also be utilized as a means of localized drug delivery, though typically of a shorter duration than that achievable with solid paving.

The gel paving process is illustrated in Figure 3 in a series of photographs taken during an *in vitro* gel paving experiment. A thermoreversible hydrogel is formed *in situ* on an arterial wall (Figure 3D), with maintenance of a patent lumen in the paved vessel through use of a mold-core catheter system. A baseline bovine coronary artery is seen in Figure 3A. A mold is created *in situ* within the arterial lumen at the designated polymer deployment site, with the core of the mold being formed by the centrally-positioned catheter and the outer mold wall by the arterial endoluminal surface (Figure 3B). A liquid polymer solution is instilled (Figure 3C), which upon a local temperature change is converted to a hydrogel. The central catheter core is removed and the vessel is left "gel paved" (Figure 3D) with a thin endoluminal rim or layer of hydrogel adherent to the underlying arterial intimal surface.

Several catheter systems have been designed for localized *in situ* formation of both thin and thick hydrogel paving layers. The catheter systems vary depending upon the nature of the flowable baseline material utilized for hydrogel formation as well as the chemical or physical means utilized to locally convert the pre-gel constituents to a gel locally. For the thermoreversible gel system, a modified dual balloon catheter system has been developed which contains two compliant (proximal and distal) occlusion balloons with an interposed shaft or third expanding

mold-core balloon. Recently, a novel gel paving catheter system with a contained fiber optic illuminating element has been developed allowing for *in situ* photopolymerization of polyethylene-glycol-lactide thin hydrogel paving layers (44,49).

Liquid Paving

The third form of paving, liquid paving, involves use of flowable polymeric, macromeric, or pre-polymeric solutions which have varying levels of avidity for the underlying tissue surface. Interactions may range from non-specific, i.e., weak Van der Wall, electrostatic, or hydrogen bonding types, to more specific receptor-ligand interactions or potentially to locally formed covalent

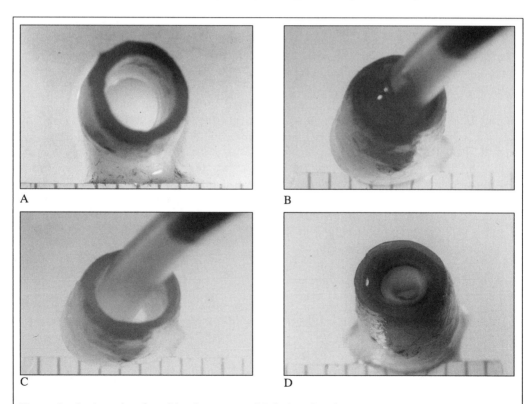

Figure 3. *In vitro* gel paving with a thermoreversible hydrogel paving system.
A) Bovine coronary artery segment in cross section.
B) Catheter positioned in artery lumen to act as a "mold-core".
C) Liquid polymer is instilled and fills cavity of "mold" - the walls of the mold defined by the central, lumen-obstructing (and preserving), catheter and the arterial endoluminal surface.
D) Upon removal of mold-core catheter, a layer of hydrogel, paving the endoluminal surface, remains.

interactions. Interactions may also occur due to physical intercalation or trapping. When fluids for liquid paving are applied locally they interact, coat, or adhere to the underlying tissue surface and act as a short-term thin chemical interface layer. This type of paving may function as a means of transiently changing tissue surface charge, porosity, or lubricity, modifying cellular avidity to overflowing or contacting molecules or cells, or as a means of short-term local drug delivery.

REVIEW OF EXPERIMENTAL STUDIES

Solid Paving

Early studies with solid polymer paving examined the acute efficacy of *in situ* endoluminal deployment of tubes or sheets of polymers as thermoformed thin films. Paving efficacy was examined both *in vitro* and acutely *in vivo*, with efficacy defined in terms of the ability to apply polymer to the vessel wall with maintained wall adherence yet without significant polymer residue remaining attached to the deployment catheter upon its removal. To date, over 100 canine, porcine, bovine, and human vessels have been paved. In all, the polymer has been reliably deployed with maintained polymer tube or sheet expansion and adherence to the underlying vessel wall (38). The conformal nature of an endoluminal paving layer may be appreciated from histologic cross-section of a paved bovine coronary artery (Figure 4). In this case, a solid sheet of poly(ε-caprolactone) was applied to the endoluminal surface. The applied polymer is seen as a wavy refractile layer in intimate contact with the vessel endoluminal surface. Of note, the architecture of the vessel wall underlying the paving zone is preserved with an intact media despite application of the paving layer.

The structural stability and support capability of endoluminal polymer films have been examined extensively both *in vitro* and *in vivo*. In an early study a variety of vessels were purposely over-distended from a base-

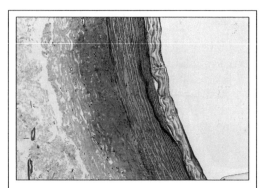

Figure 4.   Paved normal bovine coronary artery in cross section (x100). Paving layer of poly(ε-caprolactone) is visible in intimate contact with the underlying arterial wall. Arterial wall architecture is preserved, with an intact media and adventitia, despite polymer application.

line diameter at 70 mm Hg by 30 to 60%. Despite over-distension, vessels remained dilated at the balloon-dictated, post-deployment dimension without any evidence of polymer compression or collapse acutely. Control dilated and "sham paved" vessels (i.e., without polymer application), however, did not remain dilated, manifesting vessel recoil (37). A dramatic example of the structural stability of a thin endoluminal polymer layer can be seen in Figure 5. On the left, a dilated unpaved vessel is compared with a polymer-

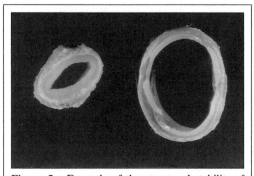

Figure 5.   Example of the structural stability of endoluminal solid paving layer. Baseline bovine coronary artery *(left)*. Contiguous segment of identical bovine coronary artery dilated and paved at balloon:artery ratio > 2:1. Note thin endoluminal polymer paving layer supports vessel wall, resisting recoil and collapse, despite the significant over-dilatation.

lined vessel paved at a dimension of balloon:artery ratio > 2:1 (right). Even at this over-distended dimension the vessel remains dilated without collapse or buckling of the endoluminal paving layer. These studies demonstrated that over a wide range of balloon (paving):artery ratios (range, 1-2.5:1, a range greater than that which would be used clinically), thin endoluminal polymer films are capable of functioning in a stent-like capacity, providing local wall support and maintaining vessels effectively at selected diameters.

Recently, the ability of polymer films to resist *in vivo* vasospasm was examined. It was demonstrated that despite clear induction of spasm with vasoconstrictors, with a detectable rise in blood pressure and an accompanying reduction in arterial caliber, paved zones did not change diameter; rather, they demonstrated adequate structural stiffness to resist *in vivo* spasm-induced recoil.

The hemocompatibility of various biodegradable thermoplastics for potential use in polymer paving has been examined both *in vitro* and *in vivo*. *In vitro*, thin films of several biodegradable polymers were spin cast, placed in a flow chamber, and subjected to overflowing blood at known, controlled shear rates. All biodegradable polymers tested had reduced thrombogenicity compared to Mylar and glass controls. Of the polymers tested, poly(lactic acid):poly(glycolic acid) co-polymer and poly(ε-caprolactone) were less thrombogenic, with relatively less platelet adherence, compared to polylactic acid alone (50).

In vivo hemocompatibility of polymers has been examined as well using both dog and pig implant models. In all cases of successful polymer deployment in which conformal contact of the polymer sheet with the vessel wall was achieved, polymer paved zones were patent without gross thrombus as detected by angiography and follow-up stereomicroscopy of explanted arterial segments, both acutely, i.e., at 2 hours post-deployment, as well as at 1 week post-deployment.

The ability of polymer films to mold and conform *in vitro* to a variety of irregular atherosclerotic plaque surfaces, both *de novo* as well as following angioplasty, has been examined *in vitro* (51). Freshly isolated plaque containing human coronary and carotid arteries were either paved primarily or following balloon dilatation. In all vessels, polymer molding to conform to underlying plaque irregularities was detectable at the polymer-intima interface, while the polymer endoluminal surface remained smooth. Lesion protrusion through the polymer into the vessel lumen was not detected in calcified or non-calcified lesions.

Several *in vivo* studies examining paved vessel patency have been undertaken (38,52). In early studies, small tubes of polymer were deployed in canine carotid arteries and followed serially over a 6-month period. In greater than 75% of cases, patency of paved vessels could be achieved beyond 6 months. In general, at 1 day and 1 week follow-ups, arteries were angiographically patent in cases of successful polymer application. By 1 month, mild lumen narrowing was noted at the polymer zone consistent with either mild intrapolymer thrombus or neointimal hyperplasia. Typically, by 3 months this lumenal narrowing stabilized with partial regression by 6 months. This behavior is consistent with early neointimal hyperplasia and eventual resolution that accompanies endoluminal implant passivation and vessel wall incorporation as is seen with conventional stents (24). In our experience to date, mild endoluminal amorphous proteinaceous fouling or non-occlusive thin thrombus build-up has been observed within the first month following implantation. No appreciable infiltration of polymorphonuclear leukocytes, monocytes, or macrophages has been detected, either adjacent to the polymer or within the underlying vessel wall. In studies by other investigators, an inflammatory response was reported following implantation of a metal stent-polymer hybrid implant in porcine coronary arteries (53). This has not been our experience to date. Similarly, investigators at Duke, examining the tissue response to poly (L-lactide) stents, have not seen an appreciable inflammatory response in stent-implanted vessels examined serially for over 18 months (40). The inflammatory response seen in metal-polymer hybrid implants may relate to specific factors associated with this model including the chronic expansile wall stress and injury associated with the co-implanted metal stent scaffolding holding polymer films in place, polymer impurities unique to the preparation of the implanted films, and biologic differences between the porcine and canine model, with an accentuated inflammatory response typical in the porcine model.

We have recently developed a new system for local endoluminal application of polymers. Initially, solid polymer paving was achieved using generalized heating balloons capable of *in situ* thermoforming polymer tubes or sheets. This first generation system with generalized heating balloons achieved polymer melting with simultaneous heating of tissues adjacent to the polymer. To avoid unnecessary tissue heating in regions adjacent to a paving zone, an alternative means of polymer paving — "photothermal paving" — was developed (42). In this approach a polymer film containing interspersed photo-absorbent dye is locally illuminated while being simultaneously mechanically deformed. The wavelength of light is specifically selected to match the absorbance characteristics of the interspersed dye, resulting in maximal optical energy absorption with resultant heating and melting of the polymer. This method affords less total heat input into surrounding non-colorized arterial walls, with less subsequent tissue thermal injury (41). An example of the photothermal polymer paving catheter system is shown in Figure 6. Recently, the ability of this method to line and support normal and dissected canine carotid arteries was examined both *in vitro* and *in vivo* (54). Endovascular dissection flaps were confirmed with intravascular ultrasound. Following photothermal paving, all vessels remained

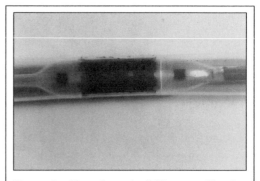

Figure 6. Photothermal solid "structural" paving catheter. Note pre-deployed, fenestrated, dye-containing poly(ε-caprolactone) paving thin film on central deployment balloon. Illuminated central fiber optic may be seen.

dilated with circular cross-sectional profiles. In all cases, photopaving successfully tacked dissections with complete flap sealing; an example of a typical case can be seen in Figure 7. The acute efficacy, structural stability, and patency of photothermally paved arteries was then examined *in vivo* (42). In all animals, photothermal paving led to successful polymer film deployment in carotid arteries *in vivo*. In all paved carotids, intraluminal ultrasound allowed visualization of the applied polymer, distinguishing complete deployment from partial deployment as evidenced by incomplete apposition of the polymer to the underlying vessel wall. All regions of incomplete deployment were subsequently successfully deployed through additional local illumination and polymer dilatation. Photothermal paving led to a significant increase in vessel diameter versus baseline (4.2 ± 0.3 mm versus 3.3 ± 0.6 mm, p = 0.02). Further, photothermal paving led to a significant increase in diameter beyond that achieved with sham deployment (4.2 ± 0.3 mm versus 3.8 ± 0.3 mm, p < 0.05). There was no difference between the baseline vessel diameters of either the sham or paved carotids. At 1 hour post-paving, both paved and sham carotids had detectable blood flow confirming acute vessel patency.

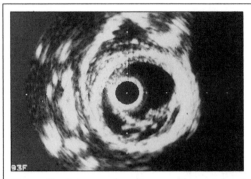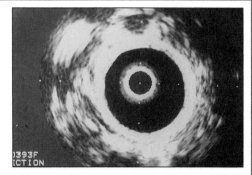

Figure 7. Intravascular ultrasound image of canine carotid artery with large intraluminal dissection flap *(left)*. Identical vessel following endoluminal solid paving *(right)*. Note endoluminal polymer paving layer has tacked dissection flap and reestablished a generally circular patent lumen.

We recently examined the ability of solid paving to function as a local endoluminal depot sustained release drug delivery device (55). Films (100 μ) of poly(ε-caprolactone) (PCL) containing 2 mg of heparin (including 600 mg ^{35}S-heparin) were applied via balloon dilatation and illumination (photothermal paving) to bilateral iliac arteries in six dogs. At 1 and 7 days post-paving, drug levels in the arterial wall, heart (distant organ), and polymer were determined. Trans-wall drug distribution was assessed from *en face* serial sections. Drug was detected at 1 and 7 days post-paving with distribution transmurally across the artery wall. At 7 days, > 40% of the drug remained in the explanted polymer films. This initial study demonstrated that endoluminal paving of arteries with biodegradable polymer films containing drug is an effective means for locally delivering sustained high concentrations of a drug to the arterial wall. These studies have demonstrated that layers of biodegradable polymers, custom-molded and applied *in situ* as endoluminal paving layers, may function as effective endoluminal wall supports and local drug delivery devices. Development of this approach may lead to a versatile clinical technique for biodegradable stenting of vessels combined with long-term, local, high-dose, site-specific drug delivery.

Gel Paving

As outlined above, a second form of paving, gel paving, has recently been developed (43-45). Studies to date with gel paving have examined the use of several polymer systems for formation of hydrogel barriers on tissue interfaces. Both reversible and nonreversible biodegradable and bioerodible gel paving systems have been developed and studied. Using various poly(oxyalkylene) (POA) polymers, thermoreversible gels have been formed via temperature dependent physical cross-linking. These gels have been effectively applied to arterial intimal surfaces via catheter, forming a continuous coating layer (45). Studies of arteries endoluminally gel paved with POA hydrogels have revealed that applied gels remain adherent to underlying arterial surfaces for several hours depending upon polymer, solute, pH, and applied layer thickness, under conditions of controlled fluid shear (44). The *in situ* reversibility of gel formation, a means for allowing local spatial tailoring of gel application, has also been demonstrated. POA hydrogels, by virtue of their mobile constituent molecular chain properties, have been shown to be minimally platelet activating or retentive and nonthrombogenic (45).

In addition to POA polymer systems which form gels on arterial surfaces via balloon-dictated physical molding, a second form of gel paving has been developed allowing for formation of conformal hydrogels on tissue surfaces with thicknesses in the range of cellular dimensions (44,56,57). In this approach, a thin layer of hydrogel is locally polymerized via an *in situ* photopolymerization reaction. In this system a tissue surface is first stained with a photoinitiator dye. A flowable macromeric precursor of the hydrogel is then delivered via catheter to the desired location of hydrogel formation and the region is briefly illuminated via fiber optic catheter. Photopolymerization occurs at the stained tissue-macromer interface leading to the "growth", from the tissue surface outward toward the lumen of the hydrogel. This system differs distinctly from the POA gel paving system in that the components of hydrogel formation are delivered to the zone to be paved as distinct and separate components which by themselves will not gel spontaneously. Gel formation occurs as the two components are brought together and illuminated facilitating *in situ* photopolymerization. In contrast, in the POA system the locally delivered polymer possesses all the constituents necessary for bulk gel formation which then is sculpted and molded locally. These two systems are complimentary in that they allow for creation of either thin or thick gels, with differing physical properties, erosion, and degradation rates depending upon the particular clinical end-use scenario envisioned.

The biological efficacy of both POA thermoreversible and PEG-lactide photopolymerizable hydrogels have been tested *in vitro* and *in vivo* (44,45). Severely abraded rat arterial specimens with exposed thrombogenic subintima have been gel paved with both gel systems and subjected to overflowing blood at a 100^{-1} sec shear rate. Compared to unpaved controls, gel paving led to a greater than 200-fold reduction in platelet deposition. Gel paving also led to the creation of a "zero surface", i.e., a surface upon which no platelet aggregates or thrombus forms. Thus, the thrombogenicity of a highly thrombogenic substrate, the denuded arterial wall, may be almost completely abolished through thromboprotection achieved via application of non-thrombogenic physical gel paving layers.

Based on encouraging *in vitro* data, the efficacy of these systems *in vivo* was then evaluated. Using a rat carotid balloon model, acute thromboprotection of injured arterial surfaces was achieved with a thermoreversible gel system in animals injured without antiplatelet agents or anticoagulants. Figure 8 shows an example of a control and gel

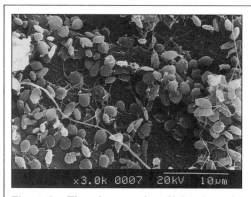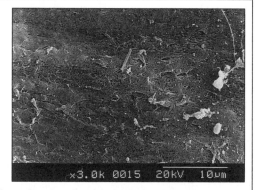

Figure 8. Thromboprotection of injured arterial surfaces via gel paving. Scanning electron micrograph of abraded rat carotid artery *(left)*. Note damaged intimal surface is coated with activated platelets and fibrin. Identical injured surface "pre-coated" with endoluminal gel paving layer subsequently exposed to overflowing blood *(right)*. Note significant reduction in platelet deposition on injured surface, gel having acted as thromboresistant physical barrier layer.

paved surface. On the left is a scanning electron micrograph of an injured control arterial intimal surface subjected to blood reflow. Of note is the significant platelet deposition. In contrast, the gel paved arterial surface shown on the right is essentially devoid of platelets. Using the PEG-lactide system and a rat carotid crush model, similar thromboprotection was also observed (34,58). Gel paving thromboprotection was also observed using PEG-lactide hydrogels despite acute balloon abrasion of the rabbit carotid (44).

With observed *in vivo* efficacy as a thromboprotection system, gel paving has provided a tool to evaluate the role of early blood-arterial wall interactions in the development of neointimal hyperplasia. In an initial study, balloon-injured rat carotid arteries were gel paved with a thermoreversible POA gel system, following injury performed under bloodless conditions. Gel paved vessels were then re-exposed to overflowing blood and animals were allowed to recover. At 14 days post-paving, gel paved carotid arteries were explanted and studied. A greater than 70% reduction in the degree of neointimal hyperplasia was observed (59). Similarly, in two different studies using a rabbit model, gel paving of balloon abraded carotid arteries, utilizing a PEG-lactide gel paving system, resulted in greater than 60% reduction in the area of neointima formed, compared to con-

trol untreated injured arteries (57,60) (see Figure 9). These observations, utilizing two differing hydrogel systems in two differing animal models, clearly suggest and reinforce the significance of early blood-arterial wall interactions as being vital initial signals which ultimately influence the cascade of events resulting in neointimal hyperplasia. These studies highlight the therapeutic potential of post-angioplasty gel paving as an interventional strategy to limit or prevent intimal hyperplasia and restenosis. If developed as a clinical therapeutic technique, gel paving may also provide an adjunct physical method for reducing surface thrombogenicity following angioplasty, thrombolytic therapy, and stent placement.

POTENTIAL CLINICAL APPLICATIONS OF POLYMERIC ENDOLUMINAL PAVING

By virtue of the customizable nature of polymer application plus the ability to utilize a variety of polymeric materials, polymer paving provides a range of endovascular therapeutic opportunities beyond mechanical stenting. Paving represents a basic form of lesion "post-modification therapy", i.e., therapy directed at facilitating or modulating lesion healing following initial lesion modification mechanically achieved to enhance ar-

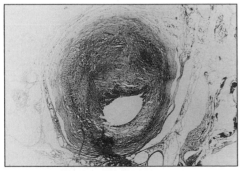 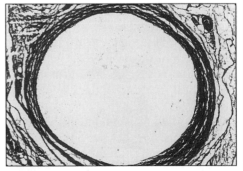

Figure 9. Reduction of neointimal thickening by application of *in situ* photopolymerized gel paving hydrogel barrier layer following injury. Control un-paved balloon injured rabbit carotid artery at 14 days post-injury *(left)*.

terial lumen patency (38). Paving may be viewed as a "bridge therapy", linking a mechanical implant device-based approach with the potential for local arterial wall biomanipulation via either additional mechanical features, i.e., barrier creation, or coupled with local pharmacologic therapy providing sustained drug delivery. It seems likely that a staged evolution will occur in the clinical development of various paving forms, and will initially examine the efficacy of implant polymers alone as custom-molded wall supports followed by combination devices containing drugs as well. Listed below are potential clinical applications for both solid and gel paving.

Solid Paving

Application of endoluminal structural supportive polymer alone may be envisioned in clinical scenarios of abrupt reclosure following failed angioplasty with accompanying wall dissection and flap generation. As outlined above, paving is highly effective in tacking and sealing wall flaps. The advantage here is that paving affords a method of flap sealing providing wall support during the period of wall healing with eventual device dissolution after healing via polymer biodegradation. This is akin to an endoluminal degradable "wall splint". Structural paving may also be utilized as a means of achieving a large sustained lumen following balloon angioplasty or other forms of percutaneous revascularization such as atherectomy or laser angioplasty. Application of a supportive paving layer will prevent recoil and facilitate maintenance of a sustained maximal cross-sectional area which has been demonstrated to be critical in reducing the likelihood for restenosis (61).

In addition to an endoluminal support role, solid paving, either alone or with interspersed drug, has significant promise as both a primary and secondary therapy aimed at reducing restenosis. As a primary therapy, such as prophylactic application immediately following percutaneous revascularization,

through maintenance of a large arterial lumen coupled with the ability to locally deliver an interspersed antiplatelet, antithrombotic, antiproliferative, antimigratory, or antimatrix agent, paving may limit intimal thickening and effectively prevent clinical restenosis. Paving may also be envisioned as a secondary therapy, i.e., applied as a treatment for restenosis, in cases of lesion recurrence following initial angioplasty. In this case local drug therapy may be tailored, as our understanding of pathophysiologic derangements particular to a given patient increase in the future, to deliver an agent appropriate to treat a given lesion phenotype.

Gel Paving

Gel paving, being a non-structural barrier form of paving, may be envisioned as a clinical therapy with a different role than solid paving. As an effective biobarrier to early blood signals, gel paving may be envisioned as a generalized prophylaxis therapy to be applied immediately following revascularization. In addition to use as a means of reducing intimal hyperplasia, gel paving may be utilized clinically as a means of limiting the thrombogenicity of a surface, e.g., to prevent rethrombosis following initial reopening of an infarct-occluded vessel, achieved via either mechanical angioplasty or pharmacologic thrombolytic therapy means. Gel paving may also be useful as a means of reducing the thrombogenicity of an arterial segment that has been stented with conventional metal stents. Gel paving may also have applicability in reducing the thrombogenicity and surface fouling of stent-grafts, bypass anastomoses, shunts, and fistulas.

In addition to serving as a short-term barrier, gel paving may also provide a means of short-term local drug delivery. Drug delivery via endoluminal hydrogels may take several forms. Delivery may be accomplished with drug interspersed throughout the hydrogel via diffusion- and erosion-based mechanisms. Additionally, the kinetics of local drug delivery from the hydrogel may be modified providing greater intraluminal residence time and more prolonged delivery through modification of the degree of cross-linking and porosity of the hydrogel layer. Drug may be bound, i.e., either via covalent or non-covalent interactions, to the polymer backbone or side chains of the gel network as well. Alternatively, the drug may be dispersed through the hydrogel in secondary incorporated microparticles or colloidal latexes. Many possible combination systems may be envisioned with endoluminal gel paving hydrogel systems to extend the time of delivery, the degree of loading, and the physicochemical nature of the drugs that may be delivered.

CONCLUSION

Solid, gel, and liquid paving are best viewed as evolving therapeutic techniques which are not mutually exclusive. Rather, they are a family of evolving approaches aimed at providing both short- and long-term means of local arterial wall biomanipulation through either the polymer alone as therapy or polymer plus drug combinations. The ultimate evolution of these approaches to practical, readily deployable, clinical interventional therapeutic methods will greatly enhance the capabilities and safety of approaches currently available to the clinical interventionalist.

ACKNOWLEDGEMENT

This work was supported in part by Grant No. RG 205N from the American Lung Association and by an Educational Grant from Focal Inc., Cambridge, MA.

REFERENCES

1. Topol EJ. Promises and pitfalls of new devices for coronary artery disease. Circulation 1991;83:689.
2. Ellis SG, Savage M, Fischman DF, et al. Restenosis after placement of Palmaz-Schatz stents in native coronary arteries: initial results of multicenter experience. Circulation 1992;86:1836-1844.
3. Hearn JA, King III SB, Douglas JS, Roubin GS. Restenosis after Gianturco-Roubin stent placement for acute closure. In: Serruys PW, Strauss BH, King SB, eds. *Restenosis after Intervention with New Mechanical Devices.* Dordrecht: Kluwer Academic; 1992;207.
4. Kuntz RE, Hinohara T, Safian RD, Selmon MR, Simpson JB, Baim DS. Restenosis after directional atherectomy: effects of luminal diameter and deep wall excision. Circulation 1992;86:1394.
5. Topol EJ, Leya F, Pinkerton CA, et al. A comparison of directional atherectomy with coronary angioplasty in patients with coronary artery disease. N Engl J Med 1993;329:221.
6. Katzen BT, Becker GJ. Intravascular stents: status of development and clinical application. Surg Clin N Am 1992;72:941.
7. Schatz RA. Introduction to intravascular stents. Cardiol Clin 1988;6:357.
8. Sigwart U, Puel J, Mirkovitch V, Joffre F, Kappenberger L. Intravascular stents to prevent occlusion and restenosis after transluminal angioplasty. N Engl J Med 1987;316:701.
9. Roubin GS, Douglas JS, Lembo NJ, Black AJ, King SB. Intracoronary stenting for acute closure following percutaneous transluminal coronary angioplasty (PTCA). Circulation 1988;78(Suppl. II):II-407.
10. Roubin GS, Cannon AD, Agrawal SK, et al. Intracoronary stenting for acute and threatened closure complicating percutaneous transluminal coronary angioplasty. Circulation 1992;85:916.
11. Sigwart U, Urban P, Golf S, et al. Emergency stenting for acute occlusion after coronary balloon angioplasty. Circulation 1988;78:1121.
12. Fischman D, Savage M, Leon M, et al. for the STRESS investigators. J Am Coll Cardiol 1994;60A.
13. Schatz RA, Baim DS, Leon M, et al. Clinical experience with the Palmaz-Schatz coronary stent: initial results of a multicenter study. Circulation 1990;83:148.
14. Serruys PW, Macaya C, de Jaegerre P, et al. for the BENESTENT investigators. Interim analysis of the BENESTENT trial. Circulation 1993;88(4 Part 2):I-594.
15. Carrozza JP, Kunt RE, Levin MJ, et al. Angiographic and clinical outcome of

intracoronary stenting: immediate and long-term results from a large single-center experience. J Am Coll Cardiol 1992;20:328.

16. Doucet B, Fajadet J, Caillard J, et al. Predictors of thrombotic occlusion following coronary Palmaz-Schatz stent implantation. Circulation 1992;86(Suppl. I):I-113.

17. Hermann HC, Buchbinder M, Clemen MW, et al. Emergent use of balloon-expandable coronary artery stenting for failed percutaneous transluminal coronary angioplasty. Circulation 1992;86:812.

18. Nath FC, Muller DWM, Ellis SG, et al. Thrombosis of a flexible coil coronary stent: frequency, predictors and clinical outcome. J Am Coll Cardiol 1993;21:622.

19. Palmaz JC. Intravascular stents: tissue-stent interactions and design considerations. Am J Radiol 1993;160:613.

20. Shaknovich A, Rocha-Singh K, Tierstin P, Lieberman S, Moses J. Subacute stent thrombosis in Palmaz-Schatz stents in native coronary arteries: time course, acute management and outcome. US multicenter experience (abstr.). Circulation 1992;86(Suppl. I):I-113.

21. Shaknovich A, Stratienko AA, Tierstein PS, Schatz RA. The Palmaz-Schatz stent. In: Vogel JHK and King SB, eds. *The Practice of Interventional Cardiology, 2nd edition*. St Louis: Mosby; 1993;320.

22. Slepian MJ. Polymeric endoluminal paving: a family of evolving methods for extending endoluminal therapeutics beyond stenting. Cardiol Clin 1994;12:14.

23. Schatz RA. A view of vascular stents. Circulation 1989;79:445.

24. Schatz RA, Palmaz JC, Tio FO, Garcia F, Garcia O, Reuter SR. Balloon-expandable intracoronary stents in the adult dog. Circulation 1987;76:450-457.

25. Rab ST, King SB, Roubin GS, et al. Coronary aneurysms after stent placement: a suggestion of altered vessel wall healing in the presence of anti-inflammatory agents. J Am Coll Cardiol 1991;18:1524.

26. Zeiher AM, Hohnloser SH. Coronary artery stents (Letter to the Editor). N Engl J Med 1991;324:1596.

27. Castleman LS, Motzkin SM. The biocompatibility of nitinol. In: Williams DF, ed. *Biocompatibility of Clinical Implant Materials*. Boca Raton: CRC Press; 1982; 129-154.

28. Duprat G, Wright KC, Charnsangavej C, Wallace S, Gianturco C. Self-expanding metallic stents for small vessels: an experimental evaluation. Radiology 1987;162:469.

29. Rodgers GP, Minor ST, Hess K, Raizner AE. Coronary artery spasm induced by stent implantation: studies in a swine model. J Intervent Cardiol 1993;6:149.

30. Baim DS. Intracoronary stenting - hope or hype? Mayo Clin Proc 1991;66:332.

31. Becker GJ. Intravascular stents: general principles and status of lower-extremity arterial applications. Circulation 1991;83(Suppl. I):I-122.

32. Hanke H, Hassenstein S, Kamenz J, et al. Prolonged proliferative response of smooth muscle cells after experimental intravascular stenting: a stent wire related phenomenon (abstr.). Circulation 1992;86(Suppl. I):I-186.

33. Karas SP, Gravanis MB, Santoian EC, Robinson KA, Anderberg KA, King SB. Coronary intimal proliferation after balloon injury and stenting in swine: an animal model of restenosis. J Am Coll Cardiol 1992;20:467.

34. Santoian EC, King SB. Intravascular stents, intimal proliferation and restenosis. J Am Coll Cardiol 1992;19:877.

35. Schwartz RS, Murphy JG, Edwards WD, Camrud AR, Vlietstra RE, Holmes DR. Restenosis after balloon angioplasty: a practical proliferative model in porcine coronary arteries. Circulation 1990;82:2190.

36. Strauss BH, Serruys PW, de Schreeder IK, et al. Relative risk analysis of angiographic predictors of restenosis within the coronary Wallstent. Circulation 1991;84:1636.

37. Slepian MJ, Schindler A. Polymeric endoluminal paving/sealing: a biodegradable alternative to intracoronary stenting. Circulation 1988;78:II-408.

38. Slepian MJ. Polymeric endoluminal paving/sealing: therapeutics at the crossroad of biomechanics and pharmacology. In: Topol EJ, ed. *Textbook of Interventional Cardiology*. Philadelphia: Saunders; 1989;647-670.

39. Slepian MJ, Habib MP, Dehdashti B, Massia SP. Polymeric endotracheal paving: a biodegradable alternative to stenting. Am J Resp Crit Care Med 1994;149:A731.

40. Zidar JP, Gammon RS, Chapman GD, et al. Short and long-term vascular tissue response to the Duke bioabsorbable stent. J Am Coll Cardiol 1993;21:439A.

41. Campbell PK, Berrigan KM, Roth L, Slepian MJ. Photothermal intravascular delivery of biodegradable materials: *in vitro* temperature measurements. Trans Soc Biomater 1991;XVII:16.

42. Slepian MJ, Berrigan KM, Roth L, Campbell PK. Endovascular photothermal paving: a new paving form - acute *in vivo* efficacy and patency. Trans Soc Biomater 1994;XVII:17.

43. Slepian MJ, Hossainy SFA, Pathak CP, Hubbell JA. Bioerodible endovascular gel paving: a new approach for reducing the thrombogenicity of injured arterial surfaces. Trans Soc Biomater 1993;XVI:235.

44. Slepian MJ, Massia SP, Sawhney A, Pathak CP, Berrigan K, Roth L. Endoluminal gel paving using *in situ* biodegradable photopolymerized hydrogels: acute efficacy in the rabbit. Circulation 1993;88(4 Part 2):I-660.

45. Slepian MJ, Hossainy SFA, Pathak CP, Sawhney A, Massia SP, Hubbell JA. Thermoreversible polyether hydrogels reduce the thrombogenicity of injured arterial intimal surfaces. Circulation 1993;88(4 Part 2):I-319.

46. Fingerle J, Johnson R, Clowes A, Majesky M, Reidy M. Role of platelets in smooth muscle cell proliferation and migration after vascular injury in the rat carotid artery. Proc Natl Acad Sci USA 1989;86:8412.

47. Harker LA. Role of platelets and thrombosis in mechanisms of acute occlusion and restenosis after angioplasty. Am J Cardiol 1987;60:21B.

48. Steele PM, Cheseboro JH, Holmes DR, Stanson DW, Badimon L, Fuster V. Balloon angioplasty in pigs: histologic wall injury as a determinant of platelet deposition and thrombus formation. Circ Res 1985;57:105.

49. Hill-West JL, Chowdhury SM, Sawhney AS, Pathak CP, Slepian MJ, Hubbell JA. *In situ* photopolymerization of thin hydrogel barriers for preventing thrombosis following vascular injury. Circulation 1993;88:(4 Part 2):I-319.

50. Slepian MJ, Hossainy SFA, Pathak CP, et al. Hemocompatibility of polymers for use in endoluminal paving: I. Structural polymers. (Submitted for publication, 1994).

51. Slepian MJ, Schindler A. Polymeric endoluminal paving/sealing: initial experience in atherosclerotic human arteries *in vitro*. J Am Coll Cardiol 1991;17:180A.

52. Slepian MJ, Schindler A. Polymeric endoluminal paving/sealing: initial *in vivo* experience in the dog. Radiology 1990;177(Suppl.):311.

53. Lincoff AM, van der Giessen WJ, Schwartz RS, et al. Biodegradable and biostable polymers may both cause vigorous inflammatory responses when implanted in the porcine coronary artery. J Am Coll Cardiol 1993;21:179A.

54. Slepian MJ, Berrigan KM, Roth L, Campbell PK. Polymeric endoluminal photo-thermal paving: initial experience in normal and dissected canine carotid arteries *in vitro*. JVIR 1994;5:10.

55. Slepian MJ, Campbell PK, Berrigan K, et al. Biodegradable endoluminal polymer layers provide sustained transmural heparin delivery to the arterial wall *in vivo*. Circulation 1994;90(4 Part 2):I-20.

56. Hill-West JL, Chowdhury SM, Slepian MJ, Hubbell JA. Thin hydrogel barriers for prevention of thrombosis and intimal thickening after balloon injury. J Am Coll Cardiol 1994; Feb. Special Issue:5A.

57. Hill-West JL, Chowdhury SM, Slepian MJ, Hubbell JA. Inhibition of thrombosis and intimal thickening by *in situ* photopolymerization of thin hydrogel barriers. Proc Natl Acad Sci 1994;91:5967.

58. Rousseau H, Puel J, Joffre F, et al. Self-expanding endovascular prosthesis: an experimental study. Radiology 1987;164:709.

59. Slepian MJ, Massia SP. Delayed re-exposure of injured arterial subintima to blood via erodible hydrogel barriers limits neointimal hyperplasia. J Am Coll Cardiol 1994; Feb. Special Issue:18A.

60. Slepian MJ, Sawhney A, Path CP, et al. *In situ* photo-polymerized thin hydrogel barriers applied following arterial injury reduce intimal thickening. J Am Coll Cardiol 1994; Feb. Special Issue:473A.

61. Kuntz RE, Safian RD, Levine MJ, Reis GJ, Diver DJ, Baim DS. Novel approach to the analysis of restenosis after the use of three new coronary devices. J Am Coll Cardiol 1993;19:1493.

Percutaneous Endovascular Graft Placement

Andrew H. Cragg

Division of Interventional Vascular Medicine,
Fairview Riverside Medical Center, Minneapolis, MN USA

INTRODUCTION

We first reported on a technique for percutaneous placement of a vascular graft in 1984 (1). The graft consisted of a closely wound nitinol wire coil. Using this device, we were able to demonstrate the obliteration of experimental aortic and iliac aneurysms. We have also investigated the use of intraluminal stents for the treatment of occlusive vascular disease (2,3) and have recently reported our initial clinical results using a nitinol stent of our own design in the iliac arteries (4). This stent is currently being used in Europe and has been applied to a wide range of vascular and nonvascular applications.

Approximately 2 years ago, we began investigating a technique for percutaneous placement of a femoropopliteal bypass graft (5) (Figure 1). The purpose of this technique was to treat patients who had long segment femoropopliteal occlusive disease which was not amenable to angioplasty or conventional stenting because of the high restenosis rate with these techniques. Our technique involves endoluminal placement of a bypass graft across the diseased segment of a peripheral artery. Our initial experience with this technique as well as a modification of our initial technique using a new dacron-covered, self-expandable stent graft are described here.

To date, this procedure has been applied on a limited basis to patients with long segment iliac and femoropopliteal stenosis or occlusion, femoropopliteal aneurysms, arteriovenous fistulas, and venous stenoses. Due to regulatory restrictions in the United States, our experience has been limited to the use of polytetrafluoroethylene (PTFE) graft

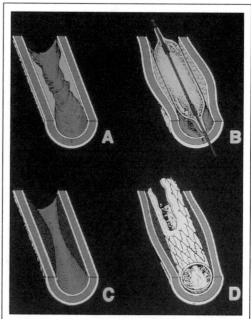

Figure 1. Restenosis after balloon angioplasty (A, B) is usually the result of intimal hyperplasia (C). Endoluminal graft placement may limit the ingrowth of intimal hyperplasia and improve the long-term patency of percutaneous revascularization.

material (Gore and Associates, Flagstaff AZ). In Europe, however, we are acquiring a great deal of experience with a stent-graft of our own design which employs heparin-impregnated polyester graft material.

MATERIALS AND METHODS

Our first percutaneous femoropopliteal graft placement was accomplished using thin-walled PTFE supported by a nitinol stent of our own design. The patient was a 63-year-old male with severe left calf claudication. He had occlusion of his left superficial femoral artery which did not respond to thrombolysis or angioplasty. A 6 mm x 10 cm intraluminal graft was placed with excellent vascular reconstruction. The graft remains patent 2 years after placement (Figure 2).

Because our stent was not yet available for general use in the United States, we began investigating the use of Palmaz™ stents (Johnson & Johnson Interventional Systems Co., Warren NJ) and Wallstents™ (Schneider, Inc., Minneapolis MN) to support an intraluminal femoral graft. To prepare the graft, we removed the spiral outer wrap on the graft material itself. This allowed the graft to be slightly thinned out and also allowed the graft to be dilated by 1 to 2 mm if necessary once it had been placed. At present, our preferred stent-graft combination involves suturing of two Palmaz stents, one on each end of the graft using interrupted 6-0 polypropylene sutures. The compressed stents are placed inside the graft with only a short length of stent protruding outside of the graft. The graft is then mounted on a 6 mm x 10 cm

angioplasty balloon and the stents crimped in place.

After performing conventional angiography and angioplasty via an antegrade puncture, a long 12 Fr sheath is placed across the segment of the femoral artery to be treated. The balloon graft assembly is loaded into a short segment of 12 Fr sheath material which is then back-loaded over a wire onto the hemostasis end of the 12 Fr sheath. The balloon and stent-graft combination are subsequently advanced into the sheath and down to the site of intended deployment. The 12 Fr sheath is then withdrawn and the balloon inflated to deploy the stents and graft. A major pitfall with this technique is that friction inside the sheath tends to force the crimped stents off of the balloon. We have been able to deploy these stent-grafts through 11 Fr sheaths but find that the 12 Fr sheath minimizes the friction and allows more reliable deployment.

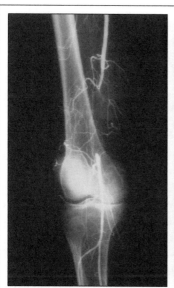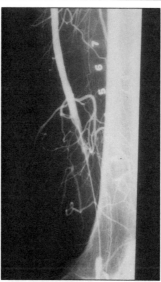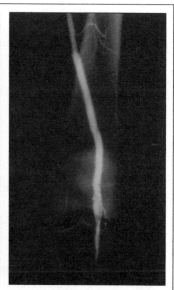

Figure 2. Femoral artery graft. Preliminary angiogram *(left)* shows a 10-cm occlusion of the superficial femoral artery. After thrombolysis and angioplasty, the artery remains occluded *(middle)*. Approximately 1 year after placement, the graft and artery remain widely patent *(right)*.

An alternative implantation technique has been utilized for the PTFE material using Wallstents. This technique requires a popliteal puncture and a through-and-through wire. The graft is pulled into the femoral artery using tethers attached to each end of the graft. Once in position, the graft is opened by angioplasty and stents. While this technique has the advantage of allowing placement of a flexible stent (which is desirable in the femoral artery), it is cumbersome to place grafts using this technique and therefore is no longer performed.

A number of limitations to use of conventional stent and graft technology were encountered in our initial experience. These included crushing of rigid stents and the need for large introducing sheaths. To overcome these limitations, we have recently begun investigating a new stent-graft combination which is presently in clinical trials in Europe. It is a nitinol self-expandable stent which is covered by heparin-impregnated dacron graft material (Mintec Inc., La Ciotat, France) (Figure 3). The graft material is ultrathin (0.1 mm) and allows deployment of the stent-graft through a 9 Fr sheath. The graft comes loaded in a 9 Fr cartridge which is back-loaded on a 9 Fr sheath and placed across the intended delivery site. The graft is advanced to the point of delivery using a 9 Fr introducing catheter. The sheath is then withdrawn to deploy the graft. The graft can then be dilated after placement using conventional angioplasty balloons.

RESULTS

Our initial technique using PTFE graft material has been applied to a small cohort of 12 patients. Technical success was achieved in 11 of the 12 patients and all had grafts placed in the femoropopliteal segment. Ten of the 12 patients had favorable clinical responses with normalization of ankle/brachial indices and symptomatic relief. After a mean follow-up period of 12 months, the primary patency rate was 50% (6 of 12) and the secondary patency

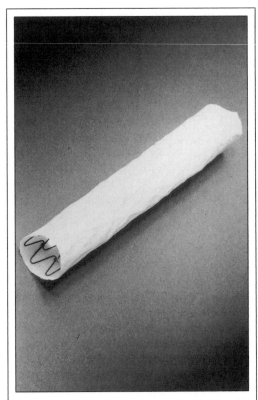

Figure 3.   Cragg endoluminal graft. A self-expandable nitinol stent is covered by ultrathin dacron material. The graft is covered by ultrathin dacron material. The graft is compressed and delivered through a 9 Fr sheath.

rate was 75% (9 of 12). Four patients had thrombosis of their graft during the follow-up interval and underwent successful thrombolysis. One patient thrombosed twice and subsequently had a femoropopliteal bypass. The cause of thrombosis in two patients was thought to be stenosis due to compression of a Palmaz stent placed in the adductor canal region. We now favor the use of flexible stents in this location. In one patient, intimal hyperplasia occurred at both ends of a Wallstent placed in the graft. One patient had thrombosis of the graft without apparent stenosis.

Long-term follow-up data using our nitinol/dacron graft system is not yet available. The graft has been used, however, for the treatment of aneurysmal and occlusive disease of both the arterial and venous systems (Figures 4-6). A randomized trial of the dacron/nitinol graft comparing it to conventional femoropopliteal bypass is also being organized in Europe; a U.S. clinical trial is pending. A bifurcated aortic prosthesis is currently available and preliminary clinical investigations are underway. Coronary graft placement is anticipated before the end of 1994.

DISCUSSION

During the past 10 years, multiple techniques have been investigated whose aim has been to improve the long-term success of balloon angioplasty. Balloon angioplasty is known to have suboptimal results in the treatment of long-segment disease, particularly in the infrainguinal vessels (6). In this situation, dilatation of lesions greater than 7 cm in length has a high rate of restenosis. Alternative therapy such as laser and atherectomy have been vigorously applied to treatment of this subset of patients, also with suboptimal results (7,8). Any technique which could improve on the high restenosis rate of long-segment femoropopliteal revascularization would find application as an alternative to surgical bypass.

Late restenosis after angioplasty is usually due to intimal hyperplasia and plaque progression. When long segments are treated, the chance of this occurring at some point along the segment increases, thus making the restenosis rate of these lesions higher than is seen with short-segment disease. The technique of endoluminal graft placement is intuitively appealing since it may allow isolation of the diseased segment and prevent the ingrowth of intimal hyperplasia or plaque responsible for restenosis. In this situation, the graft may act as a barrier to the development of intimal hyperplasia.

In our preliminary experience, the technique of percutaneous vascular graft placement has suffered several pitfalls. Conven-

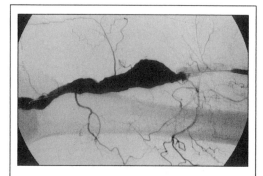

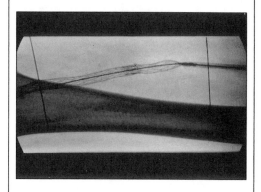

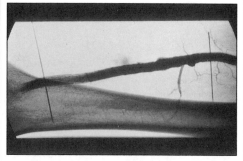

Figure 4. Femoral artery graft. Preliminary angiogram *(top)* shows a large aneurysm of the distal superficial femoral artery. Partial deployment of the graft *(middle)*. Angiogram immediately after deployment *(bottom)* shows exclusion of the aneurysm.

Case is courtesy of Dr. Albrektsson, Lund, Sweden.

tional graft material is bulky and requires large introducing sheaths. With rigid stents, there is a risk of compression following placement in the infrainguinal vessels. This

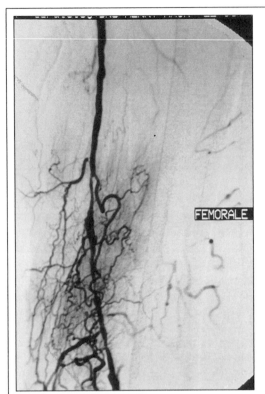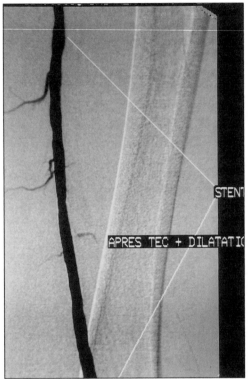

Figure 5.   Femoral artery graft. Preliminary angiogram *(left)* shows a long stenosis of the superficial femoral artery. After graft placement, the artery is widely patent *(right)*.

Case is courtesy of Dr. M. Henry, Nancy, France.

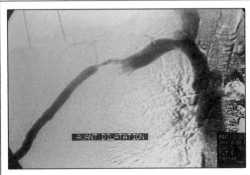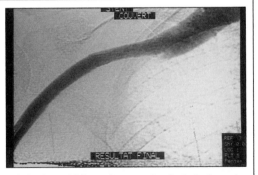

Figure 6.   Subclavian vein graft. Preliminary venogram *(left)* shows high grade stenosis of subclavian vein. After graft placement, the vein is widely patent *(right)*.

Case is courtesy of Dr. Gauthier, Saint Laurent, Du Var, France.

occurred in two patients in our preliminary series. We also observed intimal hyperplasia at the end of one of the stent-grafts.

It is likely that these grafts will suffer from the same problems associated with affecting surgical anastomoses, such as turbulence, pannus formation, and restenosis. The graft size must also be matched to the size of the inflow and outflow vessels. Development of tapered grafts and grafts with varying diameters may expand their use in this regard. As with surgical bypass grafting, the status of the inflow and outflow vessels will likely play a significant role in determining the long-term patency of individual grafts.

Future applications of this technique which are currently being investigated include the use of grafts in transjugular intrahepatic portosystemic shunting (TIPS). Graft material on a stent may limit tissue ingrowth which is a common cause of restenosis after this procedure. The use of stent-grafts for aneurysmal disease is well underway. Percutaneous coronary graft placement may favorably affect the high restenosis rate of angioplasty and stent placement in this vascular bed.

This is an exciting area of interventional therapy which is still in its infancy. Its role has not been determined as of yet but the author encourages the use of judicious clinical trials to establish the role of this technique in clinical practice.

REFERENCES

1. Cragg A, Lund G, Rysavy J, Salomonowitz E, Castaneda-Zuniga W, Amplatz K. Percutaneous arterial grafting. Radiology 1984;150:45-49.

2. Cragg A, Lund G, Rysavy J, Castaneda F, Castaneda-Zuniga W, Amplatz K. Nonsurgical placement of arterial endoprostheses: a new technique using nitinol wire. Radiology 1983;147:261-263.

3. Cragg A, DeJong S, Barnhart W, Landas S, Smith T. Nitinol intravascular stent: results of preclinical evaluation. Radiology 1993;189:775-778.

4. Hausegger K, Cragg A, Lammer J, et al. Iliac artery stent placement: clinical experience with a nitinol stent. Radiology 1994;190:199-202.

5. Cragg A, Dake M. Percutaneous femoropopliteal graft placement. Radiology 1993;187:643-648.

6. Murray R Jr, Hewes R Jr, et al. Long segment femoropopliteal stenoses: is angioplasty a boon or a bust? Radiology 1987;162:473-476.

7. Huppert P, Duda S, Helbert U, Karsch K, Claussen C. Comparison of pulsed laser-assisted angioplasty and balloon angioplasty in femoropopliteal artery occlusions. Radiology 1992;184:363-367.

8. Katzen B, Becker G, Benenati J, et al. Long-term follow-up of directional atherectomy in the femoral and popliteal arteries. JVIR 1990;3:38-39.

Transfemoral Endoluminal Exclusion of Artificially-Generated Aortic Aneurysm in Dogs by Means of Self-Expandable Stent-Grafts

Bernd Hagen[1], Bernd M. Harnoss[2], Stefan Trabhardt[3],
Matthias Ladeburg[4], Holger Fuhrmann[5], Claudia Franck[1]

[1]Department of Radiology, [2]Department of Abdominal and Vascular Surgery,
Martin Luther Hospital, Berlin, Germany
[3]Department of Surgery, Steglitz Clinic, Berlin, Germany
[4]Central Animal Laboratory of Berlin University, Berlin, Germany
[5]Small Animal Clinic, Berlin, Germany

Double-knitted, self-expandable nitinol stents were implanted transfemorally in nine dogs, single-knitted stents in two dogs, and a steel-wire mesh stent in one dog as endoluminal prostheses in artificial Dacron and polyurethane aneurysms which had previously been implanted in the infrarenal aorta. Both catheter angiography and computed tomographic angioscans showed immediate exclusion of the aneurysms after placement of stent-grafts with a pore width of under $0.65 \, mm^2$, but only partial thrombosis of the aneurysms by stents with a pore width of more than $0.85 \, mm^2$. The follow-up observation period was 4 to 15 months for 11 dogs. Macroscopic and microscopic examination of the autopsy specimens of these animals showed that the thrombus was consolidated to a large extent by typical organization tissue in the close-meshed stents. The stent-grafts were patent at all times during the follow-up period and histological examination showed homogeneous neointima of 100 to 200 μm thickness with incomplete endothelial lining. Exclusion of artificial aneurysms in dogs is effectively guaranteed by close-meshed stent grafts. However, the validity of treating human aortic aneurysms by porous stent-grafts is currently unclear since unsolved technical and logistical problems prevent their clinical application.

INTRODUCTION

Aortic aneurysms occur in older people with an incidence in autopsy studies of between 1.8 and 6.6% (1,2) and a clinical incidence of approximately 5% (3). Rates in selected patient populations may vary between 5 and 20% (4).

Since Dubost's first aneurysm resection with replacement by a homologous graft (5), surgical treatment of the aortic aneurysm as the method of choice has become an established procedure for both elective and emergency interventions. According to modern statistics, lethality in elective intervention in cases of asymptomatic aneurysms is under 5% (6), but rises dramatically in old (7) and multimorbid patients (8). Lethality is approximately 10% in cases of symptomatic aneurysms. In emergency interventions performed at the rupture stage, operative lethality has not substantially decreased over the past three decades (9), despite improved anaesthesiological conditions. For patients in hemorrhagic shock, it remains approximately 50% (10,11), but is reduced to 20% for patients without shock occurrence.

In order to avoid the operative risk, particularly in cases of symptomatic aneurysm and in patients with cardiorespiratory and renal diseases, less invasive alternatives for the treatment of aneurysms are clinically attractive. Experience has shown that neither intraluminal thrombosis with foreign materials (12,13) nor wrapping the aortic aneurysm with a textile has successfully prevented a fatal rupture (14).

The development of minimally-invasive, endovascular therapy offers a different, more promising method: the transfemoral exclusion of aortic aneurysms by means of an endoluminal bypass (15-25). These trials involved the implantation of either stented grafts (or steel attachment stent-graft systems) or stent-grafts (with the stent wrapped in microporous, synthetic material). Our own experiments on animals were intended to show whether an open stent with defined pore width could effectively exclude an artificial, infrarenal aortic aneurysm in dogs.

Further, long-term trials, including macroscopic and histologic examination of the autopsy material, were conducted in order to provide information on patency, biocompatibility, and healing and on the nature of the thrombus in an excluded aneurysm.

MATERIALS AND METHODS

Laparotomy was performed on 15 dogs (weight, 28 to 35 kg) under general anaesthesia, and the infrarenal aorta was exposed after endotracheal intubation. The aorta was clamped approximately 2 cm below the origin of the renal arteries and 1 cm above the bifurcation. All side branches within that segment were ligated. A 4-cm long aortic segment was resected and replaced by a sacciform, artificial aneurysm with a diameter of 3.5 cm. Four Dacron and 11 polyurethane aneurysms (Figure 1) were implanted in this manner. Four weeks after aneurysm implantation, double-knitted, self-expandable nitinol stents (Boston Scientific Corp., Denmark) were placed transfemorally in nine dogs and single-knitted, self-expandable nitinol stents in two other dogs via a special sheath system so that they fully bridged the aortic aneurysm. A self-expandable, woven, close-meshed steel stent (Schneider, Zurich, Switzerland) was implanted in another dog.

Nitinol wires (0.1 mm thick) were knitted in the manner of the Strecker stent using an industrial knitting machine, with stents of single-knitted wires having 16 loops with a pore width of approximately 0.85 mm^2. By doubling the wire, a close, macroporous network was available with a pore width of approximately 0.65 mm^2 in the 8-cm long, 8- to 10-mm wide, double-knitted nitinol stent. Pore width was 0.6 mm^2 in the steel-wire mesh stent. The stents were fluoroscopically positioned with subsequent angiography.

Implantation Technique

In the first four experiments, the stent was wrapped around the guidewire, compressed and inserted in a 45-cm long sheath with an inner diameter of 12 Fr and an outer diameter of 14 Fr. After removing the guidewire, the stent was expressed by means of a steel obturator with a piston-like plastic tip (Figure 1). In a second series, the stent was coaxially mounted on a wire and compressed using a crochet loop technique. This led to a reduction of sheath caliber, a better expansion ratio (1:3), and a more accurate placement due to the controlled release of the stent. The crochet loop technique allowed reduction of the outer sheath diameter to 11.5 Fr and enabled the percutaneous, transfemoral Seldinger technique to be performed.

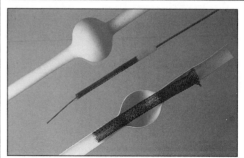

Figure 1. Experimental design: polyurethane aneurysm *(top)*; compressed stent-graft in a teflon sheath with piston-style plastic pusher *(center)*; expanded, double knitted, nitinol stent-graft *(bottom)*.

Follow-Up

One dog died of a suture infection 2 weeks after aneurysm implantation, and a second dog died of volvulus 24 hours after stent implantation. In two dogs, the (polyurethane) aneurysm had spontaneously thrombosed after only 3 months so that stent implantation could no longer be performed.

Two dogs were again examined angiographically after 6 to 12 weeks, the others underwent computed tomography (CT) scans after 4 to 16 weeks. Those scans recorded time-density graphs over a period of 12 minutes at three standardized locations within the excluded aneurysm (Figure 2). Eleven dogs were sacrificed at different times (4 to 15 months); autopsy specimens were removed and examined macroscopically and microscopically.

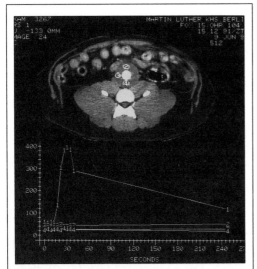

Figure 2. CT of the abdominal canine aorta after stent-graft implantation: time-density graph within the stent-graft (1), and above three points (2,3,4) in the excluded, thrombosed aneurysm.

RESULTS

Taking into account one misplacement, all close-meshed stents excluded the aneurysm, as shown by angiography and CT scans

conducted immediately after implantation (Figures 3, 4). In two cases involving coarse-meshed prostheses (single-knitted nitinol stents), there was no immediate exclusion of the aneurysm and only partial exclusion at the follow-up observation by a non-organized thrombus (Figure 5).

An autopsy performed on one dog after 24 hours (cause of death: volvulus) revealed a smooth, thin, fibrin thrombus layer which completely covered the inside of the stent (Figure 6). Fresh thrombotic deposits were discovered in the excluded aneurysm. Macroscopic and histological examination of the other autopsy specimens revealed the following. The close-meshed stents exhibited typical neointima between and over the stent filaments, while the histological picture was dominated by collagenous fibrils, smooth muscle cells, fibroblasts, monocytes, and small vessels (Figure 7). The covering layer of neointima was approximately 200 μm thick at the proximal and distal ends of the stent (Figure 8), i.e., in the direct vicinity of the native aorta, and approximately 100 μm or less (Figure 9) in the free segments bridging the aneurysm. A relatively homogeneous layer of spiral endothelial cells covered the stent at the proximal and distal ends (Figure 7), with finger-like projections reaching to the more central segments. A fibrin thrombus layer of differing thickness could be seen between these isolated endothelial areas. The aneurysms excluded by the close-meshed stents were more or less completely filled with low-cell, organized thrombus tissue (Figure 10), which was loose in some places and exhibited lacunar defects or accumulations of fresher thrombus. In the aneurysms bridged by coarse-meshed stents, the thrombus was not organized, and larger lacunae were in some cases filled with fresh blood (Figure 11) so that circulation was probable in those non-excluded areas.

DISCUSSION

Transfemoral and intraluminal placement of stent-graft systems to exclude aneurysms is

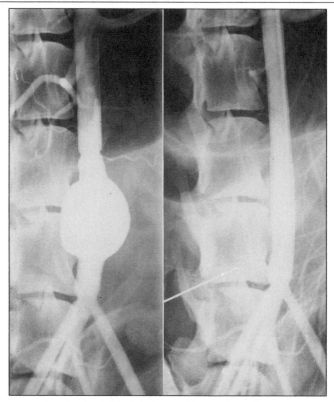

Figure 3. *Left*: aortography after implantation of a sacciform polyurethane aneurysm. *Right*: aortography immediately after implantation of a double-knitted, nitinol stent-graft with exclusion of the aneurysm.

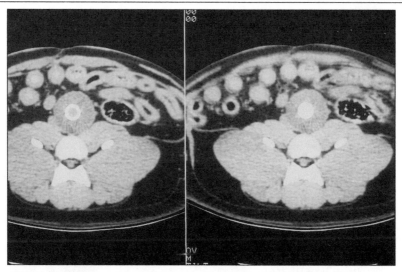

Figure 4. CT with artificial aneurysm and close-meshed stent-graft before *(left)* and after *(right)* bolus with contrast medium. Complete exclusion of the aneurysm.

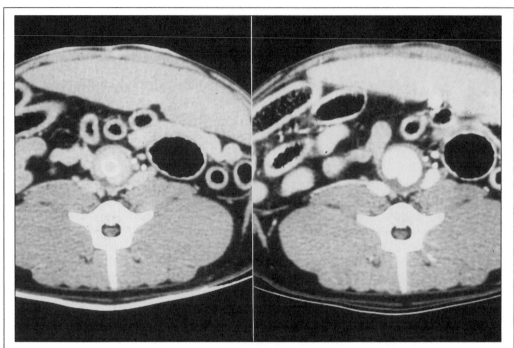

Figure 5. CT with artificial aneurysm and close-meshed stent-graft before *(left)* and after *(right)* bolus with contrast medium. Contrast medium depot in the only partially thrombosed aneurysm.

a revolutionary interventional concept which has developed from initial animal experiment studies (18,19) to a clinically established procedure within just one decade. The aim was to develop alternative therapies which were less invasive than surgical techniques in order to achieve significant reductions in mortality and peri-operative morbidity. In 1991 Parodi and Palmaz first presented the results of five patients whose infrarenal aortic aneurysms had been successfully treated with a dacron stent-graft (15).

In principle, a distinction should be made between stented grafts and stent-grafts. The models presented to date and used experimentally and clinically involve compositions of metallic and textile components. Technical problems can arise in the manual, suture-style fixation of the wrapping textile to the stent filaments, with the danger of partial stripping of the prosthesis if there are impediments during passage. Moreover, the placement of a stented Dacron graft can lead

to wrinkling, torsion, or collapse immediately after implantation (probably a "Venturi" effect) with the risk of early thrombosis (16). Affixing the prosthesis with two steel attachments can cause the graft to kink because of shrinking and scar processes of the aneurysm wall or aneurysm content.

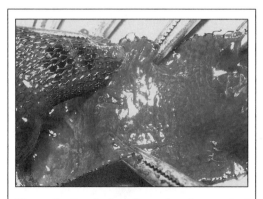

Figure 6. Luminal surface of a close-meshed nitinol stent-graft. Homogeneous fibrin thrombus layer 24 hours after implantation.

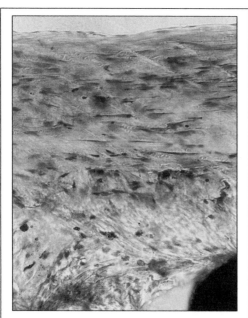

Figure 7. Histological section through a stent-graft showing nitinol wire. Typical neointimal tissue (250 μm thick) with luminally-limiting endothelial layer (Giemsa, original magnification x325).

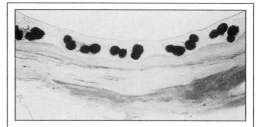

Figure 8. Histological section through the native aorta with implanted, double-knitted, nitinol stent-graft (proximal limitation). 200-250 μm thick neointima (Giemsa, x50).

In order to eliminate technical problems and to ensure better biocompatibility of the implanted material, we used close-meshed, all-metal stents as endovascular grafts in our studies. The close mesh of these nitinol and steel stents had a pore width of under 0.7 mm^2. In the application of nitinol stents, we could utilize the specific "superelastic" properties of this material by applying a special annealing process. The thermosensitive behavior of this alloy propagated by Dotter (18) and Cragg (19) was to be relegated to the background in our studies, as the application procedure in ice-cold water appeared inconvenient. New manufacturing technologies and a fixed conversion temperature of between 25° and 35° C, however, suggest improved feasibility. Thus, there is nothing to prevent the use of the nitinol-specific "thermal memory" in future applications.

Figure 9. Histological section through the low-cell organization tissue of an excluded aneurysm. *Top*: nitinol wires with surrounding neointima (100 μm thick). *Bottom*: wall of dacron aneurysm (Giemsa, x30).

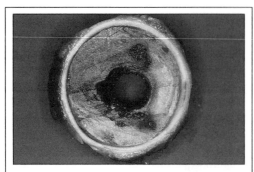

Figure 10.   Macrophoto (x3) of a cross-section of a polyurethane aneurysm with almost completely organized thrombus. Open lumen of the close-meshed nitinol stent.

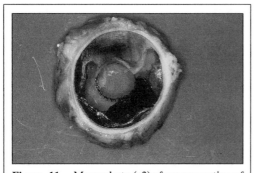

Figure 11.   Macrophoto (x3) of a cross-section of a partially thrombosed polyurethane aneurysm. Open lumen of the close-meshed nitinol stent.

Angiography and CT scans using the contrast-medium bolus technique showed both exclusion of the aneurysm as well as patency of the stent-graft during the follow-up period. Advantages compared with combined stent-textile grafts lie in the flexibility of the model, which helped to prevent kinking and compression, and in the use of 10- to 11-Fr sheaths which allowed percutaneous examination. In two stents with coarse mesh (pore width approximately 0.85 mm^2), there was neither direct nor delayed exclusion of the aneurysm, but only partial thrombosis.

The artificial aneurysm model (Dacron and polyurethane) in animal experiments as applied in our studies can by no means be extrapolated to the conditions in human aneurysm. Both the biological reaction of the native vessel wall, as well as facultative maintenance of blood circulation in the human aneurysm by open lumbar arteries or by the inferior mesenteric artery, present unsolved problems.

Macroscopic and microscopic examination demonstrated the good biocompatibility of the material used, with fast coverage of the stent by a homogeneous fibrin thrombus layer discernible after only 24 hours. Microscopic examination after 6 to 12 months showed a smooth, neointimal tissue layer over the entire stent surface, with a thickness of 200 μm in the proximal and distal sections adjacent to the native aorta and approximately 100 μm in the free segments. Endothelialization progressed from the proximal and distal ends of the stent (26) to the central parts, where in contrast to synthetic materials, the endothelialization of metallic stents described by Palmaz was also noticeable in our model (Figure 7).

From our examinations we deduce that the exclusion of artificial aortic aneurysms in dogs is guaranteed by the intraluminal placement of close-meshed stent-grafts. System efficacy has been proven in four clinical cases of peripheral aneurysms. Whether the system presented is also suitable for the treatment of aortic aneurysms appears to be a matter for speculation at present, since as yet unsolved technical and logistical problems still prevent clinical application in the aorta.

REFERENCES

1.   Mc Farland M. The epidemiologic necroscopy for abdominal aortic aneurysm. JAMA 1991;265:2085-2088.
2.   Fowkes FGR. The prevalence of aortic aneurysm. In: Greenhalgh RM, Mannick JA, Powell JT, eds. *The Cause and Management of Aneurysms.* London: WB Saunders; 1990;19-28

3. Melton LJ, Zickerstaff LK, Hollier LH, et al. Changing incidence of abdominal aortic aneurysms: a population based study. Am J Epidemiol 1984;120:379-386.

4. Collin J, Leandro A, Walton J, et al. Oxford screening programme for abdominal aortic aneurysm in men 65 to 74 years. Lancet 1988;2:613-615.

5. Dubost Ch, Allary H, Oeconomos N. Anéurysme de l'aorte abdominale traité par résection et greffe. Arch Mal Coeur 1951;44:848.

6. Sayers RD, Thompson MM, Bell PRF. Endovascular stenting of abdominal aortic aneurysms. Eur J Vasc Surg 1993;7:225-227.

7. Plecha FR, Bertin VJ, Plecha EJ, et al. The early results of vascular surgery in patients 75 years of age and older: an analysis of 3,259 cases. J Vasc Surg 1985;2:769-774.

8. Gardner RJ, Gardner NL, Tarnay TJ, Warden HE, James EC, Watne AL. The surgical experience of a one - to - sixteen-year follow-up of 227 abdominal aortic aneurysms. Am J Surg 1978;135:226-230.

9. Budd JS, Finch DRA, Carter PG. A study of the mortality from ruptured abdominal aortic aneurysms in a district community. Eur J Vasc Surg 1989;3:351-354.

10. Crawford ES. Ruptured abdominal aortic aneurysms: An editorial. J Vasc Surg 1991;13:348-350.

11. Häring R, Diermann J. Langzeitprognose und Spontanverlauf beim intrarenalen Bauchaortenaneurysma. Chirurgische Gastroenterologie 1992;8(Suppl I):61-69.

12. Blakemoore A. Progressive, constrictive occlusion of the abdominal aorta with wiring and electrothermic coagulation: one-stage operation for arterio-sclerotic aneurysm of the abdominal aorta. Ann Surg 1951;133;447-462.

13. Kwaan JHM, Dahl RK. Fatal rupture after successful surgical thrombosis of an abdominal aortic aneurysm. Surgery 1984;95:235-237.

14. Schanzer H, Papa MC, Miller CM. Rupture of surgical thrombosed abdominal aortic aneurysm. J Vasc Surg 1985;2:278-280.

15. Parodi JC, Palmaz JC, Barone HD. Transfemoral intraluminal graft implantation for abdominal aortic aneurysms. Ann Vasc Surg 1991;5:491-499.

16. Laborde JC, Parodi JC, Clem MF, et al. Intraluminal bypass of abdominal aortic aneurysm: feasibility study. Radiology 1992;184:185-190.

17. Dake MD, Stanford CA, Semba CP, et al. Endovascular stent-graft treatment of thoracic aortic aneurysms. Paper and Poster presented at the 79th Scientific Assembly and Annual Meeting of the RSNA, Chicago; 1993.

18. Dotter CT, Buschmann RW, McKinney MK, Rösch J. Transluminal expandable nitinol coil grafting: preliminary report. Radiology 1983;147:259-260.

19. Cragg AH, Lund G, Rysavy JA, Salomonowitz E, Castaneda-Zuniga WR, Amplatz K. Percutaneous arterial grafting. Radiology 1983;150:45-49.

20. Maass D, Zollikofer Ch, Largiader F, et al. Radiological follow up of transluminally inserted vascular endoprostheses: an experimental study using expanding spirals. Radiology 1984;152:659-663.

21. Balko A, Piasecki GJ, Shah DM, Carney WL, Hopkins RW, Jackson BT. Transfemoral placement of intraluminal polyurethane prosthesis for abdominal aortic aneurysm. J Surg Res 1986;40:305-309.

22. Lawrence DP, Charnsangavey C, Wright KC, Gianturco C, Wallace S. Percutaneous endovascular graft: experimental evaluation. Radiology 1987;163:357-360.

23. Yoshioka T, Wright KC, Wallace S, Lawrence DP, Gianturco C. Self-expanding endovascular graft: an experimental study in dogs. AJR 1988;151:673-676.

24. Mirich D, Wright KC, Wallace S, et al. Percutaneously placed endovascular grafts for aortic aneurysms: feasibility study. Radiology 1989;170:1033-1037.

25. Hagen B, Harnoss BM, Trabhardt S, Ladeburg M, Fuhrmann H, Franck C. Self-expandable macroporous Nitinol stents for transfemoral exclusion of aortic aneurysms in dogs: preliminary results. Cardiovasc Intervent Radiol 1993;16:339-342.

26. Palmaz JC. Intravascular stents: Tissue-stent interactions and design considerations. AJR 1993;160:613-618.

Extraction of Misplaced or Occluded Endovascular Stents

D. Liermann[1] and M. Zegelmann[2]

Departments of [1]Radiology and [2]H.T.G. Surgery,
J.W. Goethe University Hospital, Frankfurt am Main, Germany

INTRODUCTION

Every use of technology harbors an inherent risk of technical failure. The aim of this study was to illustrate possible remedies or means of preventing complications in the event of failure. The use of metallic endoprostheses in the vascular system, trachea, biliary ducts, gastrointestinal tract, or urethra is now possible largely without complications. Since 1987 we have implanted over 100 metallic endoprostheses in the vascular system for the treatment of arterial occlusive disease (AOD) without any significant complications (1-3). Owing to the special nature of the vascular system, there is considerable interest in how to retrieve a misplaced stent from a vessel and whether stent implantation would prevent or exclude further surgical procedures such as thromboendarterectomy (TEA).

The literature contains numerous references to cases of imprecisely placed, inadequately released, partially expanded, or dislocated vascular endoprostheses (2,4-6). In all of these cases the situation could normally be remedied by the implantation of additional stents. A better procedure, however, would appear to be retrieval of the misplaced stent and the implantation of a new stent. An essential factor for stent retrieval is appropriate flexibility of the stent material, allowing the stent to be deformed and pulled into the sheath without damaging the vascular wall. Based on our experience with the use of the tantalum stent in a cross-over technique, and owing to its high flexibility in joint-spanning locations, we considered this type of stent to be suitable for our planned attempts at retrieval (7). Irie and colleagues also reported on a new design of a modified Gianturco stent that allows extraction of the stent again after implantation (8). A new type of retrieval forceps which allows easier extraction of foreign bodies as well as stents from the vascular system, urogenital tract, and biliary ductal system was developed by Selby and colleagues (9). These developments indicate the obvious general interest in the possibility of extracting stents and/or making them extractable.

MATERIALS AND METHODS

The materials available were ordinary tantalum stents (Strecker™, Boston Scientific Corp., Denmark) with diameters between 8 and 11 mm and lengths between 3 and 8 cm, affixed to a 5 Fr Meditech balloon catheter (Watertown MA). These stents were positioned according to vascular anatomy and the degree of stenosis using an 8 or 9 Fr Terumo sheath (Tokyo, Japan) which was also used to extract the stents to be retrieved. Stent implantation was preceded by angiography using a contrast medium and, on evidence of stenosis, by probing using a guidewire and dilatation with a customary balloon catheter. The stent was then released in the ordinary manner by balloon insufflation via a pressure syringe. This procedure was followed by four different experimental test series.

In the first series, 10 stents were implanted in cadaver arteries and removed using special retrieval forceps. The cadaver arteries were supplied by the pathological institute of our own clinic after reviewing the case history and autopsy findings. For our we used only stenotic pelvic arteries of patients known to have had AOD. The following procedure was performed on all four test series subject to x-ray monitoring. After positioning the stent, we carefully inserted the retrieval forceps through the sheath and pushed it into the stent area. The three gripping arms could be opened by pulling back on a handle located on the back of the forceps. The tip and outside of these arms are rounded in order to prevent damage when used inside a vessel, but the inside has a sharp hump which catches in the mesh of the stent when the open forceps is pushed forwards. After the forceps have caught, the grip arms are closed by pushing the grip forward and the stent is carefully retracted into the sheath. It does not matter in which part of the stent the forceps catch. When using the relatively stable Terumo sheath, we always succeeded in pulling the stent and forceps combination fully into the sheath without destroying the latter, although strong traction was sometimes required. The use of a soft or thin-walled sheath can lead to an undesired concertina effect which subsequently requires surgical removal under anaesthesia. Extraction of the stent forceps combination through the sealing valve of the sheath regularly damaged the valve. In routine cases, we recommend inserting a new sheath via the wire in order to avoid blood loss.

With the same preliminary conditions in a second series, after positioning the stents we attempted 10 pelvic TEAs using a ring stripper. Customary ring strippers were used, with the diameter chosen in each case so that it was larger than that of the three implanted stents. After incision at the level of the common femoral artery and threading the ring stripper via the atheromatously transformed inner vascular layers, a cylinder could be peeled out of the vessel by carefully pushing the ring stripper forward. In the test series, the aim was to advance the ring stripper through the stented segment and subsequently extract the stent from the pelvic artery together with the excised vascular cylinder.

In the third and fourth test series, stents were placed in the pelvic artery during routine vascular surgery on the pelvic area conducted under anaesthesia. In the third series, the placed stent was extracted through a 9 Fr Terumo sheath using retrieval forceps before the operation itself in a total of five cases. In the fourth series, a stent was implanted intraoperatively in five other patients and removed via TEA as the actual aim of the operation. While the third series involved an additional period under anaesthesia of about 10 minutes per patient, in the fourth series an additional period under anaesthesia of only 5 minutes was sufficient, since the aim of the operation was extraction of the intimal cylinder by TEA. Simultaneous execution of both methods on the same patient was ruled out to avoid an unnecessary increase in the risk of anaesthesia.

RESULTS

In performing experimental stent extraction from cadaver arteries using retrieval forceps and the Terumo sheath, we had a 100% success rate. With the exception of damage to the Terumo sheath valve and dents to the tip of the sheath, no damage was detected. All stents could be completely extracted and there was no damage to the vascular wall in any of the extraction attempts. Seven stents were located in the common iliac artery and three in the external iliac artery. All the deceased were known to have suffered AOD, although the degree of atherosclerosis in the pelvic artery did not always correspond to the clinical classification of Fontaine. There were six cases of minor and four cases of severe change. In the patients' case histories, clinical findings were reported as stage II according to Fontaine in seven cases, stage III in two cases, and stage IV in one case (Table 1, Figure 1).

The use of a ring stripper to extract the stents within the course of TEA did not reveal any therapy failure in any of the 10

Table 1. Experimental Implantation of Stents in Iliac Cadaver Arteries:
Stent Extraction with Special Retrieval Forceps

Sex	Age	Localization	Atherosclerosis Severity	Fontaine Stage	Complete Extraction?	Damage to Vascular Wall?
Male	72	I. com.	Severe	III	Yes	No
Male	78	I. com.	Minor	II	Yes	No
Female	65	I. com.	Severe	II	Yes	No
Male	78	I. ext.	Minor	II	Yes	No
Male	75	I. com.	Severe	IV	Yes	No
Female	70	I. com	Severe	II	Yes	No
Female	68	I. ext.	Minor	II	Yes	No
Female	82	I. com.	Severe	II	Yes	No
Female	70	I. com.	Minor	II	Yes	No
Male	89	I. com.	Severe	III	Yes	No

Key: I. com. = common iliac; I. ext. = external iliac

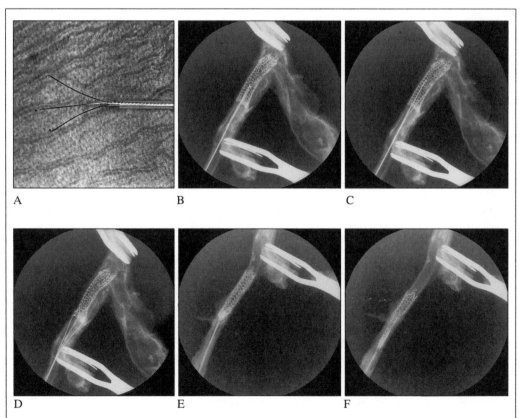

Figure 1. Experimental removal of a Strecker stent from the iliac artery of a human cadaver using forceps (see page 373).

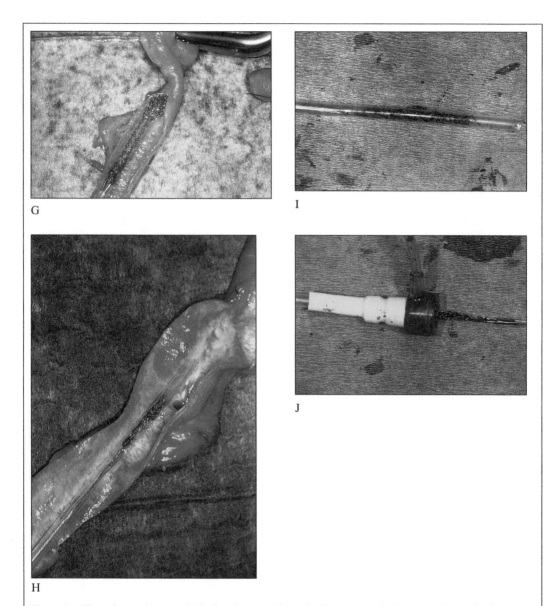

Figure 1. Experimental removal of a Strecker stent from the iliac artery of a human cadaver using forceps.

A) Three-armed forceps in open state with arms rounded on the outside and recognizable hooks on the inside of the arm tips to avoid damage to the vascular wall.
B) The closed forceps was inserted in the stent to be recovered.
C) The arms were opened to ensnare with the mesh of the stent.
D) The forceps was moved back and forwards with open arms until it had ensnared the stent filaments.
E) The stent became ensnared in the forceps, the branches were closed, and the stent was deformed to a cone at its distal end.
F) The stent was pulled into the sheath, deforming its shape.
G) Forceps and stent were drawn into the sheath of the slit preparation.
H) The stent was pulled into the sheath.
I) Forceps and wrinkled stent at the tip of the deformed sheath.
J) The stent was removed through the sheath valve.

individual attempts. The stent could easily be removed together with the incomplete intimal wall cylinder, even in two cases in which the stent was not or only partly covered by intimal material. All stents could be extracted completely and no damage to the vascular wall could be detected. Six stents were implanted in the common iliac artery and four in the external iliac artery. In that series, the AOD changes found in the pelvic artery section also did not correspond to the clinical stage according to Fontaine. In a total of 10 patients, we detected four cases of minor and six cases of severe atherosclerosis of the vascular wall. Seven patients had stage II according to Fontaine, two had stage III, and one had stage IV (Table 2, Figure 2).

The third and fourth series of experiments were conducted under anaesthesia in the operating theater during the course of other planned vasosurgical interventions. The primary aim of these series was to work as fast as possible in order to keep the anaesthetic risk to the patient low. We succeeded in performing the implantation with subsequent forceps extraction through the sheath with an average of an additional 10 minutes under anaesthesia. An average of only 5 minutes was required for implantation with subsequent TEA. All attempts at intraoperative

stent extraction were also completed without loss of material or damage to the vascular wall. In the third series, two stents were implanted in the common iliac artery and three in the external iliac artery. The degree of AOD in the pelvic area was substantial in all five cases; the degree of clinically known obstruction was assessed at stage II in one case, stage III in three cases, and stage IV in one case (Table 3).

All intraoperatively-implanted stents in the fourth series could successfully be extracted during the course of a TEA without any indication of damage to the vascular wall or loss of material. Two stents were implanted in the common iliac artery and three in the external iliac artery. All patients showed severe atherosclerotic changes to the vascular wall. Clinical findings indicated stage II disease in one case, stage III in three cases, and stage IV in one case (Table 4, Figure 3).

DISCUSSION

A success rate of 100% in the extraction of stents in all experimental series suggests that, because of its good flexibility and deformation properties (7), the tantalum stent can be extracted whenever necessary without

Table 2. Experimental Implantation of Stents in Iliac Cadaver Arteries: Stent Extraction During the Course of Thromboendarterectomy

Sex	Age	Localization	Atherosclerosis Severity	Fontaine Stage	Complete Extraction?	Damage to Vascular Wall?
Male	70	I. com.	Minor	II	Yes	No
Male	87	I. com.	Severe	III	Yes	No
Male	64	I. ext.	Severe	III	Yes	No
Female	72	I. ext.	Minor	II	Yes	No
Female	78	I. ext.	Severe	II	Yes	No
Female	74	I. com	Severe	II	Yes	No
Male	70	I. com.	Minor	II	Yes	No
Female	65	I. ext.	Minor	II	Yes	No
Male	74	I. com.	Severe	IV	Yes	No
Female	82	I. com.	Severe	II	Yes	No

Key: I. com. = common iliac; I. ext. = external iliac

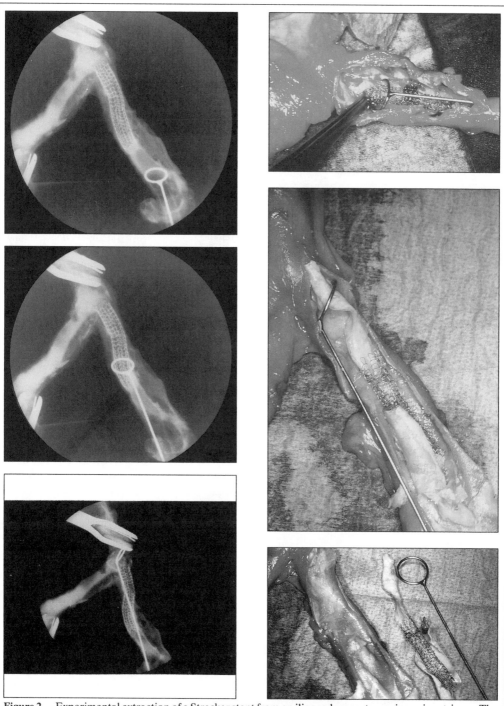

Figure 2.   Experimental extraction of a Strecker stent from an iliac cadaver artery using a ring stripper. The ring stripper was threaded *(top left)*, and pushed over the stent *(middle left)* without deforming or dislocating the stent *(bottom left)*. The open site revealed the position of the stripper *(top right)* and the cylinder of the wall which partially enclosed the stent *(middle right)*. Cylinder and stent lie alongside the vessel following extraction *(bottom right)*.

Table 3. Stent Extraction With Special Retrieval Forceps

Sex	Age	Localization	Atherosclerosis Severity	Fontaine Stage	Complete Extraction?	Extraction Operative Time	Vascular Wall Damage?
Male	72	I. com.	Severe	II	Yes	12 min.	No
Male	66	I. com.	Severe	III	Yes	11 min.	No
Male	73	I. ext.	Severe	III	Yes	9 min.	No
Female	75	I. ext.	Severe	IV	Yes	10 min.	No
Female	67	I. ext.	Severe	III	Yes	9 min.	No

Key: I. com. = common iliac; I. ext. = external iliac

Table 4. Stent Extraction During the Course of Thromboendarterectomy

Sex	Age	Localization	Atherosclerosis Severity	Fontaine Stage	Complete Extraction?	Extraction Operative Time	Vascular Wall Damage?
Male	72	I. com.	Severe	II	Yes	6 min.	No
Male	66	I. com.	Severe	III	Yes	6 min.	No
Male	73	I. ext.	Severe	III	Yes	4 min.	No
Female	75	I. ext.	Severe	IV	Yes	5 min.	No

Key: I. com. = common iliac; I. ext. = external iliac

major complications through a Terumo sheath using a retrieval set. When using this type of stent, a misplaced stent can be rectified simply by replacing it with a new one. The unsatisfactory method of rectifying misplaced stents by implanting additional stents (2,4-6) is thus superfluous in most situations. Although the tests were conducted primarily in order to find possibilities of extracting endoprostheses from the particularly sensitive vascular system, the extrapolation of these positive results to other organ systems nevertheless appears justified (9-12). The development of specially relocatable stents (8) indicates the need for, and interest in, the possibility of retrieving implantable metallic endoprostheses.

Suggested indications for the extraction of stents are incompletely expanded stents in cases of balloon rupture, problems in stent release, misplacements, dislocation of a stent from the stenotic area when too small a stent diameter has been selected, and infection caused by a stent or maintenance of an infectious process by the stent. The last indication plays a more decisive role in the trachea than in the vascular system. There is also the question of a temporary stent implantation to eliminate dissections. In the treatment of dissections in the distal superficial arteries, the temporary implantation of a stent and its subsequent extraction may be of interest as the risk of restenosis in the stented vessel segment due to intimal hyperplasia must be assessed as particularly high (1-3,5). In the scope of our studies, the unimpeded extraction of a tantalum stent within the course of TEA also appears to cause no problems and permits vascular surgeons to perform a TEA even in cases where a stent has been occluded for a longer interval and lysis is out of the question. Such prerequisites are seldom the case but could be observed when non-compliance to anticoagulation therapy occurred. In such cases it is particularly important for the vascular surgeon to know that, despite stent implantation, the possibility of a TEA still exists before a bypass is performed.

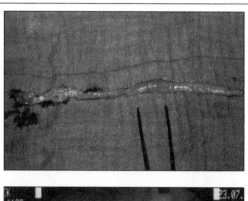
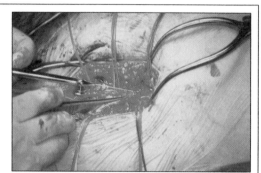
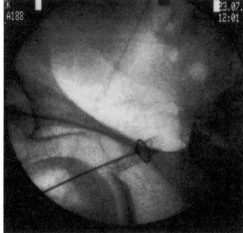
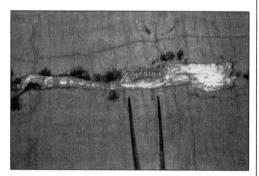

Figure 3. Intraoperative stent implantation with subsequent extraction of the stent using a ring stripper in the course of planned pelvic TEA. The femoral artery was exposed and held in the inguinal region *(top left)*. The ring stripper was easily passed the implanted stent *(bottom left)*. The stent was peeled out of the vessel together with the cylinder of vascular wall *(top right)*. Position of the stent in the vascular wall cylinder *(bottom right)*.

REFERENCES

1. Liermann D, Strecker EP, Vallbracht C, Kollath J. Indikation und klinischer Einsatz des Strecker-Stents. In: Kollath J and Liermann D, eds. *Stents ein aktueller Überblick*. Konstanz: Schnetztor Verlag; 1990;24-37.

2. Strecker EP, Liermann D, Barth KH, et al. Expandable tubular stents for treatment of arterial occlusive diseases: experimental and clinical results. Radiology 1990;175:97-102.

3. Liermann D, Strecker EP, Peters J. The Strecker stent: indication and use in iliac and peripheral arteries. J Cardiovasc Interv Radiol 1992;15:298-305.

4. Vorwerk D, Günther RW. Klinische Erfahrungen mit der Implantierung selbstexpandieren der Stents. In: Kollath J and Liermann D, eds. *Stents ein aktueller Überblick*. Konstanz: Schnetztor Verlag; 1990;138-41.

5. Triller J, Mahler F, Do D, Thalmann R. Behandlung der femoro-poplitealen Verschlußkrankheit mit vaskulärer Endoprothese oder alleiniger PTA: ergebnisse einer prospektiven Langzeitstudie. In: Kollath J and Liermann D, eds. *Stents ein aktueller Überblick*. Konstanz: Schnetztor Verlag; 1990;42-49.

6. Richter GM. Theoretische Grundlagen des ballonexpandierbaren Palmaz Stents. In:

Kollath J and Liermann D, eds. *Stents ein aktueller Überblick*. Konstanz: Schnetztor Verlag; 1990;50-57.

7. Strecker EP, Ber G, Schneider G, Freudenberg N, Weber H, Wolf RD. A new vascular balloon expandable prosthesis: experimental studies and first clinical results. J Interv Radiol 1988;3:59-62.

8. Irie T, Furui S, Yamauchi T, Makita K, Sawada S, Takenaka S. Relocatable Gianturco expandable metallic stents. Radiology 1991;178:575-578.

9. Selby JB, Tegtmeyer CJ, Bittner MG. Experience with new retrieval forceps for foreign body removal in the vascular, urinary and biliary systems. Radiology 1990;176:535-538.

10. Dotter CT, Rösch J, Bilbao MC. Transluminal extraction of catheter and guidewire fragments from the heart and great vessel: 29 collected cases. AJR 1971;111:467-472.

11. Coleman CC, Kimura Y, Castaneda-Zuniga WR, et al. Interventional techniques in the ureter. Semin Interv Radiol 1984;1:24-37.

12. Bedogni G, Meinero M, Barbieri I, et al. Foreign bodies of the biliary tract: endoscopic management. Dig Dis Sci 1986;31:1100-1104.

Atherectomy and Histology in Stented Arteries

D. Liermann, G. Herrmann, C. C. Haudenschild

Departments of [1]Radiology and [2]Pathology,
J.W. Goethe University Hospital, Frankfurt am Main, Germany

INTRODUCTION

A certain degree of ingenuity is required when taking histological samples from the vascular system of a person because the hole through which the instrument is inserted must not be too large, it must be possible to control the instrument being introduced over a relatively long distance, the instrument must be visible by x-ray, and as far as possible, the instrument must be thromboresistant. A further requirement is to obtain the largest possible quantity of histological material with only a minimal traumatic effect on the vascular wall and stent material. The histological material may not be damaged by the sampling process to such an extent that analysis is no longer possible, and the time required for obtaining the material must be kept within reasonable limits.

Development of an instrument satisfying all of these conditions would involve considerable costs in time and money, which could not be justified in view of the series of studies which have already been carried out in this context. This is the reason why we tried to cope with existing material and equipment for biopsies in various organ systems. Our choice was restricted to equipment which could take biopsies in hollow organs, and the possibilities were soon exhausted. We were left with the endoscopic biopsy forceps which have several disadvantages. They have a relatively large diameter and can only be introduced directly by means of a 9 Fr or 10 Fr sheath and have no protective sheath within the blood vessel and can thus cause injuries to the vascular wall. In addition, they cannot be brought to the required location by means of a positioned guidewire; the forceps device also cannot be guided in such a way as to allow material to be retrieved from the vascular wall in a 90° technique and safely removed from the blood vessel without embolic risk to the distal vascular section.

This finally led us to consider using an instrument which is not actually intended for sampling histological material, but rather is used for reducing vasoconstriction by removing the changed wall tissue which has caused the constriction as part of arterial occlusive disease (AOD)(1,2). This instrument, developed by Simpson, was designed as an alternative to balloon angioplasty mainly for reducing eccentric plaque. We used it under our study conditions to sample histological material from certain vascular wall sections (1,3-7). The purpose of this study was to see whether the instrument could satisfy our requirements for obtaining material without traumatic or thrombogenic consequences, without damaging the vascular walls, and by achieving an adequate quality of the sample (8) within a reasonable time. We also wished to see whether it would be possible to take samples from relatively unchanged vascular walls without perforating the blood vessel. The actual study consisted of a series of experiments following tests of the catheter in cadaver arteries in order to ensure that no serious injuries would be caused to the vascular wall while taking samples from vascular sections without plaque formation.

MATERIALS AND TECHNIQUES

The Simpson atherectomy catheter we used is an instrument intended to remove atheromatously-changed wall tissue caused during AOD. The instrument is an alternative to other recanalizing measures such as percutaneous transluminal angioplasty (PTA) or laser treatment. Its principle is based on cutting off or away changed tissue from the vascular wall within lumen-stenosing plaques. For this purpose, its tip is designed with a collection chamber and a cutting chamber. The collection chamber in the front is completely enclosed, whereas the cutting chamber has a window on one side in which a motor-driven blade can be moved perpendicular to the axis by means of a cable control. On the side opposite the sample there is a balloon which can be blown up with a maximum of 3 atm and which presses the window chamber against the plaque. The blade cuts one tissue cylinder after another out of the plaque while the instrument is being pulled back along the axis so that deposits on the vascular wall are systematically removed. Part of the material is pushed forward into the collection chamber so that as much material as possible can be removed in one process. After the fixing balloon has been deflated, the chamber with retracted blade is removed from the blood vessel, emptied, and reused. The catheter shaft conceals the cable-shaped shaft between the blade on the distal pole of the catheter and the motor unit on the proximal pole. The battery-driven motor is only started up to cut out each particular piece of tissue after pressure is applied by the contralateral balloon, with the blade being pulled backwards. At the same time, the blade is carefully drawn back by pulling a lever. The first prototypes had a flexible point on the lower chamber for guidance through the vascular system, but newer versions can also be guided to the desired location by means of a guidewire, reducing the risk of possible dissections or perforations. We used a 7 Fr or 8 Fr version, depending on the required diameter of the cutting instrument. Following corresponding preliminary tests, histological samples were taken from vascular sections treated with stents in the case of recurrences, or following endovascular irradiation in the technique described above. The samples were taken directly from the stent region and from superimposed, unaffected, or non-irradiated sections of the blood vessel in the femoral or popliteal region, bedded in formalin, and analyzed.

EXPERIMENTAL STUDIES

Vascular Material and Test Method

We selected a vascular section within an atheromatous change due to known AOD. The preparation was stretched out on a wooden board; after puncture at the common femoral artery, a 9 Fr sheath was laid and an 8 Fr Simpson atherectomy catheter was introduced and used in areas with arteriosclerotic plaque and also in areas with unaffected vascular walls. Altogether six different points were treated and analyzed after removal of the material. The test was carried out under x-ray control; after the test, the blood vessel was slit open and examined (9).

Results

In the experiments performed on the human cadaver arteries to examine the cutting behavior of the Simpson atherectomy catheter, material was cut out of the plaque in all three tests without causing damage to the vascular wall itself. The quantity and quality of the samples were adequate for histological analysis. Four cuts were made in the healthy vascular wall. In one case it was not possible to obtain any material, in one case the quantity of retrieved material was negligible, and in two cases it was not possible to obtain sufficient quantities of material. The instrument had cut through the layers of the vascular wall to the media, but without reaching the adventitia. Inspection of the vascular preparation revealed corresponding defects in the individual sections of the vascular wall but no serious damage. The preliminary tests ruled out any risk of serious damage to the vascular walls and produced histological material which was inadequate. Apart from one case with a tear instead of a cut in the preparation in the plaque area, the system's mechanism functioned reliably in all tests.

CLINICAL STUDIES

Indications

Indications for obtaining tissue samples for histological analysis using the Simpson atherectomy catheter on humans after completion of the experimental tests covered cases which were intended for renewed treatment in the stent region because of stenosis recurrence (Figure 1). Tissue was to be removed for histological analysis above and within the constricted stent region before a renewed PTA and application of prophylactic endovascular irradiation with iridium 192 HDR in an afterloading technique. It was then forwarded to the pathology center. Some of the patients required treatment for second stenoses that occurred at different times in areas outside the treated stent region; this allowed us to inspect the irradiated area by taking tissue samples for histological analysis during the necessary re-treatment of these stenosis. In addition to these cases, indications for use of the Simpson atherectomy catheter also included patients treated with stents where a recurrence was evident in other sections of the same blood vessel following freedom from stenoses for longer periods of time.

Patient Population

The patients included two elderly women (78 and 80 years of age) with reocclusion after 3 or 4 months, respectively, caused by a faulty anticoagulation protocol. The stent localization in both cases was the distal femoral artery. In one case, the closed, stented segment measured approximately 8 cm with two stents; in the other patient it measured approximately 12 cm with three stents. The original blood vessel diameter, reconstructed on the basis of the used stents, was 6 mm in both cases.

Additionally, there were 20 patients with restenosis in the stent after periods of time ranging from 6 to 54 months, with an average recurrence time of 7 months. This other group included 13 patients before PTA revision and endovascular afterloading irradiation therapy with iridium 192 HDR. The 20 patients consisted of 12 men and 8 women aged between 60 and 82 years (mean, 73 years). The stents were all localized in the area of the superficial femoral artery. The stented vascular sections had different lengths of stenosis (3 to 14 cm), with between one and four stents. The diameter of the stented region was 5 to 7 mm measured according to the stent diameter, but measured less than 1 to 3 mm because of the current stenosis.

The third group consisted of three patients who required further examination of the stented area following another episode of stenosis underneath or above the stented recurrence treated by PTA and endovascular afterloading. These patients included an 80-year-old woman with stenosis above the stented region. The stented region measured just 10 cm with three implanted stents. The therapy, a combination of PTA and endovascular irradiation therapy, had taken place 12 months previously and the angiogram showed clear passage through the stent region. The second patient was 68 years old; he suffered from stenosis in a 8-cm long vascular section between two stented segments in the superficial femoral artery. The one stented segment measured approximately 4 cm in length corresponding to the length of the implanted 6-mm stent, and the second segment had a length of 8 cm corresponding to the length of the implanted 6-mm stent. Both segments had been treated 9 months previously because of recurrences by means of PTA and endovascular irradiation therapy with iridium 192 HDR. An angiogram showed clear passage through the stented segments. The third patient was a 74-year-old man with stenosis above a recurrence that had been

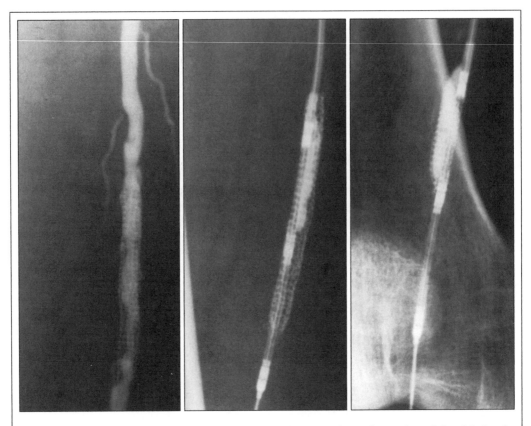

Figure 1. The angiogram shows a clear hyperplasia in the stented vascular section of the right-hand superficial femoral artery *(left)*. The illustration shows the Simpson atherectomy catheter in the stented area during the treatment *(middle)*. Insufflation of a balloon fixes the catheter to press it against the vascular wall during the cutting procedure. This makes it possible to cut out a corresponding quantity of tissue material from the vascular wall for histological analysis. This illustration *(right)* shows an atherectomy catheter taking samples in the area of a tantalum stent in the adductor canal.

treated by PTA and endovascular afterloading 14 months previously in an 8-cm long section of the superficial femoral artery treated with two stents. An angiogram of this segment treated with two 6-mm stents showed clear passage.

Results

Under clinical conditions, isolated problems were encountered when using both the 6 Fr and 8 Fr catheter. As a general rule, the 6 Fr catheter did not supply sufficient quantities of the material required for histological analysis. In three cases, material faults re-

sulted in the shaft breaking so that the relatively expensive instrument had to be replaced. There were no serious problems in all 22 cases of serious stenoses in the stented region for the first and second group of patients and sufficient quantities and qualities of sampled material were retrieved. Problems did arise, however, in obtaining material from the stented regions which had previously been subjected to irradiation treatment. The apparently relatively thin layer of cells on the inside of the stented region facing the lumen produced considerable difficulties in collecting sufficient quantities of histological material suitable for analysis. There were numerous futile attempts which failed to obtain any material. Several attempts were required in all three cases before sufficient material for histological analyses could be collected. In two cases, this resulted in interaction with the stent filaments (Figure 2), as demonstrated by retrospective evaluation of the pictures in comparison to the condition before using the Simpson catheter. Isolated filaments were cut out of the structure of the tantalum stent which deformed the design with threads of filaments protruding into the lumen. Tantalum particles were also found in the histological samples (Figure 3). No cases of thrombosis occurred following injuries to the vascular wall during the sampling process or exposed stent filaments during peri-interventional anticoagulation or Marcumar® therapy. Follow-up examinations up to 12 months after treatment also indicated no further restenosis in spite of the defects in the stent design. The patients reported discomfort during treatment with the Simpson atherectomy device. The time required for the treatment was significant, ranging from 30 minutes to 2 hours depending on the number of samples taken.

DISCUSSION

These preliminary experimental tests suggest that severe damage is improbable when using the Simpson atherectomy catheter, and that sufficient quantities of histological material can be sampled from areas of vascular walls with thicker changed tissue. However, it is scarcely possible to obtain adequate quantities of material from relatively normal wall structures (9,10). Although this is positive from the point of view of the actual use of the instrument, i.e., removal of atheromatous plaque, it is in fact a disadvantage, if not a limiting factor, for our purpose of obtaining histological material from sections of the vascular wall lined with only thin layers of cells. The lack of viable alternatives led us to use this method for clinical tests which worked quite satisfactorily for the majority of the 22

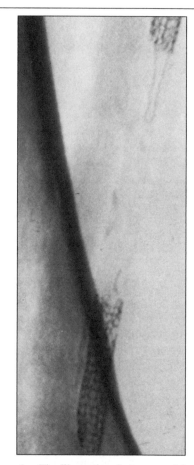

Figure 2. The illustration shows a condition following atherectomy with clear destruction of parts of the stent design and stent filaments in the adductor canal, taken during a 12-month check-up following re-PTA and endovascular irradiation, possibly due to dilatation of another stenosis in the same blood vessel. Practically no wall lining was visible in the stent area, which resulted in interaction during the atherectomy with the filaments.

patients. Negative factors included the high percentage of catheters (N=3) with material faults and the inadequacy of the 6 Fr atherectomy catheters' collecting capacity. Apart from the price of the catheter, the time required for each individual treatment is relatively long in spite of the learning curve, which makes it impossible to use the catheter for routine sampling in research work in the context of intimal hyperplasia (8,11-14). The

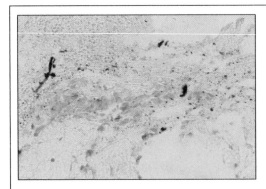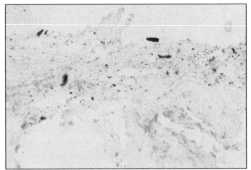

Figure 3. The histological samples of tissue material taken from the stented region *(left and right)* reveal scattered black inclusions among the cell material consisting of tantalum particles sliced from the stent during the atherectomy. These are histological samples from the same patient whose atherectomy is featured in Figures 1 and 2 with macroscopic defects.

average time for using the instrument was still longer than 50 minutes per patient.

At the moment there is no alternative device which can be used for collecting tissue samples from the vascular system for histological analysis (2). The question therefore arises whether one should simply manage without taking samples from these areas, or whether the results are so important that one should accept the considerable disadvantages of the method. In our opinion, there is no justification for simply managing without this method, particularly in view of the fact that we have practically no information from the functioning symplasma and organism about endovascular afterloading irradiation treatment with iridium 192 HDR. There is only limited experience available from other applications and experimental trials in cell cultures (15,16), but there is none from a transferable animal model (17,18). We must know about the real effects of irradiation treatment before we can use this method on patients as part of a random study.

The damage caused to the stent filaments by using the Simpson atherectomy catheters gives a reason for concern as such damage could pose a risk of thrombosis should the cells fail to grow back again sufficiently and given the rough surface. The changes in the stent design promote turbulences in blood flow, which in turn leads to the generation of new stenoses. Growth over the naked stent filaments would progress only very slowly because of the desired effect of reduced activity of the myofibroblast apparatus. But until this happens, the filaments will remain thrombogenic, creating a need for Marcumar therapy as long-term treatment.

REFERENCES

1. Simpson JB, Zimmermann JJ, Selmon MR, et al. Transluminal atherectomy: initial clinical results in 27 patients. Circulation 1986;74:2-203.
2. Wholey MH, Levitt RG, Fein-Millar D. Transluminal endarterectomy catheter (TEC). In: Castaneda-Zuniga WR and Tadavarthy SM, eds. *Interventional Radiology*. Baltimore: Williams and Wilkins; 1992;543-552.
3. Graor RA, Whitlow PL. Transluminal atherectomy for occlusive peripheral vascular disease. J Am Coll Cardiol 1990;15:1551-1558.
4. Maynar M, Reyes R, Cabrera V. Percutaneous atherectomy as an alternative treatment for postangioplasty obstructing intimal flap. Radiology 1989;170:1029-1032.
5. Maynar M, Reyes R, Pulido-Duque JM, et al. Directional atherectomy with the Simpson

atherocath. In: Castaneda-Zuniga WR and Tadavarthy SM, eds. *Interventional Radiology*. Baltimore; Williams and Wilkins; 1992;527-543.

6. Schwarten DE, Katzen BT, Simpson JB, Cutcliff WB. Simpson catheter for percutaneous transluminal removal of atheroma. AJR 1988;150:799-801.

7. Selmon MR, Robertson GC, Simpson JB, et al. Retrieval of media and adventitia by directional coronary atherectomy and angiographic correlation. Circulation 1990;82(Suppl III):624.

8. Sandritter W, Thomas C, eds. *Histopathologie*. Stuttgart: Schattauer; 1977.

9. von Pölnitz A, Backa D, Nehrlich G, Höfling B. Histological evaluation of "Vessel Biopsies" obtained with the Simpson atherectomy catheter. J Am Coll Cardiol 1989;13:2-149.

10. Iyer S, Zaitoun R, Dorros G. Lesion recurrence following directional atherectomy in peripheral vascular disease. Circulation 1990;82(Suppl III):623.

11. Bauriedel G, Höfling B. Adjunctive angioscopy during percutaneous atherectomy. J Am Coll Cardiol 1989;13:2-4A.

12. Hsu SM, Raine L, Fanger H. Use of avidin-bioptin-peroxidase complex (ABC) in immunoperoxidase techniques: a comparison between ABC and unlabeled antibody (PAP) procedures. J Histochem Cytochem 1981;34:148-151.

13. Leclerc G, Isner JM, Kearny M, et al. Evidence implicating non-muscle myosin in restenosis: use of *in situ* hybridization to analyze human vascular lesions obtained by directional atherectomy. Circulation 1992; 85:1-11.

14. Wilcox JN. Analysis of local gene expression in human atherosclerotic plaques by *in situ* hybridization. Trends Cardiol Med 1991;1: 17-24.

15. Narayan K, Cliff WJ. Morphology of irradiated microvasculature: a combined *in vivo* and electron microscopic study. Am J Pathol 1982;106:47-62.

16. Sholley MM, Gimbrone MA, Cotran RS. Cellular migration and replication in endothelial regeneration: a study using irradiated endothelial cultures. Lab Invest 1977;36:18-25.

17. Schwartz RS, Murphy JG, Edwards WD, Camrud AR, Vliestra RD, Holmes DR. Restenosis occurs with internal elastic lamina laceration and its proportional to severity of vessel injury in a porcine coronary artery model. Circulation 1990;82(Suppl III):656.

18. Schwartz RS, Koval TM, Edwards WD, et al. Effect of external beam irradiation on neointimal hyperplasia after experimental coronary artery injury. J Am Coll Cardiol 1992;19:1106-1113.

Magnetic Resonance Examination of Implanted Endovascular Prostheses in Vessels: Initial Results

D. Liermann and J. Berkefeld

Department of Radiology, J.W. Goethe University Hospital, Frankfurt am Main, Germany

INTRODUCTION

Adequate documentation of the follow-up for stent implantation in the peripheral vascular system must consist of more than pure clinical documentation including ankle-arm index (AAI), walking distance, and the clinical stage according to Fontaine's classification. Problems arise in this context on commencement of restenosis in the stent area, with continuing supply through collateral blood vessels causing a deceptively unchanged situation compared to the initial status with regard to the AAI and painless walking distance. A further difficulty is encountered in determining the cause for deteriorating clinical findings, as it is not possible to clearly differentiate between restenosis in the stent or at another point in the same vascular section. Angiograms are indispensable here to achieve precise localization. It is possible to relieve some of the strain on the patient by performing an intravenous (iv) digital subtraction angiography (DSA) instead of the more costly intraarterial angiogram; however, this still does not reduce the dose of radiation received. The increasing sensitivity of the general public to x-rays and radiation exposure makes it difficult to perform close-meshed angiograms using DSA techniques. Therefore, we began to look for viable alternatives. In addition to the color-coded Doppler, there is the possibility of using magnetic resonance (MR) tomography (1-3).

MATERIALS AND METHODS

A Magnetom 1.0 Teslar (Siemens) with conventional screening was selected. The ac-tual reconstructions and measurements within the study itself were preceded by numerous preliminary tests, some with phantoms and some with patients (4,5). In the initial tests, reconstructions were carried out in T1- and T2-weighted sequences in sagittal, axial, and coronary sections for stents of varying materials. In addition, different coils were tested for imaging quality. Furthermore, on the basis of the first animal experiments carried out by Matsumoto et al (6), fast flow-sensitive sequences (so-called Fast Low Angle Shoot or FLASH sequences) were tested with differing flip angles. These gradient echo sequences with a low flip angle have TR repetition times under 1 msec, with TE echo times of approximately 20 msec (7-11). Depending on the choice of tested flip angle, the TR/TE times also differ with different flip angles. Finally, a special MR angio-program for the Magnetom 1.0 Teslar unit was tested on a few selected patients.

Following the experimental investigations, 48 examinations were then carried out on 25 patients at different time intervals under standardized study conditions. In order to guarantee a strictly observed follow-up protocol after stent implantation in the vascular system, it is necessary for angiograms to be performed at 3, 6, and 12 months and at yearly intervals thereafter, or when clinical data indicate the need to avoid early recurrent stenosis in the stented area (12,13). In view of the already high radiation exposure during the course of treatment, patients were selected for the MR examination who had either undergone multiple percutaneous transluminal angioplasties (PTA) with subsequent recurrence, particularly after stent implantation, and patients whose recurrent condition following intimal hyperplasia had been treated with endovascular afterloading therapy. In the latter group, it was anticipated that additional information about the tissue surrounding the blood vessels could be collected.

Not considered for this examination were patients with a first stent implantation following PTA, patients with metal splinters in the skull/brain area or other unfavorable localizations, patients with pacemakers, and patients with a history of claustrophobia (4,5,14,15). Artificial hip or knee joints were not a contraindication for an MR examination.

Study conditions were based on the results of the earlier tests. This part of the study considered only patients with tantalum stents for reasons explained in the RESULTS section (16,17). Patients were allowed to assume the most relaxed position to avoid any movement artefact. The examination was carried out without administering contrast medium using sagittal, coronary, axial, and parasagittal sections for the renal stents. Examination of these stents was carried out with the assistance of the vertebral column coil or, in the case of an adipose patient, using the body coil. Following a T1-weighted survey series with a coronary section, all registrations were carried out using a FLASH gradient echo sequence with a flip angle of 30°.

Registration for stents in the iliac vascular system was carried out in sagittal, parasagittal, coronary, and axial sections using the body coil. Again, in addition to the T1-weighted survey series, all registrations were carried out in FLASH gradient echo sequences with a flip angle of 30°. Examination of stents in the femoropopliteal vascular section was usually carried out using a cervical coil; a head coil was used for patients with particularly large thighs or for stents having a relatively proximal position. Registration was again in sagittal, parasagittal, coronary, and axial sections in a T1-weighted survey series

and FLASH gradient echo sequences had a flip angle of 30°. An iv DSA was carried out in parallel on the same day before or after the MR tomogram. In five cases, an additional angio-MR was performed, usually in the coronary section.

RESULTS

Experimental Investigations

Initially, tantalum (Strecker™; Boston Scientific Corp., Denmark), Palmaz™ (Johnson & Johnson Interventional Systems Co., Warren NJ), and Wallstents™ (Medinvent, Lausanne, Switzerland) were examined in various phantom models as these are the most frequently used endoprostheses. Marked artefact were obtained for the steel Palmaz and Wallstents which were caused by the stents themselves, regardless of the chosen sequence, flip angle, or coil (2,4,14). We were, therefore, unable to assess the stent lumen. Verification in two patients confirmed these experimental results.

This finding limited the examination of techniques to tantalum stents since this material did not cause any notable artefact due to the stent itself. Experimental results indicated that, with regard to resolution, the vertebral column coil was best suited for the renal vascular system, the body coil for the iliac vascular system, and the cervical coil for the femoropopliteal vascular system. Variations were required for the renal arteries in adipose patients with the body coil used instead of the vertebral column coil. In addition, for femoropopliteal arteries, a head instead of a cervical coil was necessary for patients with voluminous thighs or in cases where stents were in a proximal position in the thigh.

While the coronary, sagittal, and axial sections were adequate for stents located in the femoropopliteal vascular segment, stents in the renal and iliac arteries also required an additional parasagittal section. Given the choice of corresponding sequences, the T1-weighted sequences were relatively unsuitable, as they illustrated the stent but did not allow for adequate evaluation of the stent lumen. As far as the gradient (FLASH) echo sequences with short repetition times were concerned, variation led to the discovery of a FLASH echo sequence with useful imaging quality. Variation of the flip angle between 10° and 90° revealed that a flip angle of 30° produced the best resolution. The time required for these examinations was reduced from an average of 2 hours at the beginning of the tests to approximately 20 minutes.

Clinical Investigations

Capacity problems meant that it was not possible to include all stent patients for the MR study. From a total of 100 stent patients, only 30 were included in the MR examinations as part of the follow-up in the femoropopliteal vascular segment, 10 for the iliac vascular system, and 8 for the renal artery system. The follow-up period covered the intervals up to the 12-month examination from the time of re-PTA in the stent area. The patients were between 50 and 84 years of age (mean, 78.2 years). Forty-eight examinations were performed on 25 patients (11 women, 14 men). As a rule, patients with stent implantation in the renal artery did not suffer from arterial occlusive disease (AOD) as the cause for stent implantation, whereas AOD was the reason for stent implantation in all patients with stents in the iliac artery or femoropopliteal vascular segment. Eighty percent of the patients abused nicotine, 30% had hypertension, and 20% were diabetic. The length of the implanted stents in the renal arteries ranged from 2 and 2.5 cm with a length from 5 to 6 mm. In the iliac arteries, the stents were between 4 and 12 cm in length with diameters between 8 and 11 mm, while stents implanted in the femoropopliteal arteries were between 4- and 14.5-cm long with a diameter between 5 and 7 mm. With the exception of the renal arteries, which also included post-examination of non-recurrences, all other localizations had at least one recurrence in the stented area.

Ten of the 25 patients had undergone endovascular afterloading therapy with 192 iridium HDR as a prophylactic measure to prevent intimal hyperplasia in the peripheral vascular segments. Here the examination also intended to evaluate the perivascular tissue before and after irradiation.

The MR examinations performed under the standardized conditions described above lasted an average examination time of 20 minutes for femoropopliteal examinations and not less than 30 minutes for renal or iliac vascular systems. For the comparison with the DSA, the results of all sections were drawn together for analysis in FLASH gradient echo sequence with a flip angle of 30°. This resulted in better imaging with the DSA for all eight examinations with renal stents (Figure 1). The lumen of the stented region could not be evaluated in all segments. There was no incorrectly positive or negative results on the basis of the MR examination. The parasagittal sections produced only a very slight resolution with considerable interference and could not be evaluated. All examined stents showed no constrictions in the follow-up.

The 10 iliac examinations were only partly evaluable and their quality was clearly inferior to the comparative DSA examinations. An acute occlusion of the right common iliac artery following intraoperative dissection prior to recanalization and stent implantation was detected by the MR. The remaining iliac vessels were patent. The examinations of the femoropopliteal vascular segment revealed the same degree of information as the DSA about patency of the stent region and neighboring vascular segments. Five stenoses were detected in 30 examinations, four of which had occurred in the stent region and one which was approximately 5 cm above the stented vascular segment.

Apart from the one stenosis above the stented region, all patients treated with endovascular afterloading were evaluated as recurrence-free on the MR tomograms. The subsequent comparative DSA confirmed these MR results. A perivascular tissue reaction

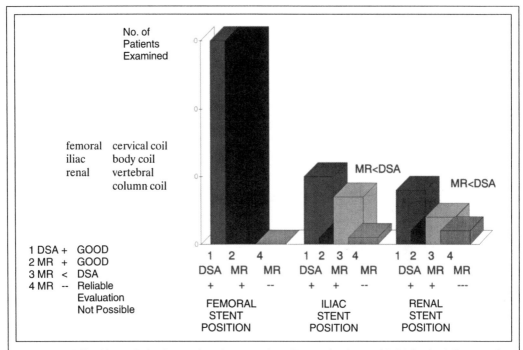

Figure 1. Lifetable analysis. Comparison between the MR examination and DSA in the follow-up after stent implantation in the vascular system. The MR examination was carried out on a 1.0 Teslar Magentum with FLASH gradient echo sequences, flip angle 30° in axial, sagittal, coronary, and parasagittal sections.

after endovascular afterloading could not be detected in the controls performed to date. The five examinations carried out using angio-MR techniques revealed adequate evaluation of the lumen both for the four cases in the femoropopliteal vascular region and the one case in the iliac vascular region.

Relative to the rest of the examination technique, one negative aspect was the inability to detect the localization of the stent, since the angio-MR technique can only illustrate flow artefact. The software available for the angio-MR for our MR tomography (Magnetom 1.0 Teslar) was also relatively user-unfriendly. In spite of tolerable adjusting and measuring times, a second workplace was required for processing the extensive data and this was a time-consuming procedure (Figures 2-4).

DISCUSSION

One of our targets was the complete replacement of the DSA, not only to improve compliance between doctor and patient while maintaining the necessary follow-up for stent patients, but to avoid additional accumulation of the total radiation dose received. This goal was only partly achieved. The artefact formation by steel stents such as the Palmaz stent or Wallstent ruled out the use of MR as part of follow-up examinations for these stent types. The results of examinations on various materials published by others confirm our experimental results (2,4,14-18). Thus, only the tantalum stent remained as a viable possibility for routine control in MR tomography, and our experimental investigations enabled

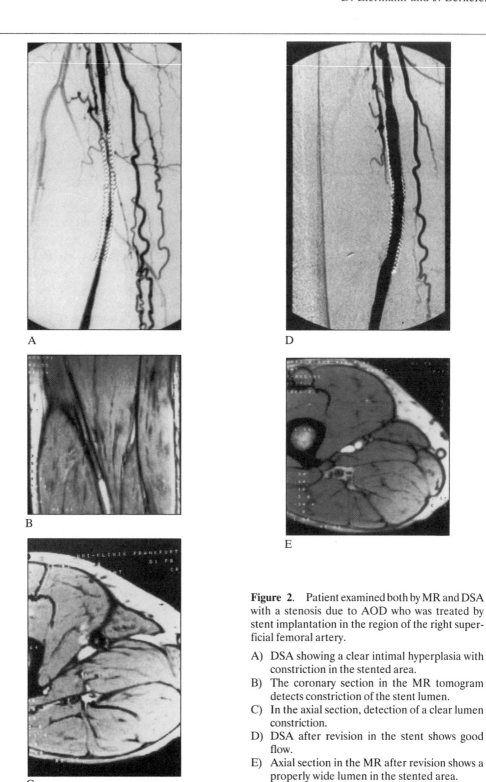

Figure 2. Patient examined both by MR and DSA with a stenosis due to AOD who was treated by stent implantation in the region of the right superficial femoral artery.

A) DSA showing a clear intimal hyperplasia with constriction in the stented area.

B) The coronary section in the MR tomogram detects constriction of the stent lumen.

C) In the axial section, detection of a clear lumen constriction.

D) DSA after revision in the stent shows good flow.

E) Axial section in the MR after revision shows a properly wide lumen in the stented area.

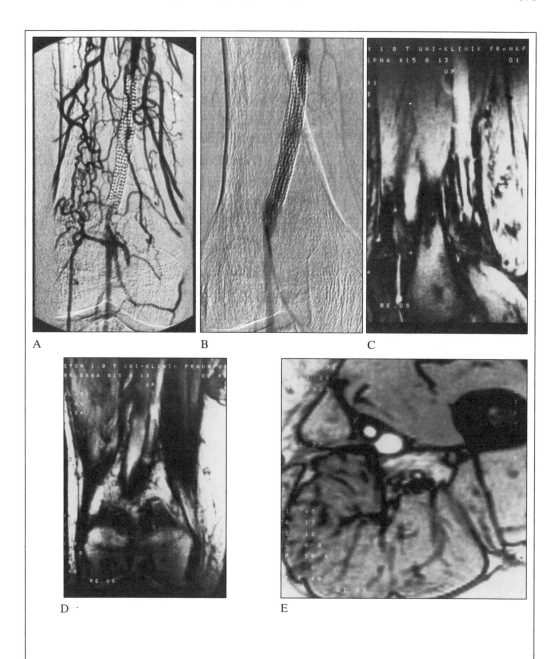

Figure 3. An 80-year-old female patient with recurrent occlusions in the right superficial femoral artery. Her last treatment consisted of endovascular irradiation using an afterloading technique.

A) DSA before revision of reocclusion in the stent.
B) DSA one year after revision and afterloading with free flow.
C) MR tomogram in sagittal section with free flow in the stent.
D) MR tomogram in coronary section with free stent lumen.
E) MR tomogram in axial section with free passage.

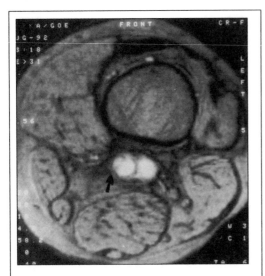

Figure 4. Using magnetic resonance tomography, the section through the artery clearly shows a dissection after PTA in the area of the superficial femoral artery (see arrow).

us to establish standard settings and sequences for this kind of control.

Our present results suggest that the only unrestricted indication and justification for MR use apply to the femoropopliteal vascular region. This corresponds to results obtained by other authors using the angio-MR with newer software (19,20). Results for examinations in the iliac or renal vascular systems using fast flow sequences of different variations (1,7,9-11,21) remained unsatisfactory and were not suitable replacements for DSA. The development of newer software programs compatible with the newer generation of MR equipment may offer an alternative to DSA for the kidneys, abdomen, and iliac region (18,22-25). Further development of software for newer MR types makes the use of angio-MR a serious alternative to DSA for other vascular segments with and without implanted stents, as the reconstruction times are faster and imaging quality good with a relatively uncomplicated procedure. The advantage of the FLASH gradient echo sequences and coil choice we selected for ex-

amination of the stented vascular segments is the fact that these examinations can be carried out with good results for stented peripheral vascular segments using older MR equipment which does not yet have a sophisticated angio-MR program.

In the non-x-ray examination of the vascular system, the color-coded Doppler is an alternative to MR tomography (18,25-27). An experienced operator is certainly capable of producing adequate images of the vascular regions using the color-coded Doppler even after stent implantation. In contrast to the MR tomogram, the color-coded Doppler can be used regardless of the material properties of the implanted stent. One drawback to color-coded Dopplers is their relatively high expense. Moreover, the MR examination appears indispensable compared to the color-coded Doppler when the purpose of the examination is to evaluate both the patency of the stented vascular segments and any changes in the perivascular tissue following stent revision and endovascular afterloading.

REFERENCES

1. Bradley Jr WG, Waluch V. Blood flow: magnetic resonance imaging. Radiology 1985;154:443-450.
2. Moneta GL, Strandness DE. Peripheral arterial duplex scanning. JCU 1987;15:645-651.
3. Zierler RE. Duplex and color-flow imaging of the lower extremity arterial circulation. Semin Ultrasound CT & MR 1990;11:168-179.
4. Shellock FG, Crues JV. High-field strength MR imaging and metallic biomedical implants: an *ex vivo* evaluation of deflection forces. AJR 1988;151:389-392.
5. Shellock FG. Biological effects and safety aspects of magnetic resonance imaging. Magn Reson Q 1989;5:243-251.
6. Matsumoto AH, Teiltelbaum GP, Barth KH, Carvlin M, Savin MA, Strecker EP. Tantalum vascular stents: *in vivo* evaluation with MR imaging. Radiology 1989;170:753-755.
7. Buxton RB, Edelman RR, Rosen RR. Contrast in rapid MRI: T1 and T2-weighted

imaging. J Comput Assist Tomogr 1987;11: 7-16.

8. Gullberg GT, Wehrli FW, Shimalawa A, Simons MA. MR vascular imaging with a fast gradient refocusing pulse sequence and reformatted images from transaxial sections. Radiology 1987;165:241-246.

9. Haase A, Frahm J, Matthei D. FLASH imaging: rapid NMR imaging using low flip angle pulses. J Magn Reson 1986;67: 258-266.

10. Podolak MJ, Hedlund LW, Evans AJ, Herfkins RJ. Evaluation of flow trough simulated vascular stenoses with gradient echo magnetic resonance imaging. Invest Radiol 1989;24:184-189.

11. Winkler ML, Orthendal DA, Mills TC. Characteristics of partial flip angle and gradient reversal MR imaging. Radiology 1988;166: 17-26.

12. Liermann D, Strecker EP, Vallbracht C, Kollath J. Indikation und klinischer Einsatz des Strecker-Stents. In: Kollath J and Liermann D, eds. Stents ein aktueller Überblick. Konstanz: Schnetztor Verlag; 1990:24-37.

13. Liermann D, Strecker EP, Peters J. The Strecker stent: indications and results in iliacal and femoropopliteal arteries. Cardiovasc Interv Radiol 1992;15(5):298-305.

14. Shellock FG, Curtis JS. MR imaging and biomedical implants, materials and devices: An updated review. Radiology 1991;180: 541-550.

15. Teitelbaum GP. MR imaging safety and artefacts. Radiology 1990;175:855-859.

16. Teitelbaum GP, Ortega HV, Vinitski S. Low artefact intravascular devices: MR imaging evaluation. Radiology 1988;168:713-719.

17. Teitelbaum GP, Raney M, Carvlin MJ, Matsumoto AH, Barth KH. Evaluation of ferromagnetism and magnetic resonance imaging artefacts of the tantalum vascular stent. Cardiovasc Intervent Radiol 1989; 12:125-127.

18. Mulligan AS, Matsuda T, Lanzer P, Gross GM. Peripheral AOD: prospective comparison of MR angio and color duplex US with conventional angiography. Radiology 1991;178:695-700.

19. Haacke EM, Masaryk TJ, Wielopolski PA. Optimizing blood vessel contrast in fast three-dimensional MRI. Magn Reson Med 1990;14:202-221.

20. Lewin JS, Laub G, Hausmann R. Three-dimensional time-of-flight MR angiography: applications in the abdomen and thorax. Radiology 1991;179:261-264.

21. Gullberg GT, Wehrli FW, Shimalawa A, Simons MA. MR vascular imaging with a fast gradient refocusing pulse sequence and reformatted images from transaxial sections. Radiology 1987;165:241-246.

22. Kim D, Edelmann RR, Kent KC, Porter DH, Skillmann JJ. Abdominal aorta and renal artery stenosis: evaluation with MR angiography. Radiology 1990;174:727-731.

23. Liermann D, Spreer J, Goetz F, et al. Magnetresonanztomographie von Gefäßen nach Stentimplantation. In: Kollath J and Liermann D, eds. Stents II ein aktueller Überblick. Konstanz: Schnetztor Verlag; 1992:153-163.

24. Powers TA, Lorenz CH, Holburn GE, Price RR. Renal artery stenosis: in vivo perfusion MR imaging. Radiology 1991;178:543-548.

25. Dousset V, Wehrli FW, Louie A, Listerud J. Popliteal artery hemodynamics: MR-imaging-US correlation. Radiology 1991;179:437-441.

26. Kohler TR, Nance DR, Cramer MM, Vabdenburghe N, Strandness DE. Duplex scanning for diagnosis of aortoiliac and femoropopliteal disease: a prospective study. Circulation 1987;76:1074-1080.

27. Sacks MD, Robinson ML, Marinelli DL, Perlmutter GS. Evaluation of the peripheral arteries with duplex US after angioplasty. Radiology 1990;176:39-44.

The Future of Cardiologic Stents

Marino Labinaz, R. Phillips, Richard S. Stack, James P. Zidar, Brigitta Brott

Division of Cardiology, Department of Medicine,
Duke University Medical Center, NC USA

Coronary angioplasty is limited by abrupt vessel closure and late restenosis. Metal stents have shown some promise in treating both of these conditions. Several limitations exist with metal stents, however. They are permanent, costly, and are associated with increased hemorrhagic complications. Furthermore, impregnation of metal stents with genetic and pharmaceutical agents to reduce thrombus deposition and neointimal formation is unlikely to be technically feasible. To overcome these limitations, biodegradable stents have been developed. Early results from animal experiments are encouraging and with continued work, the treatment of coronary artery disease with biodegradable stents will occur in the not too distant future.

INTRODUCTION

In the 15 years since the introduction of percutaneous transluminal coronary angioplasty (PTCA), catheter-based revascularization has steadily grown in importance as a treatment for coronary artery disease. United States statistics indicate that coronary angioplasty is more common than coronary artery bypass grafting (CABG) (1). Randomized studies have recently shown that PTCA is competitive with CABG in terms of symptom relief, mortality, and cost (2-5). The potential benefit of the less invasive technique, however, is limited by the problems of abrupt vessel closure and late restenosis which occur in 5 to 8% (6) and 17 to 45% (1) of all angioplasty procedures, respectively.

METALLIC STENTS

Metallic stents have provided a promising approach to the dual problems of abrupt closure and restenosis. In observational studies, metallic stents have been shown to be successful in treating abrupt and threatened closure (7,8). Early observational series have also suggested that they might have a role in reducing the likelihood of restenosis (9). In both the Benestent Trial (10) and the STRESS trial (11), patients with *de novo* lesions were randomly assigned to receive a tubular slotted Palmaz-Schatz stent or conventional angioplasty. A significant reduction in restenosis was demonstrated in patients who received stents.

Metallic stents have several limitations, however, and long-term effects of this device in the arterial wall are unknown. There has been some concern about medial atrophy with the potential for late vessel wall proliferation (12). Current designs are limited by the additional costs and increased hemorrhagic complications which are incurred by the need for systemic anticoagulation. Although coating of metallic stents to reduce thrombogenicity is technically possible, and early experimental results with stent coatings have been promising (13,14), impregnation of metallic stent materials to allow more gradual and sustained release of antirestenosis and antithrombotic medications may not be technically feasible.

POLYMERIC STENTS

Due to the limitations of metallic stents, efforts have been made to develop stents made of polymeric compounds. Polymers have had a long history of use in the cardiovascular system as vascular grafts (biostable polymers) and vascular sutures (both biostable and bioabsorbable polymers) (15). The concept of biodegradable stents has been especially appealing because these stents could provide a temporary support for the vessel wall with the ability to deliver antithrombotic and/or antiproliferative agents in a gradual, sustained fashion. Although the ideal polymeric stent could be entirely bioabsorbable, other potential designs could include combinations of metal, biostable, and bioabsorbable polymers to optimize mechanical performance and local drug delivery.

Biostable Polymer Stents

The largest experience using non-biodegradable polymers for permanent human implantation has been with polyethylene terephthalate (PET). The long-term experience using this material for intravascular grafts has been favorable. Due to these encouraging results, several investigators have implanted PET stents in animals.

Murphy and coworkers implanted self-expanding PET stents in porcine coronary arteries. Follow-up at 4 to 6 weeks revealed total occlusion of all stented segments and histologic examination revealed a chronic foreign body response surrounding the stent struts with a marked neointimal response in the center of the vessel (16). In contrast, van Beusekom and colleagues implanted PET stents in porcine peripheral arteries. At the time of follow-up, seven of eight stented segments were patent and only minimal foreign body response was noted (17). The lack of sterilization of the stents in the Murphy study and the use of peripheral arteries in the van Beusekom study may explain some of the differences noted by these investigators.

Biodegradable Stents

Several biodegradable polymers have been successfully used in humans. Polyglycolic acid and polylactic acid were the first biodegradable polymers synthesized (18,19). They have been extensively used as absorbable sutures (20) and as vehicles for the local release of antibiotics (21) and chemotherapeutic agents (22). Other biodegradable polymers that have been used clinically include polyorthesters which have been used for sustained contraceptive steroid administration (23) and polyanhydrides which have been successfully used for releasing BCNU (carmustine) locally in patients with recurrent malignant gliomas (24).

Duke Bioabsorbable Stent

In the early 1980s, the first biodegradable stent was produced at Duke University Medical Center using a specialized form of poly-L-lactide (PLLA) (25). As shown in Figure 1, a diamond braided, open-mesh, self-expanding stent was constructed of eight polymer strands. *In vitro* tests indicated that the stent had excellent crush strength and withstood 1,000 mm Hg pressure over 30 days in a 37°C saline bath (26). Sterilized stents were subsequently placed in the femoral arteries of 11 dogs (27). All animals received aspirin before stent deployment and daily until the time of sacrifice. Heparin was only used at the time of stent deployment. Follow-up data were obtained

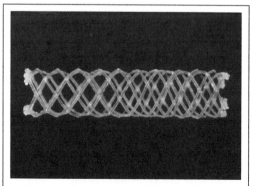

Figure 1. Duke self-expanding biodegradable stent.

Reprinted with permission from: Stack RS, Zidar JP, Waller BF, et al. A bioabsorbable intravascular stent. J Am Coll Cardiol, submitted.

variably from 2 hours to 18 months, and consisted of repeat angiography and histologic examination. All stents were found to be patent at the time of follow-up with the exception of one animal in whom stent occlusion occurred due to traumatic implantation. Of the patent stents, there was a 40% stenosis in one stented segment but only minor luminal irregularities in the remaining segments. By 2 weeks, stent struts were covered with neointima and at 12 weeks a moderate degree of medial compression was seen. The stent struts were fully absorbed at 18 months and despite some focal neointimal thickening, there was no significant encroachment of the luminal cross-sectional area (Figure 2). There was preservation of the internal elastic lamina and no significant thrombus was seen. In contrast to other studies, no significant inflammatory response was noted throughout the various follow-up intervals. These studies are summarized in Table 1.

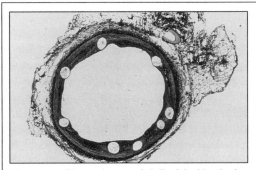 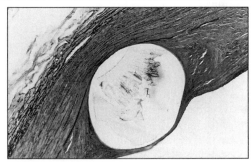

Figure 2. Photomicrograph (x5) of the histologic response at 18 months to the PLLA Duke self-expanding shunt *(left)*. High-power micrograph (x40) of a degenerated stent strut at 18 months *(right)*. There is no foreign body reaction and minimal neointimal response. The internal elastic lamina is intact and there is minimal medial thinning.

Reprinted with permission from: Stack RS, Zidar JP, Waller BF, et al. A bioabsorbable intravascular stent. J Am Coll Cardiol, submitted.

Table 1. *In Vivo* Results with Duke Biostent

Dog Number	Duration	Patent	Endothelialized	Biocompatible
1	2 hours	+	−	+
2	2 days	−	−	+
3	4 days	+	−	+
4	4 days	+	−	+
5	1 week	+	−	+
6	1 week	+	−	+
7	2 weeks	+	+	+
8	2 weeks	+	+/−	+
9	2 weeks	+	+	+
10	3 months	+	+	+
11	18 months	+	+	+

Reprinted with permission from ref. 15.